This important new publication summarises the recent exciting advances in screening for Down's syndrome. It addresses important clinical questions such as: risk assessment, whom to screen, when to screen, which techniques to use and the organisation of screening programmes nationally and internationally.

An international and authoritative team of authors has been invited to assess the latest developments in this rapidly advancing area. The volume provides a critical and much needed evaluation of the potential and limitations of new and established techniques for screening for Down's syndrome. It will serve as an essential source of information for all those involved in prenatal diagnosis and the provision of obstetric care.

SCREENING FOR DOWN'S SYNDROME

SCREENING FOR DOWN'S SYNDROME

Edited by

J. G. GRUDZINSKAS
Royal London Hospital, London

T. CHARD
St Bartholomew's Hospital, London

M. CHAPMAN
United Medical Dental School, Guy's Hospital, London

H. CUCKLE
University of Leeds

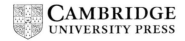

CAMBRIDGE
UNIVERSITY PRESS

Published by the Press Syndicate of the University of Cambridge
The Pitt Building, Trumpington Street, Cambridge CB2 1RP
40 West 20th Street, New York, NY 10011-4211, USA
10 Stamford Road, Oakleigh, Melbourne 3166, Australia

First published 1994

Printed in Great Britain at the University Press, Cambridge

A catalogue record for this book is available from the British Library

Library of Congress cataloging in publication data
Screening for Down's syndrome / edited by J.G. Grudzinskas . . . [et al.].
p.   cm.
Includes index.
ISBN 0 521 45271 6 (hc)
1. Down's syndrome – Diagnosis.   2. Prenatal diagnosis.
I. Grudzinskas, J. G. (Jurgis Gediminas)
[DNLM: 1. Down Syndrome – diagnosis.   2. Gonadotropins, Chorionic –
analysis.   3. Prenatal Diagnosis.   4. Genetic Screening.   WS 107 S4334 1995]
RG629.D68S37   1995
616.85′8842 – dc20
DNLM/DLC
for Library of Congress   94-2374 CIP

ISBN 0 521 45271 6 hardback

Contents

Contributors

J. R. Beekhuis
Department of Obstetrics and Gynaecology, Antenatal Diagnosis Unit, University Hospital, Groningen, The Netherlands

Z. Blumenfeld
Reproductive Endocrinology and Infertility Section, Department of Obstetrics and Gynecology, Rambam Medical Center, The Bruce Rappaport Faculty of Medicine, Technion – Israel Institute of Technology, Haifa 31096, Israel

I. Bonacchi
Department of Clinical Biochemistry, Instituti Clinici di Perfezionamento, Milan, Italy

A. Boué
INSERM U 73, Château de Longchamp, Paris, France

B. Brambati
First Institute of Obstetrics and Gynaecology, University of Milan, Milan, Italy

M. L. Brizot
35 Elmwood Rd, London SE24 9NS, UK

M. Bronshtein
Al-Kol Institute of Ultrasound, Department of Obstetrics and Gynecology, Rambam Medical Center, The Bruce Rappaport Faculty of Medicine, Technion – Israel Institute of Technology, Haifa 31096, Israel

T. Bryndorf
Chromosome Laboratory, 4051, Section of Clinical Genetics, Department of Obstetrics and Gynaecology, Rigshospitalet, Copenhagen, Denmark

T. Chard
Departments of Reproductive Physiology and Obstetrics and Gynaecology, St Bartholomew's Hospital Medical College and the London Hospital Medical College, London EC1A 7BE, UK

B. Christensen
Chromosome Laboratory, 4051, Section of Clinical Genetics, Department of Obstetrics and Gynaecology, Rigshospitalet, Copenhagen, Denmark

L. A. Cole
Department of Obstetrics and Gynecology, Yale University School of Medicine, New Haven, CT 06510, USA

H. S. Cuckle
Institute of Epidemiology and Health Services Research, University of Leeds, 34 Hyde Terrace, Leeds LS2 9LN, UK

G. C. Cunningham
Department of Obstetrics, Gynecology, Reproductive Science and Pediatrics, University of California Medical Center, San Francisco, CA 94143, USA

J. Dungan
UT Medical Group, Department of Obstetrics and Gynaecology, 853 Jefferson Ave, Memphis, TN 38104, USA

S. Elias
UT Medical Group, Department of Obstetrics and Gynaecology, 853 Jefferson Ave, Memphis, TN 38104, USA

A. R. Ellis
United Kingdom National Quality Assessment Schemes for Peptide Hormones and Related Substances, Immunoassay Section, Department of Clinical Biochemistry, Royal Infirmary, 1 Lauriston Place, Edinburgh EH3 9YW, UK

M. S. Golbus
Department of Obstetrics, Gynecology, Reproductive Sciences and Pediatrics, University of California Medical Center, San Francisco, CA 94143, USA

J. G. Grudzinskas
Academic Unit of Obstetrics and Gynaecology, The Royal London Hospital, London, UK

E. B. Hook
School of Public Health, University of California, Berkeley, CA 94720, USA

R. Iles
Departments of Reproductive Physiology and Obstetrics and Gynaecology, St Bartholomew's Hospital Medical College and the London Hospital Medical College, London EC1A 7BE, UK

L. H. Kornman
Department of Obstetrics and Gynaecology, Antenatal Diagnosis Unit, University Hospital, Groningen, The Netherlands

L. Lustig
Department of Obstetrics, Gynecology, Reproductive Sciences and Pediatrics, University of California Medical Center, San Francisco, CA 94143, USA

M. C. M. Macintosh
Departments of Reproductive Physiology and Obstetrics and Gynaecology, St Bartholomew's Hospital Medical College and the London Hospital Medical College, London EC1A 7BE, UK

J. N. Macri
NTD Laboratories Inc., 383 Old Country Rd, Carle Place, New York 11514, USA

A. Mantingh
Department of Obstetrics and Gynaecology, Antenatal Diagnosis Unit, University Hospital, Groningen, The Netherlands

T. M. Marteau
Psychology and Genetics Research Group, United Medical and Dental Schools of Guy's and St Thomas's Hospitals, Guy's Campus, London SE1 9RT, UK

A. Milford Ward
Department of Immunology, Northern General Hospital, Sheffield, UK

F. Muller
Biochemie, Ambroise Paré, Paris, France

K. H. Nicolaides
Harris Birthright Centre for Fetal Medicine, Department of Obstetrics and Gynaecology, King's College School of Medicine and Dentistry, Denmark Hill, London SE5 8RX, UK

J. Philip
Chromosome Laboratory, 4051, Section of Clinical Genetics, Department of Obstetrics and Gynaecology, Rigshospitalet, Copenhagen, Denmark

O. Phillips
UT Medical Group, Department of Obstetrics and Gynaecology, 853 Jefferson Ave, Memphis, TN 38104, USA

T. M. Reynolds
Department of Clinical Chemistry, Burton Hospitals NHS Trust, Belvidere Rd, Burton upon Trent, DE13 0RB, Staffs, UK

J. Seth
United Kingdom National Quality Assessment Schemes for Peptide Hormones and Related Substances, Immunoassay Section, Department of Clinical Biochemistry, Royal Infirmary, 1 Lauriston Place, Edinburgh EH3 8YW, UK

K. Shrimanker
Academic Unit of Obstetrics and Gynaecology, The Royal London Hospital, London, UK

L. Shulman
UT Medical Group, Department of Obstetrics and Gynaecology, 853 Jefferson Ave, Memphis, TN 38104, USA

J. L. Simpson
Department of Obstetrics and Gynecology, University of Tennessee, 853 Jefferson Ave, Memphis, TN 38103, USA

R. J. M. Snijders
66 Chaucer Rd, London SE24 0NU, UK

K. Spencer
Endocrine Unit, Department of Clinical Biochemistry, Oldchurch Hospital, Romford, RM7 0BE, Essex, UK

Y. Suzuki
Academic Unit of Obstetrics and Gynaecology, The Royal London Hospital, UK

P. Theodoropoulos
9 Deviazi 114.76, Poligono, Athens, Greece

L. Tului
First Institute of Obstetrics and Gynaecology, University of Milan, Milan, Italy

J. M. M. van Lith
Academic Medical Centre, Meibergdreef 9, 1105 AZ Amsterdam, The Netherlands

Y. Xiang
Chromosome Laboratory, 4051, Section of Clinical Genetics, Department of Obstetrics and Gynaecology, Rigshospitalet, Copenhagen, Denmark. (On leave of absence from Department of Obstetrics and Gynaecology, Peking Union Medical College Hospital, Beijing, 100730, People's Republic of China.)

1

Down's syndrome epidemiology and biochemical screening

ERNEST B. HOOK

One may consider at least four major questions about the epidemiology of Down's syndrome that are pertinent directly or indirectly to biochemical screening and prevention.

(1) What is the impact of this disorder upon society, i.e. why *should* society screen?
(2) What variables are associated with Down's syndrome that one may consider in adjusting results from screening?
(3) What are the implications for policy issues?
(4) What are the possibilities for future primary prevention?

Impact

Variation in the use of selective abortion of affected conceptuses and fertility among older mothers make it difficult to quantify the global impact of Down's syndrome, but clearly it makes a major contribution to the proportion of mental retardation. Earlier European data, in which older women (≥ 35 years) probably contributed well over 10% of livebirths to the population and prenatal diagnosis was not in use, suggest that Down's syndrome contributed about 10% of those with IQs under 20; about a third of those with IQs 20–49; and a smaller but variable proportion, about 3%, of those with moderate retardation but with IQs 50 or over. Other studies are compatible with even higher proportions among those with IQs under 50, about a third of the total. (References to earlier literature appear in Hook, 1985a.)

In recent studies, derived from populations in which there are proportionally fewer older women having children ($< 10\%$), the proportion of those with retardation diagnosed as Down's syndrome has been lower.

1

These suggest a proportion of about 10% among those 'mentally handi-capped' (e.g. Rasmussen *et al.*, 1982 cited by Webb *et al.*, 1987; Derey-maeker *et al.*, 1988). In areas in which relative fertility of older women is still high, however, the proportion is probably close to that seen earlier in European populations. For example, a study in Taiwan notes 18% Down's syndrome (Li *et al.*, 1988) among retardates. A recent study in Malaysia reports 32% of Down's syndrome in a group of retardates (Noor *et al.*, 1987) and published data for 1986–7 suggest 12% of mothers aged 35 years or over are affected (Boo *et al.*, 1989). (See also below.)

Mental retardation is not the only consequence of this condition. The increased frequency of other malformations, leukemia, etc. also puts a disproportionate burden on medical delivery systems. About 50% of these individuals have congenital heart defects (Fabia and Drolette, 1970), and about 12% of all livebirths with a congenital heart defect have a cytogenetic abnormality, about 75% of these being Down's syndrome (Ferencz *et al.*, 1987). With medical advances and social changes, these individuals receive more intensive and effective medical and surgical therapy in many jurisdictions, prolonging life and changing the life-span (e.g. Fabia and Drolette, 1970; Jones, 1979; Baird and Sadovnick, 1987, 1988, 1989). Data on differences in these trends appear in Mastroiacovo (1985); Malone (1988); Bell *et al.* (1989); Mastroiacovo *et al.* (1990). Despite the diminishing prevalence, either because of maternal age trends or because of more effective prenatal diagnosis, the economic impact of those affected who *are* born with the condition is likely to increase.

One economist estimated the excess economic cost to society of each Down's syndrome child over and above that of a normal child at $144 000 US (1985), discounted to the time of birth (Conley, 1985). This figure varies with factors such as health care practices and costs, mortality, special education, lost employment opportunity, and reimbursement, all of which obviously differ among jurisdictions and over time within areas. Assuming this figure is correct, in the USA, with a current expected livebirth prevalence rate of perhaps 1.2 to 1.3 per 1000 in the absence of prenatal diagnosis, society could justify (economically) spending up to $180 of such (1985) dollars for *each* pregnancy screened to detect *and prevent* a case. In the UK, with about the same background rate (Cuckle *et al.*, 1991), costs of £90 000 have been estimated (Gill *et al.*, 1987) implying a boundary of about £110. In areas such as Ireland (North or South) in which relative fertility is still high among older mothers (Radic, 1986; Dolk and Nevin, 1990) and the expected livebirth rate of Down's syndrome children is likely to be closer to 1.5 per 1000 (or even higher;

see, for example, Coffey and McCormick, 1977; Radic, 1986), even higher expenditure per pregnancy should be economically justified assuming the same baseline cost. This also assumes that a case diagnosed prenatally would be 'terminated', which is unlikely in a country without provision for selective abortion, let alone any abortion. Non-termination of pre-natally diagnosed cases is an important but usually neglected factor in these analyses. Efforts targeted at older mothers would have even greater economic support, and one that increases with age and risk.

Epidemiological issues related to screening

Apart from maternal serum analytes, selected abnormalities found in fetal imaging or fetal 47, +21 genetic material in maternal circulating blood, the only generally recognized *definitive* risk factors for a Down's syndrome livebirth are (elevated) maternal age, the birth of a previous affected individual, and the presence in one parent of a 47, +21 line or a structural rearrangement that will contribute a double dose of the responsible 21q region to a gamete. Individuals with the last two risk factors usually proceed immediately to prenatal cytogenetic diagnosis (at least in California), although biochemical screening results might diminish the need for that procedure in this group as well.

Age is the most ubiquitous risk factor for which adjustment of results from biochemical screening is required. The *relative* risks associated with observed values of maternal serum screening markers are multiplied by the baseline maternal age specific risk to derive an adjusted risk. (e.g Cuckle *et al.*, 1987; Palomaki and Haddow, 1987a; Tabor *et al.*, 1987; Miller *et al.*, 1991). But other biological and environmental factors have been proposed as associated with Down's syndrome. These could be used to adjust further the results from biochemical screening. Here I will address some of these but with particular focus on maternal age.

For historical reasons, women aged 35 years and over have been labeled 'high' risk and those under 35 years as 'low' risk for having a Down's syndrome infant. This goes back to the era when rates were calculated by 5-year intervals and a simple graph of rates imprinted on the viewer's eye an apparent quantum jump at 35 years (e.g. Penrose and Smith, 1966, p. 151, or Fig. 1.1.) The boundary is of course arbitrary (if we had six fingers, the boundary would have been 36). Moreover, when plotted by 1-year intervals, the rate changes gradually and continuously (Fig. 1.2). Nevertheless, the age 35 boundary point has been so imprinted in the

E.B. Hook

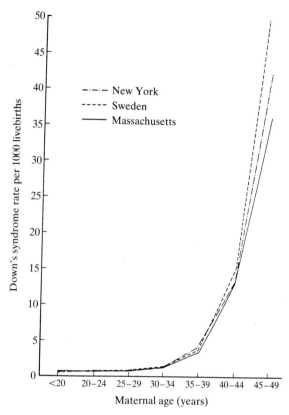

Fig. 1.1. Rates of Down's syndrome in three studies by 5-year maternal age intervals plotted on a linear scale. Note the abrupt change at 35–39 years.

medical mind that in many, but not all jurisdictions, it has been accepted as the established risk figure for provision of prenatal cytogenetic diagnosis. For example, in England, Scotland and Wales in 1991, of 97 Local Health Districts or Boards which did not perform serum screening (of a total of 200), two had a criterion of age ≥ 32 years, two a criterion of age ≥ 34 years, 49 at ≥ 35 years, $8 \geq 36$ years, $31 \geq 37$ years, and $5 \geq 38$ years (Wald *et al.*, 1992). The upper criteria are chosen, or may be chosen, to limit the impact upon diagnostic laboratories.

This has had a subtle, perhaps unappreciated, effect upon the significance of published risk figures by maternal age. For example, when I and others published risk figures by 1-year intervals, we viewed them as only rough guides to the magnitude of risk. Some disputes arose which focused on the major differences between, for example, rates in amniocentesis and in

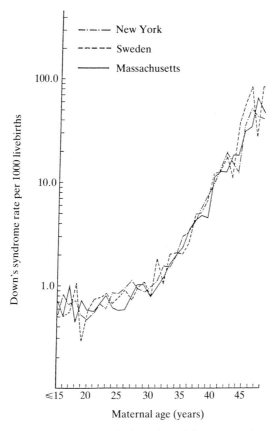

Fig. 1.2. Rates in the same population plotted by 1-year intervals on a log scale. Note no abrupt change at 35 years. (Reprinted with permission from Hook, 1982.)

livebirths (e.g. Ferguson-Smith, 1978; Hook, 1978). But all recognized that any point estimate will show variation.

Subsequent publications implied a variation in risk of Down's syndrome. But whether the rates at age 35 years were 1/350 or 1/400 or anywhere in this range did not affect the decision to have amniocentesis. The age not the risk figure provided the boundary. In the USA, for women under 35 years, the risk schedules were primarily of value because they gave women an indication of how close they came *relatively* to the risk at the generally agreed boundary.

Prenatal biochemical screening and 'at risk' projections derived from these results have changed the picture. Precise risk figures by maternal

age have become very important (or more accurately, the *ratios* of risk
figures at various ages to the risk figure at age 35 (or whatever age
boundary is chosen) has become critical). If a risk criterion is missed by
a decimal point an amniocentesis may not be performed. In one sense, of
course, age is just as arbitrary. A day or a month might decide for or
against an amniocentesis. Age can be measured precisely, but not risk for
age; there is an uncertainty about any cited risk figure for any particular
woman. And precisely what maternal-age risk schedule should be used is
still a matter of concern.

There is considerable variation in published risk figures by maternal
age for livebirth risk, and the rate schedules in use are based upon
extensive data only from those of European (or European ancestral)
origin. In the USA, no one makes any adjustment for racial or ethnic
variables in risk counseling for Down's syndrome, but the presumption
that the published maternal age-specific risk figures derived from the
mostly European populations (or rather, the ranges in those figures) apply
to the average individual of that age in any ethnic and racial group
remains a presumption. There are very few good studies of those of
non-European background. Some workers, mostly from an earlier era,
have implied lower maternal age-specific rates in some non-European
groups (for review of earlier studies see Hook and Porter, 1977). These
results are almost certainly attributable to underassessment in non-
Europeans. For American Blacks, the best, though small, study found
slightly higher rates than in American Whites (Sever *et al.*, 1970; see also
Kashgarian and Rendtorff, 1969). There are very few adequate studies in
Asians. An interesting study in Malaysia (Boo *et al.*, 1989) compared rates
in Malays, Chinese, and Indians but the database was small. Recent data
on three racial groups in Birmingham UK (Knox and Lancashire, 1991)
appear in Table 1.1. These do not adjust for losses due to prenatal
diagnosis but do include stillbirths. They provide some reassurance that
rates are likely not to be *higher* in Pakistani or Afro-Caribbeans than in
UK whites. Perhaps the UK National Register on Down's syndrome
(Mutton *et al.*, 1991) will eventually provide large scale useful data on
this issue in the non-European groups in the UK.

Wilson *et al.* (1992) make a plausible case for higher 5-year maternal
age-specific rates in Latinos (primarily natives of Mexico and Central
America) in Los Angeles than in those of European background. I have
recently looked for such trends in all California livebirths by 1-year
maternal age interval in data from the California Birth Defects Monitoring
Program. The rates appear no higher than the published rates for those

Table 1.1. *Down's syndrome in stillbirths and livebirths in three ethnic groups in Birmingham, UK, 1964–84*

Maternal age (years)	Caucasians		Asians		Afro-Caribbean	
	DS/births	Rate	DS/births	Rate	DS/births	Rate
<25	91/120 231	0.76	15/23 538	0.64	8/11 738	0.68[a]
25–29	73/79 789	0.91	19/14 948	1.27	8/6045	1.32
30–34	58/41 456	1.40	17/7906	2.15	4/4258	0.94
35–39	80/17 323	4.62	12/4011	2.99	6/2515	2.39
≥40	61[b]/5371	11.41[b]	15/2339	6.41	8/994	8.05
Total	363[c]/264 170	1.37[c]	78/52 742	1.48[d]	34/25 550	1.33[e]

From Knox and Lancashire (1991) with modification. The rates given here are, with exceptions noted, from Table 3.5 (p. 53) of Knox and Lancashire (1991). The denominator in each age category is from Appendix 2.2, Table iv, (p. 38) and the totals given are the calculated sum in each category. The number of Down's syndrome cases given at each age is calculated, with the exceptions noted, from the age specific rates given in Table 3.5 of this reference and livebirths in each age group.

[a] The entry in the reference (1.74) appears to be a misprint.
[b] The given rate actually 'predicts' 61.3 cases in the number of livebirths given.
[c] Table 3.2 of this reference gives 354 total cases in Caucasians (denominator not specified) and a rate of 1.383 per 1000. The number and rates for other defects in the table imply a denominator about 255 920 total births, smaller than the total of 264 490 cited elsewhere in this reference. The overall difference in rates is trivial, but the two tables imply a difference of at least $363 - 354 = 9$ cases in whites total.
[d] 1.47 in the original report (p. 52).
[e] From p. 51 of original report.

of European background, but the available Latino data do not include any prenatal terminations. Prenatal cytogenetic utilization is relatively low in this population for religious and social reasons; underestimates from this loss may not be serious, but there is still a residual uncertainty.

There is evidence for higher rates of Down's syndrome, in the middle part of the maternal age range, in Israeli Jews of Asian or African origin compared with those of European origin (Hook and Harlap, 1979). A problem with both the study in Israel and in Los Angeles is that the data available for reanalysis have been based only upon 5-year intervals (see Table 1.2 for rates in these two groups). Therefore, there is no group which can be confidently stated to have lower maternal age-specific rates than Europeans. Equally, on present evidence, one cannot assume that the average livebirth rates must be the same for all ethnic and racial groups.

Table 1.2. *5-year maternal age-specific rates and ratios of Down's syndrome in two non-European populations per 1000 and ratio to rates in Sweden*

Maternal age (years)	Sweden	'Latinos'/LA	Ratio to Swedish rates	Non-European Jews in Israel	Ratio to Swedish rates
15–19	0.59	0.74	1.3	—	—
20–24	0.74	0.80	1.1	0.60	0.8
25–29	0.88	1.02	1.2	1.23	1.4
30–34	1.45	2.35	1.6	2.65	1.8
35–39	3.74	4.85	1.3	6.53	1.7
40–44	14.96	24.22	1.6	16.54	1.1

Modified from data in Hook and Harlap (1979) and Wilson *et al.* (1992).

A number of other 'demographic risk' factors have been proposed. The effects of any of these, at least within those of European ancestry, are unlikely to be large. This does *not* exclude the possibility of small effects (certainly of relative risks between 0.5 and 2.0) *nor* the possibility that there are smaller subgroups within intensively studied populations or larger groups in other populations in which these or other factors are associated with large magnitude effects. Inbreeding in Kuwaitis (Alfi *et al.*, 1980) but not in most other groups may be one example and could be explained by recessive genes in *this* particular population which predisposed to non-disjunction. Another possible example is the history of a prior spontaneous (unkaryotyped) abortion, but only in very young women (Hook and Cross, 1983).

An intriguing observation in many studies is the suggestion of a negative association of maternal cigarette smoking (Cuckle *et al.*, 1990; Kline *et al.*, 1993). Though Cuckle tends to dismiss the trend, the summary table appears to provide some supporting evidence consistent with a relative risk of about 0.7 to 0.8. The issue is further complicated by the fact that maternal smoking is associated with higher maternal serum α-fetoprotein (MSAFP) levels (about 3%) and lower human chorionic gonadotropin levels (about 23%) (Palomaki *et al.*, 1993). If cigarette smoking *per se is* established as a (negative) risk factor, then because of the large but variable proportion of smokers in different populations, it will be necessary to re-examine published livebirth rates to estimate how much of the residual variation may be attributable to differences in smoking habits. This would greatly complicate the application of maternal age-specific rates.

Maternal serum thyroid auto-antibodies are a plausible associated risk (Cuckle *et al.*, 1988) but this is an expensive test relative to its likely contribution. There is also evidence (Khoury *et al.*, 1989) that a maternal history of thyroid disease is a risk factor (relative risk 1.5). This is compatible with the trends with thyroid auto-antibodies and the information would be easy to collect. Similarly, the modest association (1.3- to about 2-fold increase) of maternal bleeding and Down's syndrome that has been reported in several studies (see Cuckle and Wald, 1987 for review) appears plausible. If confirmed and defined more precisely, this could also become an 'adjustment' factor.

One of the most perplexing variables is maternal preconceptual exposure to ionizing radiation. There are some highly suggestive studies in the literature and support from studies in lower organisms. But there are also highly convincing negative results (for review, see Kline and Stein, 1985.) Observations from Hiroshima and Nagasaki argue against an association because there is a (non-significant) *negative* trend (Schull and Neel, 1962). Discrepancies among the radiation studies have spawned a number of hypotheses explaining the differences on the basis of timing or dosage. However, a positive history cannot presently be used to adjust risk. Other factors with at least suggestive associations with Down's syndrome include oral contraceptives and spermicides, but neither has been confirmed (references in Kline and Stein, 1985; Kline *et al.*, 1989).

A separate issue is the 'fine tuning' of estimates of risk derived from existing methods of screening. Each of these issues has been a source of lively controversy, for example:

(1) Do we analyze serum markers using Multiples of the Median (MoMs) or by observed values of MSAFP and other serum proteins adjusted for known sources of variability within a particular laboratory (see Reynold *et al.*, 1993; Wald, 1993)?

(2) Existing methods of risk projection presume not only independence of each of these markers with age and each other over the entire range but also multivariate 'normal', i.e. Gaussian, distributions of the serum markers. Are these assumptions proven? The evidence may (or may not) be *consistent* with such assumptions. A sensitivity test to test the *range* would be worthwhile. (See discussion and references in Hook, 1988, 1989.)

(3) Which *relative* risk schedules for MSAFP and Down's syndrome (i.e.

lists of rates projecting the change in risk associated with a particular MSAFP value) should be used? Three different rate schedules from three different countries, USA, England and Denmark have appeared (Cuckle *et al.*, 1987; Palomaki and Haddow, 1987 and unpublished supplement to this paper; Tabor *et al.*, 1987). The USA group is now using the English schedule (Wald *et al.*, 1989). But it is not clear which is appropriate if there are regional variations. Most workers appear to be using the English reference series, e.g. Zeitune *et al.* (1991), (which has modified the schedule for all trisomies).

(4) How precisely do we derive the estimate for spontaneous losses between amniocentesis and term birth? And should we assume rates under age 20 years continue to decline or level out (Zeitune *et al.*, 1991; Hook, 1985b)?

There is no doubt that biochemical screening enhances risk estimates. But the extent to which some women who would otherwise *receive* amniocentesis are inappropriately deemed as low risk remains a point of concern. The accumulation of data on older women within screening programs will allow evaluation of these projections.

Some policy issues

Serum screening is improving prenatal detection of affected conceptuses and, with new markers or other prenatal observations, may become even more efficient. One further factor which should be considered is variability in termination.

This pertains to an individual's perception of the risks of amniocentesis and views on pregnancy termination. Among women at risk because of advanced age or other risk factors before the advent of biochemical screening, the proportion in whom Down's syndrome was diagnosed by amniocentesis but who were not effectively terminated was 2–3% in New York State (E.B. Hook, unpublished data). Later studies have reported proportions closer to 10% (e.g. Vincent *et al.*, 1991), but these include cases diagnosed as at risk through maternal serum screening as well as just age. In California, preliminary data suggest that the proportion of non-terminations of Down's syndrome is much higher among women initially detected through serum screening than among those who had amniocentesis only because of age. There may well be social differences between women identified through screening and those who go directly to amniocentesis (or chorionic villus sampling, CVS) because of risk factors such as age. Probably women in whom the diagnosis is made in the first trimester (CVS) are more likely to terminate (Verp *et al.*, 1988).

Why would a pregnant woman place herself and her fetus at unnecessary risk, merely to get information that she would not act upon? Several factors might operate. First, some obstetricians probably underestimate the excess risk of fetal loss in discussion with their patients. The best controlled studies, from Europe, suggest an excess risk due to amnio-centesis of 1% (Tabor, 1988). Some in the USA have questioned the local applicability of these results. A risk of 1/200 is often cited (Platt and Carlson, 1992) although some centers claim an even lower risk, of the order of 1/400. Second, insurers or taxpayers often pay for these procedures. Given an opportunity to have, free of charge, a diagnostic procedure that might be harmless, a women might elect to undergo a procedure which will provide some information about the pregnancy outcome, irrespective of what she intends to do about it.

Some years ago when I helped set policy on these issues for the New York State Department of Health, Ruth Berini, then head of the National Genetics Foundation, suggested that prenatal diagnosis should only be paid for by the State if the woman promised to have a termination if a Down's syndrome fetus was diagnosed. However, while that made sense economically, the Health Department supported personal autonomy. In effect, the statement really meant 'We're having enough trouble getting money from the legislature to subsidize prenatal diagnostic services. We can only defend this by just providing useful information to the patients, not encouraging, let alone requiring, an advance agreement to act on this information (i.e. abort) as a precondition of the services.' But there was a legal response to this suggestion as well. Whatever promissory note a woman might sign about her intended behavior after a prenatal diagnosis of Down's syndrome, USA courts would probably find that a woman always has the right to change her mind.

Nevertheless, there are other ways to achieve this goal. For example, insurance companies (or the taxpayers) could *lend* a woman the money for prenatal diagnosis. The loan is to be forgiven *if* (i) a normal fetus is diagnosed or (ii) a Down's syndrome (or other cytogenetically abnormal conceptus) is diagnosed *and* the pregnancy is terminated. Some view this as an unpleasant scenario and it may well indeed be unacceptable in many political environments. Others may see it as an efficient method to avoid wasting scarce health funds particularly with increasing 'health rationing'.

Prospects for primary prevention

To result in *prevention*, prenatal detection requires both timely diagnosis and selective abortion; one or both are unavailable to large segments of the world's population. Prenatal diagnosis/selective abortion is only an interim solution until more acceptable and less interventionist strategies are developed. One obvious, almost trivial, method is illustrated in Table 1.3, which correlates the proportion of women aged 35 years or over

Table 1.3. *Correlation of the proportion of older mothers having livebirths of infants with Down's syndrome and estimated impact of prenatal diagnosis programmes on rates in selected countries*

Country and period of study	Proportion of mothers ≥ 35 years (%)	Down's syndrome expected rate per 1000 births	Down's syndrome 'observed' rate per 1000 livebirths[a]	Likely rate reduction attributable to prenatal diagnosis[b] (%)
Czechoslovakia (1980–4)	3.6	1.07	1.06	<1
New Zealand (1980–5)	4.6	1.22	1.24	0
USA, Atlanta (1980–5)	4.8	1.18	1.06	10
Denmark (1981–5)	7.1	1.35	1.02	25
Mexico (1982–5)	7.1	1.36	1.36	0
England and Wales (1980–5)	7.3	1.37	1.23	10
Sweden (1980–5)	10.3	1.55	1.35	13
Finland (1980–5)	10.6	1.59	1.45	9
Northern Ireland (1981–5)	11.1	1.62	1.60	1

[a] The 'observed' rates are those derived in the original reference by correcting for estimated underascertainment in each reporting source.

[b] The estimate given is $(1 - O/E)/100$ if positive, where O is the 'observed' rate, and E is the expected rate. If negative, then no impact (0%) is inferred. Statistical fluctuations in the calculated number observed may of course obscure utilization of prenatal diagnosis in some jurisdictions (perhaps in New Zealand) or exaggerate it.

Calculated from data presented by Kallen and Knudsen (1989), reprinted from Hook, E.B. (1992). Chromosome abnormalities: prevalence, risks and recurrence. In *Prenatal Diagnosis and Screening*, ed. D.J.H. Brock, C.H. Rodeck and M.A. Ferguson-Smith, p. 384. Edinburgh: Churchill Livingstone.

having livebirths and the expected prevalence of Down's syndrome in the absence of prenatal diagnosis. Note that in Czechoslovakia with a 3% proportion of 'older' mothers, the predicted rate without prenatal diagnosis is almost equivalent to the achieved rate in Denmark which has prenatal diagnosis but almost twice the proportion of older mothers. And note the very high relative fertility rate in Northern Ireland, with apparently a very low uptake of prenatal diagnosis. (A separate report noted 9% of women aged 35 years and over had selective termination (Dolk and Nevin, 1990) which predicts about a 6% drop in the predicted livebirth rate in this age range and roughly a 3% decline in those of all ages compared to the drop of 1% given in the table.) The highest projected rates of which I am aware are from Brazil. Martello *et al.* (1984) reported that for births during 1970 19.7% of mothers of livebirths were aged 35 years or older; the predicted rate of Down's syndrome was 2.7 per 1000. The issue of prenatal diagnosis and prevention in different populations is discussed further by Hook (1979), Holloway and Brock (1988) and Huether (1990).

Apart from changes in fertility patterns, which can have only limited impact, there is no plausible plan for primary prevention. The most significant recent advances in epidemiology have come from molecular biology. Contrary to earlier expectations based on cytological observations, we now know that the vast majority of cases, about 95%, originate from non-disjunction in the mother (Antonarakis *et al.*, 1991). In addition, and contrary to earlier indications from scoring of cytological markers, maternal age is greater in cases in which the extra chromosome is of maternal origin than where it is of paternal origin: in 17 cases of paternal origin the maternal age was 28.7 (S.E.M. 1.3) years; in 249 cases of maternal origin the mean was 31.5 (S.E.M. 0.4) years (Sherman *et al.*, 1992; Sherman, 1992). (For 132 'maternal' cases assigned to meiosis-I origin, mean maternal age was 31.8 years (S.E.M. 0.5); for 52 cases assigned to meiosis-II origin, mean age was 30.4 years (S.E.M. 1.3); for 11 cases of inferred mitotic origin, mean age was 26.7 years (S.E.M. 2.2) suggesting that the maternal age effect is limited primarily, if not exclusively, to cases of first division maternal non-disjunction.) Thus 'relaxed selection' (i.e. preferential uterine *retention* of 47, +21 conceptuses to the time of livebirth or analogous effects such as preferential fertilization of disomic gametes in older women) cannot account for *all* of the maternal age effect and may not account for any (for references see Hook, 1985b). This ends some 15 years of puzzling observations in which there appeared to be no difference in maternal age between cases of maternal or paternal origin. These results suggest the eventual possibility of one high technology 'fix'. If young men can 'bank' their sperm, perhaps young women can in the future 'bank' their ova for reuse for a planned subsequent conception.

Of course, for vast numbers for whom this technology is unavailable, simpler methods must be sought. We still do not understand why there is a maternal age effect in humans, despite decades of intriguing work on humans and mouse and many clever suggestions. (See review in Bond and Chandley, 1983; Hook, 1985b, and also Kline and Levin, 1992 and te Velde, 1993.) Some of the most interesting observations come from molecular biology (Sherman *et al.*, 1992). Diminished recombination appears to occur in 47, + 21 cases of maternal meiosis-I origin (mean map length of 31 cM) compared with those of maternal meiosis-II origin (80 cM) or those with normal maternal 21 disjunction (99 cM). But among those of meiosis-I origin in 60 cases age 31 or younger map length is 40 cM compared with 26 cM in the 72 cases age 32 or higher (Sherman *et al.*, 1992). The latter trend, if confirmed, may lead to ultimate understanding of the maternal-age effect. While fully cognizant of the great advances that prenatal screening has brought, let us not ignore the need to search for the ultimate mechanisms of non-disjunction in humans and the hope for its primary prevention.

References

Alfi, O.S., Chang, R. & Azen, S.P. (1980). Evidence for genetic control of non-disjunction in man. *Am. J. Hum. Genet.*, **32**, 477–83.

Antonarakis, S.E. & The Down Syndrome Collaborative Group (1991). Parental origin of the extra chromosome in trisomy 21 as indicated by analysis of DNA polymorphisms. *N. Eng. J. Med.*, **324**(13), 872–6.

Baird, P.A. & Sadovnick, A.D. (1987). Life expectancy in Down syndrome. *J. Pediatr.*, **110**(6), 849–54.

Baird, P.A. & Sadovnick, A.D. (1988). Life expectancy in Down syndrome adults. *Lancet*, **2**(8624), 1354–6.

Baird, P.A. & Sadovnick, A.D. (1989). Life tables for Down syndrome. *Hum. Genet.*, **82**, 291–2.

Bell, J.A., Pearn, J.H. & Firman, D. (1989). Childhood deaths in Down's syndrome. Survival curves and causes of death from a total population study in Queensland, Australia, 1976 to 1985. *J. Med. Genet.*, **26**, 764–8.

Bond, D.J. & Chandley, A.C. (1983). *Aneuploidy*. pp. 83–91, 67–73. Oxford: Oxford University Press.

Boo, N.Y., Hoe, T.S., Lye, M.S., Poon, P.K. & Mahani, M.C. (1989). Maternal age-specific incidence of Down's syndrome in Malaysian neonates. *J. Singapore Paediatr. Soc.*, **31**, 138–42.

Coffey, V.P. & McCormick, E. (1977). Down's syndrome in Eastern Health Board area of Ireland 1953–1976. *J. Irish Med. Assoc.*, **70**(4), 140–5.

Conley, R.W. (1985). Down syndrome: economic burdens and benefits of prevention. In *Aneuploidy: Etiology and Mechanism*, ed. V.L. Dellarco, P.E. Voytek & A. Hollaender, pp. 35–9. New York: Plenum Press.

Cuckle, H.S. & Wald, N.J. (1987). Vaginal bleeding in pregnancies associated with fetal Down syndrome. *Prenatal Diagn.*, **7**, 619–22.

Cuckle, H.S., Wald, N. & Thompson, S. (1987). Estimating a woman's risk of having a pregnancy associated with Down's syndrome using her age and serum alpha-fetoprotein level. *Br. J. Obstet. Gynaecol.*, **94**, 387–402.

Cuckle, H.S., Wald, N., Stone, R., Densem, J., Haddow, J. & Knight, G. (1988). Maternal serum thyroid antibodies in early pregnancy and fetal Down's syndrome. *Prenatal Diagn.*, **8**, 439–45.

Cuckle, H.S., Alberman, E., Wald, N.J., Royston, P. & Knight, G. (1990). Maternal smoking habits and Down's syndrome. *Prenatal Diagn.*, **10**, 561–7.

Cuckle, H., Nanchahal, K. & Wald, N. (1991). Birth prevalence of Down's syndrome in England and Wales. *Prenatal Diagn.*, **11**, 29–34.

Dereymaeker, A.M., Fryns, J.P., Haegeman, J., Deroover, J. & Van den Berghe, H. (1988). A genetic-diagnostic survey in an institutionalized population of 158 mentally retarded patients. The Viaene experience. *Clin. Genet.*, **34**(2), 126–34.

Dolk, H. & Nevin, N.C. (1990). Down's syndrome and fertility in older women. *Lancet*, **336**, 511.

Fabia, J. & Drolette, M. (1970). Life tables up to age 10 for mongols with and without congenital heart defects. *J. Ment. Defic. Res.*, **14**, 235–42.

Ferencz, C., Rubin, S.D., McCarter, R.J. *et al.* (1987). Cardiac and non-cardiac malformations: observations in a population based study. *Teratology*, **35**, 367–78.

Ferguson-Smith, M.A. (1978). Maternal age and Down syndrome. *Lancet*, **2**, 213.

Gill, M., Murday, V. & Slack, J. (1987). An economic appraisal of screening for Down's syndrome in pregnancy using material age and serum alpha fetoprotein concentration. *Soc. Sci. Med.*, **24**, 725–31.

Holloway, S. & Brock, D.J.H. (1988). Changes in maternal age distribution and their possible impact on demand for prenatal diagnostic services. *Br. Med. J.*, **296**, 978–81.

Hook, E.B. (1978). Differences between rates of trisomy 21 (Down's syndrome) and other chromosomal abnormalities diagnosed in livebirths and in cells cultured after 2nd trimester amniocentesis – suggested explanations and implications for genetic counseling and program planning. In *Sex Differentiation and Chromosomal Abnormalities. Birth Defects Original Article Series*, Vol. 14, No. 6C, ed. R.L. Summitt & D. Bergsma, pp. 249–267. New York: Alan R. Liss.

Hook, E.B. (1979). Genetic counseling and prenatal cytogenetic services: Policy implications and detailed cost-benefit analyses of programs for the prevention of Down syndrome. In *Service and Education in Medical Genetics*, ed. I.H. Porter & E.B. Hook, pp. 29–54. New York: Academic Press.

Hook, E.B. (1982). Epidemiology of Down syndrome. In *Down Syndrome: Advances in Biomedicine and the Behavioral Sciences*, ed. S.M. Pueschel & J.E. Rynders, pp. 11–88. Cambridge, MA: The Ware Press.

Hook, E.B. (1985a). The impact of aneuploidy upon public health: mortality and morbidity associated with human chromosome abnormalities. In *Aneuploidy: Etiology and Mechanism*, ed. V.L. Dellarco, P.E. Voytek & A. Hollaender, pp. 7–33. New York: Plenum Press.

Hook, E.B. (1985b). Maternal age, paternal age, and human chromosome abnormality: nature, magnitude, etiology, and mechanisms of effects. In *Aneuploidy: Etiology and Mechanism*, ed. V.L. Dellarco, P.E. Voytek & A. Hollaender, pp. 117–32. New York: Plenum Press.

Hook, E.B. (1988). Variability in predicted rates of Down syndrome associated with elevated maternal serum alpha-fetoprotein levels in older women. *Am. J. Hum. Genet.*, **43**, 160–4.

Hook, E.B. (1989). Screening for Down syndrome: reply to Wald *et al. Am. J. Hum. Genet.*, **44**, 587–90.

Hook, E.B. (1992). Chromosome abnormalities: prevalence, risks and recurrence. In *Prenatal Diagnosis and Screening*, ed. D.J.H. Brock, C.H. Rodeck & M.A. Ferguson-Smith, pp. 351–92. Edinburgh: Churchill Livingstone.

Hook, E.B. & Cross, P.K. (1983). Spontaneous abortion and subsequent Down syndrome livebirth. *Hum. Genet.*, **64**, 267–70.

Hook, E.B. & Harlap, S. (1979). Differences in maternal age specific rates of Down syndrome between Jews of European origin and North African or Asian origin. *Teratology*, **20**, 243–8.

Hook, E.B. & Porter, I.H. (1977). Human population cytogenetics – comments on racial differences in frequency of chromosome abnormalities, putative clustering of Down's syndrome, and radiation studies. In *Population Cytogenetics – Studies in Humans*, ed. E.B. Hook & I.H. Porter, pp. 353–65. New York: Academic Press.

Huether, C.A. (1990). Epidemiological aspects of Down syndrome: sex ratio, incidence, and recent impact of prenatal diagnosis utilization. *Issues Rev. Teratol.*, **5**, 283–316.

Jones, M.B. (1979). Years of life lost through Down's syndrome. *J. Med. Genet.*, **16**, 379–83.

Kallen, B. & Knudsen, L.B. (1989). Effect of maternal age distribution and prenatal diagnosis on the population rates of Down syndrome – a comparative study of nineteen populations. *Hereditas*, **110**, 55–60.

Kashgarian, M. & Rendtorff, R.C. (1969). Incidence of Down's syndrome in American negroes. *J. Pediatr.*, **74**, 468–471.

Khoury, M.J., Becerra, J.E. & d'Almada, P.J. (1989). Maternal thyroid disease and risk of birth defects in offspring: a population-based case-control study. *Paediatr. Perinat. Epidemiol.*, **3**, 402–20.

Kline, J. & Levin, B. (1992). Trisomy and age at menopause: predicted associations given a link with rate of oocyte atresia. *Paediatr. Perinat. Epidemiol.*, **6**, 225–39.

Kline, J. & Stein, Z. (1985). Environmental causes of aneuploidy: why so elusive? In *Aneuploidy: Etiology and Mechanism*. ed. V.L. Dellarco, P.E. Voytek & A. Hollaender, pp. 149–64. New York: Plenum Press.

Kline, J., Stein, Z. & Susser, M. (1989). *Conception to Birth: Epidemiology of Prenatal Development.* pp. 131–7. New York: Oxford University Press.

Kline, J., Levin, B., Stein, Z., Warburton, D. & Hindin, R. (1993). Cigarette smoking and trisomy 21 at amniocentesis. *Genet. Epidemiol.*, **10**, 35–42.

Knox, E.G. & Lancashire, R.J. (1991). *Epidemiology of Congenital Malformations*, pp. 1–221, especially pp. 38, 52, 53. London: HMSO (Her Majesty's Stationery Office).

Li, S.Y., Tsai, C.C., Chou, M.Y. & Lin, J.K. (1988). A cytogenetic study of mentally retarded school children in Taiwan with special reference to the fragile X chromosome. *Hum. Genet.*, **79**(4), 292–6.

Malone, Q. (1988). Mortality and survival of the Down's syndrome population in Western Australia. *J. Ment. Defic. Res.*, **32**, 59–65.

Martello, N., Santos, J.L.F. & Frota-Pessoa, O. (1984). Down syndrome in the different physiographic regions of Brazil. *Rev. Brasil Genet. (Brazil J. Genet.)*, **7**(1), 157–73.

Mastroiacovo, P. (1985). The Italian Birth Defects Monitoring System: baseline rates based on 283 453 births and comparison with other registries. *Prevention of Physical and Mental Congenital Defects, Part B: Epidemiology, Early Detection and Therapy, and Environmental Factors*, pp. 17–21.

Mastroiacovo, P., Bertollini, R. & Corchia, C. (1990). Survival trends in Down syndrome (letter). *Lancet*, **335**, 1278–9.

Miller, C.H., O'Brian, T.J., Chatelain, S., Butler, B.B. & Quirk, J.G. (1991). Alteration in age-specific risks for chromosomal trisomy by maternal serum alpha-fetoprotein and human chorionic gonadotropin screening. *Prenatal Diagn.*, **11**, 153–8.

Mutton, D.E., Alberman, E., Ide, R. & Bobrow, M. (1991). Results of first year (1989) of a national register of Down's syndrome in England and Wales. *Br. Med. J.*, **303**, 1295–7.

Noor, P.J., Chin, Y.M., Ten, S.K. & Hassan, K. (1987). Prevalence of chromosomal anomalies of the mentally retarded – report of a study of 124 institutionalized children in Kuala Lumpur. *Singapore Med. J.*, **28**(3), 235–40.

Palomaki, G.E. & Haddow, J.E. (1987a). Maternal serum alpha-fetoprotein, age, and Down syndrome risk. *Am. J. Obstet. Gynecol.*, **156**, 460–3.

Palomaki, G.E., Knight, G.J., Haddow, J.E., Canick, J.A., Wald, N.J. & Kennard, A. 1(993). Cigarette smoking and levels of maternal serum alpha-fetoprotein, unconjugated estriol, and hCG: impact on Down syndrome screening. *Obstet. Gynecol.*, **81**, 675–8.

Penrose, C.S. & Smith, G.F. (1966). *Down's Anomaly*. p. 151. London: J and A Churchill.

Platt, L.D. & Carlson, D.E. (1992). Prenatal diagnosis – when and how? *N. Eng. J. Med.*, **327**, 636–8.

Radic, A. (1986). *Surveillance of Congenital Malformations in the Eastern Health Board Region 1979–1983*. Dublin: The Medico-Social Research Board.

Reynold, T., Nix, B. & Dunstan, F. (1993). Use of MoMs in medical statistics. *Lancet.* **341**, 59.

Sever, J.L., Gilkeson, M.R., Chen, T.C., Ley, A.C. & Edmonds, D. (1970). Epidemiology of mongolism in the collaborative project. *Ann. N.Y. Acad. Sci.*, **171**, 328–40.

Sherman, S.L. (1992). Presentation to American Society of Human Genetics, October 1992. (Update and correction of Petersen, M.B., Antonarakis, S.E., Hassold, T.J., Freeman, S.B., Sherman, S.L. & Mikkelsen, M. (1992).) Paternal nondisjunction in trisomy 21. *Am. J. Hum. Genet.*, **51**, A24).

Sherman, S.L., Freeman, S.B., Grantham, M. *et al.* (1992). Presentation to American Society of Human Genetics, October 1992: Non-disjunction of trisomy 21: comparison of centromere maps resulting from maternal meiosis I and II non-disjunction. *Am. J. Hum. Genet.*, **51**, A24.

Schull, W.J. & Neel, J.V. (1962). Maternal radiation and mongolism. *Lancet*, **1**, 537–8.

Tabor, A. (1988). Genetic amniocentesis – indications and risk. *Danish Med. Bull.*, **35**, 520–37.

Tabor, A., Larsen, S.O., Neilsen, J. *et al.* (1987). Screening for Down's syndrome using an iso-risk curve based on maternal age and serum alpha-fetoprotein level. *Br. J. Obstet. Gynaecol.*, **94**, 636–42.

te Velde, E.R. (1993). Disappearing ovarian follicles and reproductive ageing. *Lancet*, **341**, 1125–6.

Verp, M.S., Bombard, A.T., Simpson, J.L. & Elias, S. (1988). Parental decision following prenatal diagnosis of fetal chromosome abnormality. *Am. J. Med. Genet.*, **29**(3), 613–22.

Vincent, V.A., Edwards, J.G., Young, S.R. & Nachtigal, M. (1991). Pregnancy termination because of chromosomal abnormalities: a study of 26 950 amniocenteses in the Southeast. *Southern Med. J.*, **84**, 1210–13.

Wald, N.J. (1993). Use of MoMs. *Lancet*, **341**, 440.

Wald, N.J., Cuckle, H.S., Sneddon, J., Haddow, J.E. & Palomaki, G.E. (1989). Screening for Down syndrome. *Am. J. Hum. Genet.*, **44**, 586–7.

Wald, N.J., Wald, K. & Smith, D. (1992). The extent of Down's syndrome screening in Britain in 1991. *Lancet*, **340**, 494.

Webb, T.P., Thake, A.I., Bundsey, S.E. & Todd, J. (1987). A cytogenetic survey of a mentally retarded school-age population with special reference to fragile sites. *J. Ment. Defic. Res.*, **31** (Pt 1), 61–71.

Wilson, M.G., Chan, L.S. & Herbert, W.S. (1992). Birth prevalence of Down syndrome in a predominantly Latino population: a 15-year study. *Teratology*, **45**, 285–92.

Zeitune, M., Aitken, D.A., Crossley, J.A., Yates, J.R.W., Cooke, A. & Ferguson-Smith, M.A. (1991). Estimating the risk of a fetal autosomal trisomy at mid-trimester using maternal serum alpha-fetoprotein and age: a retrospective study of 142 pregnancies. *Prenatal Diagn.* **11**, 847–57.

2

Perception of risk

M.C.M. MACINTOSH

Biochemical screening for Down's syndrome provides a risk value for an individual woman. It is the perception of this risk that determines subsequent actions. The purpose of this chapter is first to present a brief history of risk and risk analysis and the incorporation of risk concepts into medicine with particular reference to obstetrics and gynaecology; and secondly to review the importance of the perception of risk with respect to Down's syndrome screening.

History

The term risk is defined as the chance of a bad outcome. The word is derived from the Greek word *rhiza* which means the hazards of sailing too close to the cliffs. However formal risk assessment was utilised in 3200 BC, long before Greek civilisation, by the Asipu, living near the Tigris and Euphrates. They provided solutions to difficult decisions (Covello and Mumpower, 1985). As they were empowered to read the signs of the gods, probability played no part in their judgement. Quantitative risk analysis was frequently used in religious settings. Arnobius, a prominent figure in the pagan church (North Africa, fourth century AD), proposed the equivalent of a 2×2 matrix to help with the decision of 'accepting Christianity' or 'remain a pagan'. He described the uncertain states 'God exists' and 'God does not exist'. This was the first published heuristic for making decisions under conditions of risk and uncertainty (Covello and Mumpower, 1985). During the Middle Ages, there was minimal under-standing of the nature of the links between hazards and harm. Witchcraft was taken seriously and bad outcomes were attributed to malign influences leading to many unjustified executions. The watershed in understanding came with the introduction of probability theory by Blaise Pascal in 1657.

Table 2.1. *Studies linking adverse health states with potential causes*

	Observer[a]	Year
Breast cancer and nulliparity	Ramazzini	1700
Scrotal cancer and chimney sweeps	Pott	1775
Cancer of the nasal passages and tobacco snuff	Hill	1782
Cholera and contaminated water	Snow	1855
Skin cancer and sunlight exposure	Unna	1894
Bladder cancer and aromatic amines	Rehn	1895

[a] From Covello and Mumpower, 1985.

Prediction became a subject for the scientist and not just the soothsayer. Commercially the insurance industry flourished. Fire insurance was established in 1666 following the Great Fire and Lloyds was founded in 1688. Life insurance followed the derivation of life expectancy tables from parish records by Graunt in 1662. Halley (best known for his comet) also contributed to life tables in 1693. The Church viewed life insurance as an immoral wager and in France it was prohibited until 1820 (Covello and Mumpower, 1985).

Within medicine, the nature of disease and adverse factors began to emerge and by the end of the nineteenth century many associations had been recognised (Table 2.1). However, the ability to demonstrate scientifically the links between a hazard and harm does not necessarily result in acknowledgement of the risk by the public or medical profession.

Misperceptions in obstetrics and gynaecology

Misperception of risk may have serious consequences and there are many such examples in the history of obstetrics and gynaecology.

In the nineteenth century puerperal sepsis was responsible for epidemics of maternal deaths. Wound infections were thought to be caused by a 'miasma' (bad air) which hung around a building. Ignaz Phillip Semmelweiss (1818–65), the first assistant in the maternity hospital, Vienna, demonstrated that puerperal sepsis was caused by the transfer of 'putrid particles' from the corpses in the dissection room via the unwashed hands of the medical staff to the women in the ward. Sadly his arguments did not convince the obstetricians of Vienna. At the same time in America, Oliver Wendell Holmes was placed in an equivalent predicament and concluded that 'medical logic does not appear to be taught or practised in our schools'.

Risks of technology

In the last 30 years, there has been a rapid development of technology and its impact is at times unforeseen. Continuous electronic fetal heart monitoring was introduced in the late 1960s. By providing more information it was assumed to be useful. As certain fetal heart rate patterns are associated with fetal hypoxia, there is a commitment to expedite deliveries in their presence. However, the relationship is not specific and there will inevitably be an increase in operative deliveries. Subsequent comparison with intermittent auscultation has shown that the only benefit is a reduction in neonatal convulsions restricted to prolonged, induced or augmented labours. Even in units where fetal blood sampling is used, the Caesarean section rate has doubled (Nielson, 1993). Despite the minimal advantages of this method of monitoring, it continues to be used inappropriately in low-risk spontaneous labours. The machine has become the companion of the woman in labour and the number of midwives has dwindled.

Risk of drugs

Today there are stringent controls within the UK concerning the use of certain drugs in pregnancy. Indeed, the Committee on the Safety of Medicines was formed as a response to recognition in 1961 of the teratogenic effects of thalidomide, a drug which had been widely recommended as an antiemetic and hypnotic in early pregnancy. In the United States the already established Food and Drugs Administration managed to prevent its use.

Vitamins and oxygen have been perceived to be harmless. With oxygen this belief led to the unforeseen hazard of retinopathy of prematurity caused by administration of high concentration oxygen (Silverman, 1980). Supplementation with folic acid if not helpful was viewed at worst as innocuous. This viewpoint (by negating the need for a study) resulted in a long delay in mounting the Medical Research Council randomised study that eventually confirmed that high dose folic acid (4 mg) can prevent recurrence of neural tube defects (NTD).

The contraceptive pill is variously blamed or credited for many of the changes that have occurred in sexual behaviour since the 1960s. Three major 'pill scares' have featured at length in the popular press. The first was in 1967 when the pill was linked to thrombosis (Platt *et al.*, 1967), then with arterial disease in 1977 (RCGP, 1977; Vessey *et al.*, 1977) and subsequently with cancer of the breast and cervix in 1983 (Pike *et al.*, 1983; Vessey *et al.*, 1983). The *Lancet* articles prompted 34 articles in the national press and 161 articles in the provincial press (Wellings, 1985). It is apparent that bad news is more newsworthy than good as a report published the previous week implying a protective effect of the pill on breast cancer received only one mention in the national press (Kalache *et al.*, 1983). The response of the public was inevitable: there was a 14% drop in prescriptions and a peak in the abortion rate 6 months later. However, despite all the scares, the pill remains the most popular form of contraception.

Perception of risk and Down's syndrome screening

The association of raised maternal age and Down's syndrome was first described by Shuttleworth (1909). The extra G chromosome in Down's syndrome was discovered in 1959 by Lejeune and subsequently identified as chromosome 21 (Lejeune *et al.*, 1959). Antenatal diagnosis by amniocentesis was introduced thereafter and was offered only to the older mother because of the 0.5% to 1% risk of miscarriage. Until 1976, maternal-age risks were cited only for 5-year intervals; therefore, no distinction in risk was made between a 35- and a 39-year-old woman. Cost–benefit analysis of prenatal diagnosis programmes and the need to provide improved genetic counselling acted as the stimuli for estimation of age-specific incidences. These were first presented by Hook and Chambers (1977) and based on birth certificate data of white babies in New York. Subsequently there have been numerous other livebirth studies estimating age-specific risks in Down's syndrome (Cuckle *et al.*, 1987).

Nearly 20 years ago, the UK Government targeted prenatal screening as a priority area for expansion and recommended the provision of amniocentesis to women aged 40 years and above and maternal serum α-fetoprotein (AFP) screening for all (DHSS, 1976). At the same time a working party of the Clinical Genetics Society reported the unequal development of these services and recommended the provision of facilities to karyotype 8% of all maternities (Clinical Genetics Society, 1978). By the early 1980s all health regions offered amniocentesis to women with age limits varying between 35 and 40 years. First-trimester diagnosis was possible after the introduction of chorionic villus sampling (CVS) in 1983.

This technique has slightly higher risks of miscarriage (1–2%) but is increasingly used. However screening for Down's syndrome on the basis of raised maternal age made little impact as the majority of Down's syndrome pregnancies (70%) occur to the under 35 group (Mutton *et al.*, 1993). In 1984 the association of low second-trimester AFP with trisomy 18 (Edward's syndrome) and subsequently Down's syndrome was recognised (Merkatz *et al.*, 1984). This led to the concept of biochemical screening as described in detail in other chapters.

The acceptability of a test depends on the balance of the perceived risks and benefits. This perception may vary greatly between all those involved, be it mother, clinician or the public health professional.

The mother's perspective

Ideally a mother makes an informed decision concerning antenatal screening. However, a sizeable proportion undergo tests with only a limited understanding of their significance. In one study, over a third of women recently delivered were unsure or incorrect as to whether they had undergone AFP screening for spina bifida and a quarter were similarly unsure with respect to amniocentesis (Marteau *et al.*, 1988). In a survey of women interviewed after amniocentesis, a quarter were unaware that there was a risk of miscarriage (Farrant, 1985).

Prenatal diagnosis is often described in a positive and simplistic way. The ethos is that screening is good and a 'perfect baby' is an attainable goal. There is pressure to undergo screening 'for the good of the baby', which is misleading as the purpose is usually to offer termination rather than palliation. There have been legal cases in the United States in which children with congential abnormalities have successfully sued the clinician for not providing antenatal diagnosis (the so called wrongful life cases). However, it is difficult to see how termination is in the baby's interest.

Many mothers view screening as a form of reassurance and fortunately this is the usual outcome. The screen-positive group for Down's syndrome are those with risks above a specified cut-off value (usually between 1 in 200 to 1 in 300). Not surprisingly, women identified as 'at risk' on the basis of biochemical screening generally experience more anxiety compared with those who had realised they were at risk before they were pregnant (Abuelo *et al.*, 1991).

The cut-off value is an administrative choice which determines the number of karyotypes performed, usually around 5% of maternities.

Traditionally amniocentesis has been offered when the risk of Down's syndrome approaches that of fetal loss as a result of the procedure (between 0.5 and 1%). This assumes that equal value is placed on the hazard of losing a normal pregnancy and that of the occurrence of Down's syndrome, which is an illogical premise. There is a wide variation in women's selection of cut-off risk for choosing amniocentesis (Thornton and Lilford, 1990) with the median value being 1 in 750. If this is so then many more women might utilise the service. A survey on women's views found that over 70% of women thought that amniocentesis should be offered to all (Tymstra et al., 1991).

A second commonly held assumption is that the actual level of risk determines the decision to proceed to amniocentesis. However, this is not equivalent to perceived risk (Marteau et al., 1991) and prospective assessments of biochemical screening programmes have shown that uptake is independent of actual risk until it becomes greater than 1 in 50 (Haddow et al., 1992; Wald et al., 1992).

Uptake rates of amniocentesis are an indirect assessment of acceptability. Most studies have focussed on the older woman and may have a bias towards those who wish to avoid an invasive procedure. Rates of 50% have been described in the UK (Knott et al., 1986; Marteau et al., 1989), USA (Crandall, 1991) and the Netherlands (Leschot, 1991). There has been increasing uptake of amniocentesis with time (Baird et al., 1985). Whether this will increase significantly above 50% is debatable, although rates as high as 85% have been recorded (Diernaes et al., 1982). High utilisation rates do not imply acceptability as there may be a component of 'anticipated decision regret' where a woman perceives the necessity to avail herself of all possible tests (Tymstra, 1991).

Conversely, failure of uptake of amniocentesis may be due to lack of awareness. Knott et al. (1986) reviewed women aged 38 years and over who had delivered at a London teaching hospital. Uptake of amniocentesis was 59%. Antenatal diagnosis was not apparently discussed in 7% and in this group there was a high proportion of Asian women. Late booking (after 20 weeks) occurred in 9%.

The uptake of serum screening is around 80% with a 75% acceptance rate of amniocentesis if the screen is positive: this results in an overall utilisation of 60% (Sheldon and Simpson, 1991; Haddow et al., 1992; Wald et al., 1992). However, much lower acceptance rates (less than 40%) have been documented in a retrospective study of a single marker AFP screening programme for Down's syndrome (Fleming and Goldie, 1992).

The clinician's perspective

It is the clinician who initially decides whether to discuss the availability of the test. In the UK there is a strong trend towards providing complete information to the individual, but it remains the clinician's right to advise the patient of what he deems is in their best interests. There is an ongoing case of a mother of a Down's syndrome baby suing her obstetrician for not informing her of the existence of the biochemical test. He expressed the widely held view that the test was anxiety provoking. In regions with no service (in 1991 this was half of the UK), many health care workers had a policy of discussing the matter only if it was initiated by the woman.

When the service is available, there are varying attitudes towards explanation of the test. Until the late 1970s, blood was taken 'routinely' for testing during pregnancy with minimal explanation to the mother. Biochemical screening for NTD introduced the need for discussion and an 'opt-in' policy as recommended by the Black Report (DHSS, Black Report, 1979). Despite this, a quarter of consultants used screening without informing the mother (Farrant, 1985).

There is also considerable divergence in the interpretation and application of test results. In one health region, 15 obstetricians have five distinct policies varying from using no particular cut-off value to the use of values ranging from 1 in 100 to 1 in 300 (Fleming and Goldie, 1992).

Debate exists over the time needed and optimum method to present the risk results. In particular some consider the specific risk value should be given rather than a result expressed as 'screen negative'. Interpretation of a result depends on the manner of the explanation. For example a 28-year-old woman with a baseline age-based risk of Down's syndrome of 1 in 1000 and a biochemical risk of 1 in 500 is not reassured by being informed that her risk is 'double' that of an average person of her age but will be reassured if the result is presented as 'negative'.

One of the major criticisms from the profession is the time-consuming need for counselling. This may be an overstated problem as only a minority (25%) of older mothers have difficulty in making a decision as to whether to have an amniocentesis (Scholz *et al.*, 1989). Therefore, in a unit with 5000 deliveries one could anticipate that 3750 women will accept biochemical screening; 190 will be screen positive and only 50 will have difficulty making a decision. There are established methods pioneered by the Paukers in the United States to help those confronted by a difficult decision (Pauker and Pauker, 1977). The technique consists of structuring

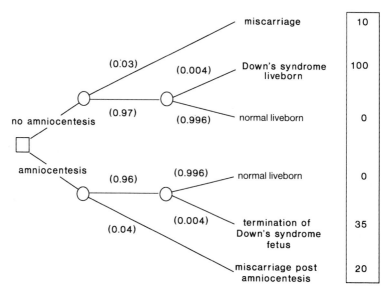

Fig. 2.1. A decision tree for undertaking amniocentesis. The numbers in the brackets are the probabilities of the chance events. In this example: 4% and 3% are the expected fetal loss rates depending on whether an amniocentesis is or is not performed, respectively; the risk of a Down's syndrome fetus is 1 in 250 (probability 0·004). The numbers in the box are the mother's relative values of the possible outcomes with 100 for the worst (the birth of a Down's syndrome child) and 0 for the best (the birth of a normal child). The cost of declining amniocentesis is 0.688 {(0.03 × 10) + 0.97 × [(0.004 × 100) + (0.996 × 0)]} compared with 0.934 {(0.04 × 20) + 0.96 × [(0.004 × 35) + (0.996 × 0)]} for proceeding with amniocentesis. The optimum decision for these values is thus to decline amniocentesis.

the problem into a decision tree comprising all possible outcomes. The patient's values are incorporated and the objective is to arrive at a course of action that maximises the benefits. Figure 2.1 is a decision tree for a woman with a positive biochemical screening test for Down's syndrome. The probabilities for the chance events are taken from the literature and the patient values are arrived at using a lottery technique in which an outcome to be valued is measured in terms of a gamble between the best and worst outcome. Although decision analysis is logical and has the merits of structuring thought processes, criticisms have been directed at its complexity in a clinical setting and at the patient-derived values. Inconsistency of patient judgment has been well demonstrated (Thornton and Lilford, 1990).

The public health priority

The objective of the public health professional is to reduce the prevalence of Down's syndrome in a cost effective manner that is acceptable to society. Approximately 1 in 12 people in the UK oppose prenatal diagnosis (Royal College Physicians, 1989). But the majority are in favour and biochemical screening for Down's syndrome has become increasingly available in the UK: 69% of all districts provided a service in 1992 (Wald *et al.*, 1991). The health districts are as diverse as the clinicians in their policies. There is still controversy over the relative merits of the various markers and which combinations to use. Comparisons of detection rates must be judged in relation to the equivalent false-positive rates and this is not always possible. Prospective trials are cited as the best method of discriminating between the various combinations but this is unlikely to succeed because the differences sought are very small. For example, to show that a 65% detection rate is significantly different from a 60% detection rate then 1471 cases of Down's syndrome are needed. All studies have softened their end points by referring to detection and not termination rates. Some 8% of women would decide to continue the pregnancy in the knowledge that they have a Down's syndrome fetus (Vincent *et al.*, 1991).

Biochemical screening effectively doubles detection rates as compared with an 'age alone' policy. Yet it remains difficult to assess accurately the cost–benefits of such programmes. The main savings are to educational and social budgets rather than health budgets. Partly as a consequence of this, a piecemeal and unequal service is developing in the UK.

Conclusion

Much debate in screening for Down's syndrome centres around the optimum choice and combination of tests. However, it is the perception of risks balanced against the benefits that will determine the utilisation of such services. It is clear that there is a wide variation in the opinions of women, clinicians and public health professionals. This diversity greatly outweighs the effect of the small increments in detection rates gained by optimising the available tests. There is a need to ensure that the anxiety inevitably engendered by screening is minimised and that women undertake tests in as fully informed a manner as possible.

References

Abuelo, D.N., Hopmann, M.R., Barsel-Bowers, G. & Goldstein, A. (1991). Anxiety in women with low maternal serum alpha-fetoprotein screening results. *Prenatal Diagn.*, **11**, 381–5.

Baird, P.A., Sadnovick, A.D. & McGillivray, B.C. (1985). Temporal changes in the utilization of amniocentesis for prenatal diagnosis by women of advanced maternal age, 1976–1983. *Prenatal Diagn.*, **5**, 191–8.

Clinical Genetics Society (1978). *The Provision of Services for the Prenatal Diagnosis of Foetal Abnormality in the United Kingdom.* London: The Eugenics Society.

Covello, V.R. & Mumpower, J. (1985). Risk analysis and risk management: an historical perspective. *Risk Analysis*, **2**, 103–20.

Crandall, B. (1991). Maternal age and amniocentesis for the identification of Down syndrome and other chromosome abnormalities. In *Screening in Prenatal Diagnosis.* ed. A. Mantingh, A.S.P.M. Breed, J.R. Beekhuis & J.M.M. van Lith, pp. 25–32. Groningen: Academic Press.

Cuckle, H.S., Wald, N.J. & Thompson, S.G. (1987). Estimating a woman's risk of having a pregnancy associated with Down's syndrome using her age and maternal serum alpha-fetoprotein level. *Br. J. Obstet. Gynaecol.*, **94**, 387–402.

DHSS, Black Report (1976). *Prevention and Health: Everybody's Business.* London: Her Majesty's Stationery Office.

DHSS (1979). *Report by the Working Group on Screening for Neutral Tube Defects.* London: Her Majesty's Stationery Office.

Diernaes, E., Filtenberg, J.A. & Hasch, E. (1982). Three years experience with prenatal diagnosis in a Danish County. *Lancet*, **2**, 1044–5.

Farrant, W. (1985). In *The Sexual Politics of Reproduction, Who's for Amniocentesis?* ed. H. Homan, pp. 96–122. London: Gower.

Fleming, C. & Goldie, D.J. (1992). Risk of Down's syndrome and amniocentesis rate. *Br. Med. J.*, **304**, 252.

Haddow, J.E., Palomaki, G.E., Knight, G.J. *et al.* (1992). Prenatal screening for Down's syndrome with use of maternal serum markers. *N. Engl. J. Med.*, **327**, 588–93.

Hook, E.B. & Chambers, G.M. (1977). Estimated rates of Down syndrome in live births by one year maternal age intervals for mothers aged 20–49 in a New York State study – implications of the risk figures for genetic counselling and cost benefit analysis of prenatal diagnosis programs. *Birth Defects: Original Article Series XIII* **34**, 123–41.

Kalache, A., McPherson, K., Barltrop, K. & Vessey, M.P. (1983). Oral contraceptives and breast cancer. *Br. J. Hosp. Med.*, **83**, 278–83.

Knott, P.D., Penketh, R.J.A. & Lucas, M.K. (1986). Uptake of amniocentesis in women aged 38 years or more by the time of the expected date of delivery: a two-year retrospective study. *Br. J. Obstet. Gynaecol.*, **93**, 1246–50.

Lejeune, J., Gautier, M., Turpin, R. (1959). Les chromosomes humains en culture de tissues. *C.R. Acad. Sci.*, **248**, 602.

Leschot, N. (1991). Unreliable detection methods: how can we tell our patients? In *Screening in Prenatal Diagnosis.* ed. A. Mantingh, A.S.P.M. Breed, J.R. Beekhuis & J.M.M. van Lith, pp. 91–100. Groningen: Academic Press.

Marteau, T.M., Johnston, M., Plenicar, M., Shaw, R.W. & Slack, J. (1988). Development of a self-administered questionnaire to measure women's knowledge of prenatal screening and diagnostic tests. *Psychsomatic Res.*, **32**, 403–8.

Marteau, T.M., Johnston, M., Shaw, R.W. & Slack, J. (1989). Factors influencing the uptake of screening for open neural-tube defects and amniocentesis to test for Down's syndrome. *Br. J. Obstet. Gynaecol.*, **96**, 739–48.

Marteau, T.M., Kidd, J., Cook, R. *et al.* (1991). Perceived risk not actual risk predicts uptake of amniocentesis. *Br. J. Obstet. Gynaecol.*, **98**, 282–6.

Merkatz, I., Nitowski, H., Macri, J. & Johnson, W. (1984). An association between low maternal serum α-fetoprotein and fetal chromosomal abnormalities. *Am. J. Obstet. Gynecol.*, **148**, 886–94.

Mutton, D.E., Ide, R., Alberman, E. & Bobrow, M. (1993). Analysis of national register of Down's syndrome in England and Wales: trends in prenatal diagnosis, 1989–91. *Br. Med. J.*, **306**, 431–2.

Nielson, J.P. (1993). Cardiotocography during labour. *Br. Med. J.*, **306**, 47.

Pauker, S.P. & Pauker, S.G. (1977). Prenatal diagnosis: a directive approach to genetic counseling using decision analysis. *Yale J. Biol. Med.*, **50**, 275–89.

Pike, M.C., Henderson, D.E., Krailo, M.D., Duke, A. & Roy, S. (1983). Breast cancer in young women and use of oral contraceptives; possibly modifying effect of formulation and age of use. *Lancet*, **2**, 926–30.

Platt Lord, R. and the Committee on Safety of Drugs (1967). A preliminary communication to the Medical Research Council by a subcommittee. Risk of thrombo-embolic disease in women taking oral contraceptives. *Br. Med. J.*, **2**, 355–9.

RCGP Oral Contraceptive Study (1977). Mortality among contraceptive users. *Lancet*, **2**, 727–31.

Royal College of Physicians (1989). *Prenatal Diagnosis and Genetic Screening. Community and Service Implications.* London: Royal College of Physicians.

Scholz, C., Endres, M., Zach, K. & Murken, J. (1989). Psychosocial aspects of the decision to utilize prenatal diagnosis, results of an empirical study. *Offentliche Gesundheitswesen* **51**, 278–84.

Sheldon, T.A. & Simpson, J. (1991). Appraisal of a new scheme for prenatal screening for Down's syndrome. *Br. Med. J.*, **302**, 1133–6.

Shuttleworth, G.E. (1909). Mongolian imbecility. *Br. Med. J.*, **2**, 661.

Silverman, W.A. (1980). *Retrolental Fibroplasia: A Modern Parable.* New York: Grune and Stratton.

Thornton, J.G. & Lilford, R.J. (1990). Prenatal diagnosis of Down's syndrome: a method for measuring the consistency of women's decisions. *Med. Dec. Making*, **10**, 288–93.

Tymstra, T.J. (1991). The imperative character of screening technologies. In *Screening in Prenatal Diagnosis.* ed. A. Mantingh, A.S.P.M. Breed, J.R. Beekhuis & J.M.M. van Lith, pp. 65–70. Groningen: Academic Press.

Tymstra, T.J., Bajema, C., Beekhuis, J.R. & Mantingh, A. (1991). Women's opinions on the offer and use of prenatal diagnosis. *Prenatal Diagn.*, **11**, 893–8.

Vessey, M.P., McPherson, K. & Johnson, B. (1977). Mortality among women participants in the Oxford/FPA contraceptive study. *Lancet*, **2**, 731–3.

Vessey, M.P., Lawless, M., McPherson, K. & Yeates, D. (1983). Neoplasia of the cervix uteri: a possible adverse effect of the pill. *Lancet*, **2**, 930–4.

Vincent, V.A., Edwards, J.G., Young, S.R. & Nachtigal, M. (1991). Pregnancy termination because of chromosomal abnormalities: a study of 26 950 amniocenteses in the southeast. *South Med. J.*, **84**, 1210–13.

Wald, N., Wald, K. & Smith, D. (1991). The extent of Down's syndrome screening in Britain in 1991. *Br. Med. J.*, **340**, 494.

Wald, N.J., Kennard, A., Densem, J.W., Cuckle, H.S., Chard, T. & Butler, L. (1992). Antenatal maternal serum screening for Down's syndrome: results of a demonstration project. *Br. Med. J.*, **305**, 391–3.

Wellings, K. (1985). Help or hype: an analysis of media coverage of the 1983 'pill scare'. *Br. J. Family Plan.*, **11**, 92–8.

3

Risk estimation in Down's syndrome screening policy and practice

H.S. CUCKLE

Screening can be defined as the selection from amongst apparently healthy individuals of those at high enough risk of a given disorder to warrant diagnostic procedures that are too hazardous or expensive to offer to all. Thus risk is implicitly at the centre of screening. The introduction of biochemical screening for Down's syndrome represents a new development in that the risk is explicitly used in the interpretation of results as positive (i.e. exceeding a cut-off risk) or negative. Many centres go further and include the individual risk on the test report. This approach enables women and their families to make informed choices regarding prenatal diagnosis, but that is not the main reason for its use. Risk is used principally as a way of combining several interrelated pieces of information, such as maternal age, family history and marker levels, into a single value. It can be shown statistically that using this value as the composite screening variable maximizes the discriminatory power or efficiency of the test. In other words, a higher detection rate (i.e. percent positive among Down's syndrome pregnancies) can be obtained for a given false-positive rate (i.e. percent positive among unaffected pregnancies) than any other way of combining the information. The two uses of risk, namely to inform individual choice and to maximize screening efficiency, are often confused in debate over screening policy. The health care system in which the policy is being implemented will also determine the weight given to the choice and efficiency aspects.

The aim of this chapter is to clarify the concept of risk in Down's syndrome screening with particular reference to ongoing policy issues. For the purposes of illustration, four markers currently being measured at 15–20 weeks of gestation will be considered. The same principles will apply to other markers and gestations. The markers are intact or total

31

human chorionic gonadotrophin (hCG), free β-subunits (β-hCG), α-fetoprotein (AFP) and unconjugated oestriol (uE_3).[1]

Individual risks

Meaning of risk

To say that the risk of having an infant with Down's syndrome is 1 in 100 is a probability statement. It is equivalent to saying that among groups of 100 similar women on average one in the group will be expected to have a baby with the disorder. Such a risk statement is an expression of imperfect knowledge. Either an infant has Down's syndrome or it does not and a diagnostic test will determine this with certainty. In contrast, the risk merely indicates whether the balance of information is inclined one way or the other. If more information is obtained the risk can be revised but that does not mean that the unrevised risk was wrong – it was the best estimate for the information available at the time. Thus the very notion of a correct or incorrect risk is flawed. Moreover it does not make sense to estimate a confidence interval around an individual woman's risk as this implies that some correct underlying risk is likely to be contained within the interval.

Calculating risk

None of the markers which have been investigated in detail so far appear to be correlated with maternal age. Consequently, the calculation of an individual woman's risk has two independent components, namely her age-specific risk and the likelihood ratio, a factor quantifying the relative increase or decrease in risk given her marker levels.

The age-specific risk can be determined directly from a large body of data on the birth prevalence of the disorder. Several studies have published prevalence figures broken down into single years of age. These have been combined in a meta-analysis and a curve fitted to allow interpolation within a year (Cuckle *et al.*, 1987). The birth prevalence (p) expressed as an odds of 1 in $1/p$ is the risk at term. The risk at the time

---

[1] Tables are derived using the parameters of Wald *et al.* (1992a) ('dates' gestation, unadjusted for maternal weight) unless otherwise stated. Risks are that of a term pregnancy and for simplicity in risk calculation all parameters have been taken to fit Gaussian frequency distributions over a range extending from 3.5 standard deviations below the mean to 3.5 above. For the estimation of detection and false-positive rates, the age distribution of 1989 and 1990 maternities in England and Wales is used (OPCS, 1991, 1992).

of the test is usually taken to be 20–30% higher due to preferential fetal losses.

The likelihood ratio cannot be determined directly because of insufficient data. Marker levels are now available from many thousands of unaffected pregnancies but from much smaller numbers of affected pregnancies. Therefore, an indirect approach is adopted using either a statistical model of the frequency distributions of marker levels in affected and unaffected pregnancies or multiple regression analysis on the observed likelihood ratio. The two methods are equivalent for markers with the same standard deviations in affected and unaffected pregnancies, but when there is a substantial difference in standard deviations, as appears to be the case, the former method is more accurate. To date only a Gaussian statistical model has been considered and it appears to be adequate at least over most of the operating range. The Gaussian model is determined by the mean and standard deviation of each marker and the correlation coefficients between markers for both the affected and unaffected distributions.

An individual woman's risk is calculated by multiplying the left hand side of the age-specific risk expressed as an odds of $p: (1 - p)$ by the likelihood ratio for the marker levels (x) and re-expressing the result as the risk 1 in $(1 - p)/px + 1$.

Distribution parameters

There are 13 sets of distribution parameters in the published literature for hCG or free β-hCG, AFP and uE_3. They have been derived from affected pregnancy samples taken at mid-trimester and tested when the outcome of pregnancy was known. This could have been soon after the sample was taken if the series was based on samples obtained prior to diagnostic testing otherwise it may not have been until after delivery. Therefore the calculation of risk rests on the unproved assumption that the marker frequency distributions are similar for infants surviving to term as for those surviving to mid-trimester.

Table 3.1 shows the risks calculated for three women aged 35 years with extreme, borderline and average marker levels using each of the parameter sets. There is considerable variability in the calculated risk. For women with extreme or average levels this would be of no practical consequence, but the 2–3-fold range of calculated risks for women with borderline levels is of conern. To avoid confusion, it would be desirable for a common set of parameters to be adopted by all centres. This could be readily done for the marker means by combining all the published

Table 3.1. *Risk of a Down's syndrome term pregnancy for three
35-year-old women with extreme, borderline and average marker levels
according to the parameter set used*[a]

	Parameter set risk (1 in)		
	Extreme	Borderline	Average
hCG, AFP and uE₃			
Wald *et al.*, 1988	30	180	1400
Nørdgaard-Pedersen *et al.*, 1990	20	350	1800
Heyl *et al.*, 1990	20	160	5800
Spencer, 1991	20	190	1300
Ryall *et al.*, 1992	40	260	1600
Wald *et al.*, 1992a[b]	55	280	1600
Spencer *et al.*, 1992	45	300	1400
Crossley *et al.*, 1993[c]	35	210	1500
Free β-hCG, AFP and uE₃			
Spencer, 1991	40	290	1500
Ryall *et al.*, 1992	55	380	2400
Spencer *et al.*, 1992	60	340	1600
Wald *et al.*, 1993[d]	45	290	1900

[a] Extreme levels of hCG (or free β-hCG), AFP and uE_3 are 2.6, 0.6 and 0.6 MoM, respectively; borderline levels are 1.8, 0.8 and 0.8; average levels are all 1.0. Risks are taken to the nearest 5, if greater that 1 in 100; nearest 10 if 1 in 100 to 1 in 1000; nearest 100 if less than 1 in 1000.
[b] Four parameter sets are specified: only that for 'dates' gestations, uncorrected for maternal weight is used here.
[c] Parameters for uE_3; the others are specified in Stevenson *et al.*, 1987 and Crossley *et al.*, 1991.
[d] Parameters for free β-hCG; the others are specified in Wald *et al.* (1992a).

sources (see, for example, Wald and Cuckle, 1992). However heterogeneity between published studies is an obstacle to doing this for the standard deviations and correlation coefficients.

Screening efficiency

The efficiency of a Down's syndrome screening test is determined by the distribution of individual risks in affected and unaffected pregnancies. The usual measures of efficiency are the detected rate, false-positive rate and positive predictive value (i.e. the average risk in those with positive results).

Comparing performance

When the efficiency of different tests is being compared there is a need to hold some factors fixed and compare the others. For example, the false-positive rate can be fixed at, say, 5% and the resulting detection rates compared. In general the cut-off risk will need to be changed as a consequence. Although this ensures that a scientifically valid judgement is made about performance *in principle* it may not be desirable to change the cut-off risk for practical reasons. Suppose the cut-off is currently 1 in 250 but the new test dictates that it should become 1 in 275. Patient information leaflets probably quote 1 in 250 and there is a general understanding that a risk below this value is negative. Unless the predicted benefits were large, it is likely that to avoid confusion and undermining confidence the cut-off will not be changed. Therefore it is worthwhile making comparisons using a fixed cut-off risk as well as with a fixed false-positive rate.

Prospective study

Prospective study is the ultimate way of determining performance. However, the results obtained in such studies are subject to arbitrary and possible local factors such as differential uptake of screening according to maternal age. Moreover, even the largest studies are likely to include less than 50 Down's syndrome pregnancies and so these results are insufficient by themselves. For policy decisions, indirect methods of estimation must be used although they will need to be tempered in the light of prospective experience.

Indirect methods

Two indirect approaches have been described, one based on statistical models (Cuckle *et al.*, 1987; Royston and Thompson, 1992) and the other based on the observed distribution of likelihood ratios (Spencer *et al.*, 1992). Both combine information on the age distribution of maternities in Down's syndrome and unaffected pregnancies with the corresponding distributions of likelihood ratios. The proportion of maternities for women at each single year of age is multiplied by the age-specific prevalence of Down's syndrome to yield the age distribution for affected pregnancies. The distribution of unaffected pregnancies is obtained by subtraction. The two methods differ in how they estimate the likelihood ratio distributions.

Model method

This estimates the likelihood ratio distributions by use of a statistical model of the underlying marker distributions in the population. In the examples published so far, a Gaussian model was used and this was assigned the same parameter set as the Gaussian model used to calculate risk. The assumption of the same parameters for the population and the risk will tend to over-estimate screening efficiency since in general the marker distributions used to calculate risk are unlikely to fit exactly the populations to which the screening test is applied. Consequently there will be a lower screening efficiency than that estimated. Table 3.2 illustrates the loss of detection that may arise using seven published parameter sets for hCG, AFP and uE_3. Assuming that a widely used parameter set (Wald *et al.*, 1992a) was applied to calculate risk in a population with markers distributed according to the different parameter sets, the estimated detection rate for a 5% false-positive rate would fall by up to 6.5%. A loss of this kind is serious, since it is of the same order of magnitude as any gain in efficiency expected by modifications to the screening protocol.

Some of the published parameters are based on stored blood samples which have been retrospectively assayed for the markers concerned. In these cases the standard deviations and correlation coefficients need to be adjusted to avoid bias. The bias arises because analytical error due to

Table 3.2. *Estimated detection rate (%) for a 5% false-positive rate according to the parameter set used to model the population and that used to calculate risk*[a]

	Population risk parameters		
	Population (a)	Wald *et al.*, 1992a (b)	(a − b)
Wald *et al.*, 1988	60.2	56.7	3.5
Nørdgaard-Pedersen *et al.*, 1990	62.2	55.9	6.3
Heyl *et al.*, 1990	68.1	61.6	6.5
Spencer, 1991	59.7	55.2	4.5
Ryall *et al.*, 1992	58.0	55.1	2.9
Spencer *et al.*, 1992	59.5	58.8	0.7
Crossley *et al.*, 1993	60.4	55.6	4.8
Wald *et al.*, 1992a	57.1	—	—

[a] For hCG, AFP and uE_3.

long-term batch-to-batch variability will be absent, leading to smaller standard deviations and greater correlation coefficients when compared with routine assay. Without adjustment, the higher precision of measurement would lead to an over-estimation of screening efficiency.

Observed likelihood ratio method

This method depends on the availability of marker levels in a series of Down's syndrome and unaffected pregnancies. They could be derived from prospective study but more likely are derived from banked serum samples which are retrieved from storage and assayed. For these purposes samples taken prior to amniocentesis or chorion villus sampling for advanced maternal age or family history can be used, assuming, as seems likely, that the marker levels will be representative of all samples. The likelihood ratio is then calculated for each sample to obtain a distribution of likelihood ratios. This approach is direct and so has the advantage of not being dependent on the fit of a model to the population. However, if derived from a retrospective series, the estimate of screening efficiency is difficult to interpret because of bias. There will be over-estimation due to the absence of long-term batch-to-batch variability and a competing tendency to under-estimation if the parameter set used to calculate risk is appropriate for a prospective series.

General features

The model method of estimating screening efficiency can also be used to predict general features of a Down's syndrome screening programme. Some features which would not otherwise be immediately obvious are considered here.

Maternal age

For a fixed cut-off risk, the detection and false-positive rates will increase with age because of the increasing prior risk (see Table 3.3). The overlap in marker distributions between Down's and unaffected pregnancies is the same at each maternal age, but the use of a fixed cut-off risk gives the optimal weighting to each age and hence maximizes screening efficiency.

The contribution of maternal age as a marker in its own right to overall screening efficiency can be obtained by comparing the estimated detection rate for a given false-positive rate with those achieved by taking all women to have the same age. For the parameter set of Wald *et al.* (1992a) and

Table 3.3. *Estimated detection and false-positive rates (%) for hCG, AFP and uE$_3$ according to maternal age*[a]

Maternal age (years)	Additional years				
	+0	+1	+2	+3	+4
15	34.8[b]	34.8	34.9	35.0	35.2
	2.1[c]	2.1	2.1	2.2	2.2
20	35.5	35.7	36.1	36.4	36.6
	2.2	2.3	2.3	2.4	2.4
25	37.5	38.4	39.8	41.4	43.2
	2.6	2.7	3.0	3.4	3.8
30	45.5	48.0	51.7	55.9	60.0
	4.3	5.0	6.2	7.7	9.6
35	64.9	69.9	74.5	79.2	83.6
	12.2	15.5	19.4	24.2	30.0
40	87.6	90.9	93.6	95.6	97.2
	36.8	44.2	51.9	59.7	67.2
45	98.3	99.0	99.4	99.6	99.8
	74.9	81.2	86.4	90.7	93.8

[a] 1 in 250 cut-off risk.
[b] Detection rate (%).
[c] False-positive rate (%).

a 5% false-positive rate, the overall detection rate is 57% but only 48% when age is fixed, so that age contributes 9% detection.

The precise contribution of maternal age is determined by the distribution in the population being screened. In general, a population with a higher proportion of older women will yield a greater detection rate for a given false-positive rate. The magnitude of this effect is not large.

Positive predictive value

One consideration when choosing a cut-off is the minimum risk that is regarded as high enough to warrant prenatal diagnosis. Another is the positive predictive value, which is important for allocation of resources since it determines the number of invasive procedures and karyotypes that need to be carried out in order to diagnose each case. Despite the use of a single cut-off, the positive predictive value is not invariate with maternal age but increases with advancing age. Table 3.4 shows this for cut-off risks between 1 in 200 and 1 in 400.

Table 3.4. *Positive predictive value for hCG, AFP and uE₃ according to maternal age and cut-off risk*

Maternal age (years)	Positive predictive value (1 in) at a cut-off risk of		
	1 in 200	1 in 300	1 in 400
15	80	115	148
20	79	115	147
25	79	114	144
30	76	109	137
35	68	93	114
40	48	61	70
45	24	26	28
Overall	61	85	107

New markers

The addition of a new marker will necessarily increase the variability of risks. If the marker has low discriminatory power when considered alone it may be thought that it will reduce overall screening efficiency by adding to random error. The markers A–F in Table 3.5 show that this is not so. For simplicity the additional markers are taken to have Gaussian distributions with the same standard deviation in affected and unaffected

Table 3.5. *Estimated detection rate (%) for a 5% false-positive rate using hCG, AFP and uE₃ with an additional marker[a]*

Additional marker	Deviation from normal[b]	Detection rate (%)
None	—	56.7
A	$\frac{1}{4}$	57.3
B	$\frac{1}{2}$	59.1
C	$\frac{3}{4}$	61.9
D	1	65.4
E	$1\frac{1}{4}$	70.2
F	$1\frac{1}{2}$	75.0

[a] Taken to have the same standard deviation in affected and unaffected pregnancies and uncorrelated with hCG, AFP and uE₃.
[b] The number of standard deviations between the mean level of the additional marker in affected and unaffected pregnancies.

pregnancies and no correlation with the existing markers. They differ only in the extent to which the mean in affected pregnancies deviates from the mean in unaffected pregnancies.

All the additional markers in Table 3.5 yield an increase in the detection rate for a 5% false-positive rate ranging from 0.6% to 18.3%. Despite the greater spread of risks with the addition of a further marker, there is an improved separation on average between affected and unaffected pregnancies. This is so even for marker A where the deviation of the affected mean from normal is small. However Table 3.5 does not take account of the fact that, as shown in Table 3.2, differences between the actual and modelled distributions will reduce the detection rate. The small predicted benefit for marker A may be counterbalanced by a deviation from fit experienced in practice.

New markers and maternal age

The benefit of adding a new marker is not uniform across all ages: a greater effect will be seen in younger women than in those who are older. This is demonstrated in Table 3.6 using marker C as an example. The explanation is related to the position of the cut-off risk in the spread of risks. At young ages the cut-off is in the upper tail of risks for Down's syndrome pregnancies. The increased spread of risks together with the greater separation between the affected and unaffected risk distributions

Table 3.6. *Estimated detection and false-positive rates (%) for hCG, AFP and uE$_3$ according to maternal age with and without marker C^a*

Maternal age (years)	Detection rate (%)			False-positive rate (%)		
	With (*a*)	Without (*b*)	(*a* − *b*)	With (*c*)	Without (*d*)	(*c* − *d*)
15	41.9	34.8	7.1	2.4	2.1	0.3
20	42.4	35.5	6.9	2.4	2.2	0.2
25	44.8	37.5	7.3	2.8	2.6	0.2
30	52.1	45.5	6.6	4.4	4.3	0.1
35	68.9	64.9	4.0	11.0	12.2	−1.2
40	88.4	87.6	0.8	31.5	36.8	−5.3
45	97.9	98.3	−0.4	65.7	74.9	−9.2
Overall	62.1	57.1	5.0	5.1	5.1	0.0

^{a} Cut-off, 1 in 250.

Restricting screening to young women and automatically offering amniocentesis to older women is another option. Some centres may wish to adopt such a policy because of the expectation, based on past practice, among women that they will be offered an amniocentesis. If biochemical screening is restricted to women aged under 35 this policy will be extremely inefficient. The overall estimated detection and false-positive rates including all women aged over 35 years as positive will be 61.3% and 11.0%, respectively, for a 1 in 250 cut-off risk. If there were sufficient resources to perform amniocentesis on 11% of women, it would be more efficient to select them by biochemical screening at all ages. The detection rate would be 70%. If women aged over 40 years instead of over 35 years are automatically offered amniocentesis there will be a more acceptable effect on detection and false-positive rates (58.6% and 5.9%, respectively) and with 45 years as the cut-off age there will be a negligible effect (57.1% and 5.2%, respectively).

Conclusions

The use of risks in biochemical screening for Down's syndrome is beneficial but because this is a new departure in medicine there is confusion among both professionals and patients. The use of statistical models can educate the interested practitioner in some of the general rules underlying Down's syndrome screening and provides an aid for planning screening policy. Whilst the parameter sets underlying the models may vary, and a variety of assumptions are made, the technique offers a reasonable way of predicting the outcome of a screening programme before it is introduced. The results of prospective studies would appear to confirm the efficacy of the model method.

References

Cheng, E.Y., Luthy, D.A., Zebelman, A.M., Williams, M.A., Lieppman, E. & Hickok, D.E. (1993). A prospective evaluation of a second-trimester screening test for fetal Down syndrome using maternal serum alpha-fetoprotein, hCG, and unconjugated estriol. *Obstet. Gynecol.*, **81**, 72–7.

Crossley, J.A., Aitken, D.A. & Connor, J.M. (1991). Prenatal screening for chromosome abnormalities using maternal serum chorionic gonadotrophin, alpha-fetoprotein and age. *Prenatal Diagn.*, **11**, 83–101.

Crossley, J.A., Aitken, D.A. & Connor, J.M. (1993). Second-trimester unconjugated oestriol levels in maternal serum from chromosomally abnormal pregnancies using an optimized assay. *Prenatal Diagn.*, **13**, 271–80.

Cuckle, H.S., Wald, N.J. & Thompson, S.G. (1987). Estimating a woman's risk of having a pregnancy associated with Down's syndrome using her age and serum alpha-fetoprotein level. *Br. J. Obstet. Gynaecol*, **94**, 387–402.

Goodburn, S.F., Yates, J.R.W., Raggatt, P.R. *et al.* (1993). Second trimester maternal serum screening using alpha-fetoprotein, human chorionic gonadotrophin and unconjugated oestriol: experience of a regional programme. *Prenatal Diagn.*, in press.

Haddow, J.E., Palomaki, G.E., Knight, G.J. *et al.* (1992). Prenatal screening for Down's syndrome with use of maternal serum markers. *N. Engl. J. Med.*, **327**, 588–93.

Heyl, P.S., Miller, W. & Canick, J.A. (1990). Maternal serum screening for aneuploid pregnancy by alpha-fetoprotein, hCG, and unconjugated estriol. *Obstet. Gynecol.*, **76**, 1025–31.

Nørgaard-Pedersen, B., Larsen, S.O., Arends, J., Svenstrup, B. & Tabor, A. (1990). Maternal serum markers in screening for Down syndrome. *Clin. Genet.*, **37**, 35–43.

OPCS (Office of Population Censuses and Surveys) (1991 & 1992). *Birth Statistics Series FM*1, Nos. 18 & 19. London: HMSO.

Phillips, O.P., Elias, S., Shulman, L.P., Andersen, R.N., Morgan, C.D. & Simpson, J.L. (1992). Maternal serum screening for fetal Down syndrome in women less than 35 years of age using alpha-fetoprotein, hCG and unconjugated estriol: a prospective 2-year study. *Obstet. Gynecol.*, **80**, 353–8.

Reynolds, T., John, R. & Spencer, K. (1993). The utility of unconjugated estriol in Down syndrome screening is not proven. *Clin. Chem.*, **39**, 2035–5.

Royston, P. & Thompson, S.G. (1992). Model-based screening by risk with application to Down's syndrome. *Stat. Med.*, **11**, 257–68.

Ryall, R.G., Staples, A.J., Robertson, E.F. & Pollard, A.C. (1992). Improved performance in a prenatal screening programme for Down's syndrome incorporating serum-free hCG subunit analyses. *Prenatal Diagn.* **12**, 251–61.

Spencer, K. (1991). Evaluation of an assay of the free β-subunit of choriogonadotropin and its potential value in screening for Down's syndrome. *Clin. Chem.*, **37**, 809–14.

Spencer, K., Coombes, E.J., Mallard, A.S. & Milford-Ward, A. (1992). Free beta human choriogonadotropin in Down's syndrome screening: a multicentre study of its role compared with other biochemical markers. *Ann. Clin. Biochem.*, **29**, 506–18.

Stevenson, J.D., Chapman, R.S., Perry, B. & Logue, F.C. (1987). Evaluation and clinical application of a two-site immunoradiometric assay for alpha-1-foetoprotein using readily available reagents. *Ann. Clin. Chem.*, **24**, 411–18.

Wald, N. & Cuckle, H. (1992). Biochemical screening. In *Prenatal Diagnosis and Screening*, ed. D.J.H. Brock & C. Rodeck, pp. 563–77. Edinburgh: Churchill Livingstone.

Wald, N.J., Cuckle, H.S., Densem, J.W. (1988). Maternal serum screening for Down syndrome in early pregnancy. *Br. Med. J.*, **297**, 883–7.

Wald, N.J., Cuckle, H.S., Densem, J.W., Kennard, A. & Smith, D. (1992a). Maternal serum screening for Down's syndrome: the effect of routine ultrasound scan determination of gestational age and adjustment for maternal weight. *Br. J. Obstet. Gynaecol.*, **99**, 144–9.

Wald, N.J., Kennard, A., Densem, J.W., Cuckle, H.S., Chard, T. & Butler, L. (1992b). Antenatal maternal serum screening for Down's syndrome: results of a demonstration project. *Br. Med. J.*, **305**, 391–4.

Wald, N.J., Densem, J.W., Stone, R. & Cheng, R. (1993). The use of free β-hCG in antenatal screening for Down's syndrome. *Br. J. Obstet. Gynaecol.*, **100**, 550–7.

4

Screening by test combination: a statistical overview

T.M. REYNOLDS

Basic mathematical principles

There are two commonly used methods for combining laboratory results into a Down's syndrome risk estimate: the likelihood method (Palomaki and Haddow, 1987) and the linear discriminant function method (Nørgaard-Pedersen *et al.*, 1990). At present most centres in the UK use the likelihood ratio method and, therefore, only the statistical background to this type of testing will be examined. The basic principle is that the population distributions for an analyte are known for the 'normal' and 'abnormal' groups. Therefore, for any given analyte concentration, the likelihood of membership of the 'normal' and 'abnormal' groups may be calculated. The likelihood is calculated as the Gaussian height for the analyte concentration based on the appropriate population mean and standard deviation (S.D.). The ratio of the heights calculated using 'normal' and 'Down's syndrome affected' population parameters is the 'likelihood ratio'. The woman's prior odds for carrying a Down's syndrome fetus are calculated using a formula derived by epidemiological studies (Cuckle *et al.*, 1987) and these are modified using the likelihood ratio to derive the posterior odds that are used as the Down's syndrome 'risk estimate'. Since a knowledge of some of the mathematics is vital to the understanding of the behaviour of the Down's syndrome risk screen, the basic equations will be considered here. Further detail may be found elsewhere (Reynolds and Penney, 1990).

First, the formula for derivation of prior odds, i.e. the risk at term of a Down's syndrome birth. For the purposes of the calculation, maternal age is the age at the expected date of delivery and the result is a value *n* such that the risk of a Down's syndrome birth is 1 chance in *n*. A graph of maternal age versus risk is shown in Fig. 4.1.

47

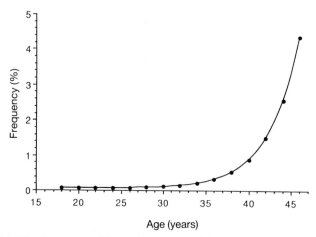

Fig. 4.1. The frequency of Down's syndrome births related to maternal age.

$$\text{Risk} = \frac{0.999373 - e^{\left((0.286 \times \text{Age}) - 16.2395\right)}}{0.000627 + e^{\left((0.286 \times \text{Age}) - 16.2395\right)}} \tag{4.1}$$

The second important concept is the likelihood ratio. In likelihood ratio Down's syndrome screening a major assumption is made: the population distribution of the biochemical results after conversion to multiples of the median (MoMs) may be transformed to approximate to a Gaussian distribution function. The usual transformation utilised is conversion to $\text{Log}_{10}(\text{MoM})$. In calculating likelihood ratios, the Gaussian 'height' is used instead of the probability: this is advantageous because the Gaussian height can easily be calculated, unlike the Gaussian probability density function (the integral of the height function). However, this reliance on a defined distribution is also a significant problem because for the method to work properly the data must conform to the Gaussian model. The first and simplest formula to consider is the univariate Gaussian equation.

$$f(x) = 1/(\sigma\sqrt{2\pi}) \cdot e^{-1/2 \cdot ((x - \mu)/\sigma)^2} \tag{4.2}$$

In this equation, $f(x)$ is the Gaussian height for the applied parameter x; μ is the population mean for parameter x and σ is the population standard deviation. The equation can be examined in three parts. On the left hand side of the equation (first part), the expression $1/(\sigma\sqrt{2\pi})$ controls the maximum height of the Gaussian peak. The central portion (second part) involving 'e' converts the output of the third section of the equation into the correctly shaped envelope. The final section (third part) $((x - \mu)/\sigma)^2$ calculates a standard deviate defining how far from the centre of the population distribution the value x lies. This value is also known as the 'Mahalanobis distance' and may be used to determine whether a result can be considered to be acceptable. When the bivariate case is considered (applied parameters x and y), an extra value ρ must be used. This is the correlation coefficient relating parameters x and y.

$$f(x, y) = 1/(2\pi\sigma_x\sigma_y\sqrt{(1 - \rho^2)}) \cdot e^{-1/2 \cdot (1/(1-\rho^2) \cdot Z)}$$

where:

$$Z = ((x - \mu_x)/\sigma_x)^2 + ((y - \mu_y)/\sigma_y)^2 - [2\rho((x - \mu_x)/\sigma_x) \cdot ((y - \mu_y)/\sigma_y)] \quad (4.3)$$

Here, the standard deviate expression (Z) is much longer than in the univariate equation and contains an expression in which the distances from the mean for both x and y are multiplied together and also multiplied by 2ρ before being subtracted from the sum of the x and y standard deviates. This procedure removes the influence of parameter x on parameter y from the composite standard deviate. If there is no correlation ($\rho = 0$), this expression is zero and no correction is made but if there is a large correlation (e.g. $\rho = 0.5$), then a large correction factor is applied. If there are more than two variables, the equation becomes too unwieldy to be written in its expanded form and the general multivariate Gaussian distribution function must be used. This utilises matrix algebra which is complex and has already been described elsewhere (Reynolds and Penney, 1990). The 'V' in the following equation represents the covariance matrix relating all of the applied parameters.

$$f(x_1, x_2, \ldots, x_n) = (2\pi)^{-n/2} \cdot |V^{-1}|^{1/2} \cdot e^{-1/2\{(x-\mu)' \cdot V^{-1} \cdot (x-\mu)\}} \quad (4.4)$$

The method of deriving the Down's syndrome risk should also be explained. Firstly, the prior odds are derived from the maternal age using the age-risk formula (e.g. a 25-year-old woman has a Down's syndrome risk of 1 in 1351 at term). Next the Gaussian heights for her serum results are determined for 'normal' and 'abnormal' population parameters (Fig. 4.2). This figure shows two scenarios: in case one, the ratio of the height on the 'normal' curve and the height on the 'abnormal' curve is approximately 4; for case two the ratio is approximately 0.25. The prior odds are multiplied by this ratio such that for the 25-year-old woman, scenario one results in posterior odds of 1 in 5404 whilst scenario two results in posterior odds of 1 in 337.

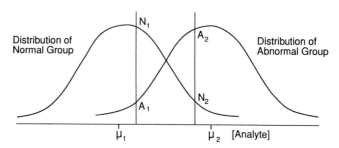

Fig. 4.2. The basis of the likelihood ratio method.

Standardisation for gestation dates and the effectiveness of conversion of patient results to conform to the Gaussian model

The concentrations of the analytes used in Down's syndrome screening change with gestation. Therefore, in order to calculate risks, either the patient results must be standardised to be unaffected by gestation age or population parameters must be derived for all possible gestations. The simpler of these methods is to standardise the results. The method of standardisation currently used in Down's syndrome screening has arisen from the methods used for α-fetoprotein (AFP) results in neural tube defect screening (the multiple of the median (MoM)). Several methods have been proposed for derivation of the medians used to calculate MoMs: gestation dating by integer weeks with medians derived for each week (weekly medians); weighted regression of week-derived medians (or their logs) against gestation dates; regression of raw patient results (or their logs) against gestation dates. These last two methods allow dates to be expressed in smaller units (i.e. days). To assess which of these methods achieves a satisfactory standardisation for gestation age, medians for AFP and human chorionic gonadotrophin (hCG) were derived using each of the above methods from a dataset of 5082 Down's syndrome screening tests and MoMs were calculated using each set of medians. The population distributions for AFP MoMs derived using each method are shown in Table 4.1.

If conversion of results to MoMs is satisfactory, the MoM value of the 50th percentile should be equal to 1 and the spread of results for all methods should be approximately the same. It can be seen that for AFP MoMs derived using regression of gestation age versus results (not log-transformed), the point at which MoM = 1 is at the 60th percentile. For hCG, this effect is also seen for weekly medians (data not shown). Therefore, neither of these methods can be considered acceptable and the

Table 4.1. *MoM distribution for 5082 consecutive AFP results*

Percentile	Weekly[a]	MoM distribution			
		Weighted regressed weekly[b]	Weighted regressed log(weekly)[c]	Regressed result	Regressed log(result)[d]
1	0.382	0.385	0.385	0.354	0.389
5	0.531	0.537	0.537	0.486	0.532
10	0.618	0.616	0.617	0.554	0.608
25	0.781	0.785	0.770	0.702	0.764
40	0.906	0.911	0.911	0.817	0.896
50	1.000	1.001	1.002	0.901	0.987
60	1.100	1.105	1.105	1.006	1.098
75	1.313	1.303	1.310	1.186	1.295
90	1.688	1.674	1.680	1.517	1.656
95	1.941	1.958	1.957	1.765	1.931
99	2.625	2.643	2.647	2.381	2.600

[a] Week-derived medians.
[b] Weighted regressed week-derived medians.
[c] Weighted regressed log(week-derived medians).
[d] Regressed log(results) where regression is against gestation date.

only derivations that generate satisfactory MoM distribution are weighted regression of weekly medians (Wald *et al.*, 1988a) or regression of gestation age against log-transformed patient results (Reynolds *et al.*, 1992a).

Both of these methods of deriving MoMs give very similar distributions. Therefore, only the results of testing of one distribution for true Gaussian form will be described (distribution tested = direct regression of gestation date versus log(results)). On probability paper, a straight line indicates that a distribution is Gaussian. Figure 4.3 shows such a graph for AFP and it can be seen that after log transformation, the results do appear to be Gaussian. However, testing with the Lillefors test for normality (Conover, 1980) gives test statistics of 0.0211 for AFP MoMs and 0.0118 for hCG MoMs (significance cut-offs: $\omega_{0.90} = 0.0113$; $\omega_{0.95} = 0.0124$; $\omega_{0.99} = 0.0145$) meaning that, although the hCG distribution can be considered Gaussian, the AFP distribution cannot be Gaussian as the test statistic is greater than the 99% cut-off. The discrepancy from a Gaussian distribution may be small but may have effects on the screening process (as yet undetermined).

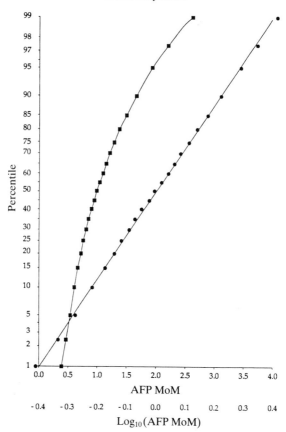

Fig. 4.3. Probability plot for raw AFP MoMs (■) and $\log_{10}$-transformed AFP MoMs (●).

Finally, to prove that conversion to MoMs removes dating dependency, MoMs may be regressed against gestation age. For the dataset described above, correlation coefficients between dates and AFP ($r = 0.0061$), and between dates and hCG ($r = 0.0056$), were not statistically significant implying that, despite the other limitations, conversion to MoMs does correct effectively for gestation date.

Deficiencies of MoMs in correction of analytical problems

Parvin *et al.* (1991) examined, both theoretically and experimentally, the effect of changing AFP assays on MoMs and on Down's syndrome risks. They showed that a change in the assay significantly altered the distribution

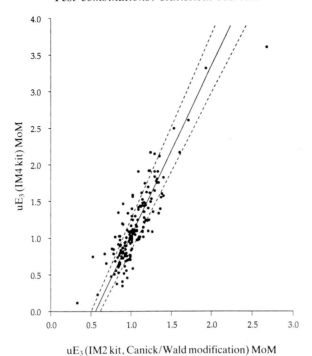

uE₃ (IM2 kit, Canick/Wald modification) MoM

Fig. 4.4. Comparison of MoMs derived from results from the Canick/Wald modified uE_3 assay with an optimised uE_3 assay (IM4). The solid line is the regression line and the dashed lines are the 95% confidence limits.

of MoMs and consequently the Down's syndrome risk estimates. The original work on unconjugated oestriol (uE_3) used an assay for uE_3 that had been designed for use in the third trimester (Canick *et al.*, 1988; Wald *et al.*, 1988b). The assay was modified for use in the second trimester by diluting the lowest standard with zero standard and by doubling the sample volume. Later, an optimised assay was developed and a comparison of the two assays was carried out (Reynolds and John, 1992) which showed that there was a large methodological bias between the two kits. Significant differences were present in the raw patient results and these were not removed by conversion to MoMs (Fig. 4.4).

The effect of this methodological bias on the population MoM distribution is extremely significant (Table 4.2). If the population standard deviation is estimated from the 10–90% distance as described in the original paper on multivariate risk screening (Wald *et al.*, 1988b), the standard deviations for the two methods are 0.1712 (modified kit) and 0.4358 ('new kit'). The original standard deviation published for unaffected

Table 4.2. *Distribution of MoMs for Canick/Wald modified uE_3 kit and optimised uE_3 kit*

	Distribution of MoM	
Percentile	Canick/Wald modified	Optimised
2.5	0.71	0.35
5	0.78	0.47
10	0.83	0.58
25	0.89	0.75
50	1.00	1.00
75	1.15	1.36
90	1.27	1.70
95	1.35	1.86
97.5	1.45	2.11

cases was 0.26. It therefore appears that the Canick modification of the third trimester kit may have caused a significant under-estimation of the population standard deviation for uE_3.

A comparison of the effect of using optimised kit MoMs and modified kit MoMs on likelihood ratios was also performed and the difference in likelihood ratios derived from the two sets of results are shown in Fig. 4.5 (Reynolds and John, 1992). It is immediately obvious that there is a massive difference between ratios derived from results of the modified kit and those from the optimised kit. This is unacceptable because it may alter the proportions of screening test results that come into the 'high' or 'low' risk categories. In the comparison study, the net result was to increase the proportion of 'high risk category' results from 4.5% using the modified kit to 6.8% with the optimised kit for a constant risk cut-off (1:300). Therefore, it is apparent that MoMs cannot correct for method differences particularly when there are large biases between two assays.

The importance of correct population parameters

Correct population parameters are vital if the algorithm used to calculate Down's syndrome risks is to give the correct result. The effect of different population parameters on Down's syndrome screening was evaluated using the original population parameters (Wald *et al.*, 1988a) and 'new' parameters that have been described for ultrasound-dated pregnancies (Wald *et al.*, 1992). In the 'new' parameters there is a log distribution and

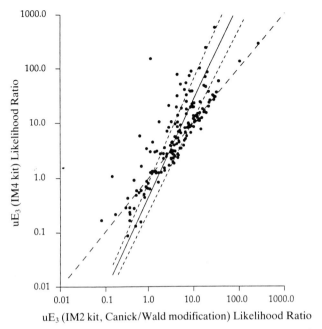

Fig. 4.5. Comparison of likelihood ratios resulting from the MoMs in Fig. 4.4. The solid line is the regression line; short dashed lines are the 95% confidence limits; and the long dashed line is the line of identity (i.e. slope = 1, intercept = 0).

a narrower S.D. for uE_3 for the unaffected group when compared to the Down's syndrome group. For scan-dated pregnancies the S.D.s suggested are: unaffected, 0.1184; Down's syndrome, 0.1741. Comparable S.D.s from a study at the University Hospital of Wales are: unaffected, 0.1861; Down's syndrome, 0.1954. The receiver operator characteristic (ROC) plot (Fig. 4.6) compares the effect of using the two sets of parameters to derive risk estimates on detection and false-positive rates for a set of 536 randomly selected unaffected pregnancies and 52 Down's syndrome pregnancies (data from University Hospital of Wales and Oldchurch Hospital, Essex). For this set of samples using the 1988 parameters, the addition of uE_3 has no benefit whatsoever when compared to 'double testing' (AFP + total hCG) and that when the 1992 parameters for scan-dated pregnancies are applied, the addition of uE_3 results in a significant loss of detection for a constant false-positive rate (Reynolds *et al.*, 1993b).

This loss of detection is because of the narrower S.D. for the unaffected group compared to the S.D. for the Down's syndrome group. This excessively narrow S.D. means that many quite unremarkable samples

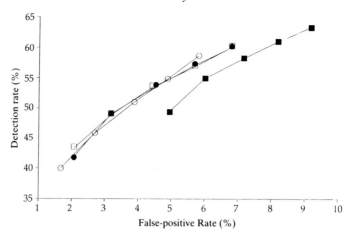

Fig. 4.6. Comparison of the effect of using different population parameters on false-positive and detection rates. 'Double' test (AFP + total hCG) (●, ○); 'triple' test (AFP + total hCG + uE$_3$) (■, □). Open symbols are population parameters from Wald *et al.* (1988a). Filled symbols are population parameters from Wald *et al.* (1992).

are interpreted by the algorithm to deviate significantly from normality. Since a large proportion of these are in the lower tail of the 'normal' group distribution, they overlap with the upper tail of the 'abnormal' group distribution. The net effect is determined by which distribution has the wider S.D. (Fig. 4.7). In the figure it can be seen that the overlap is such that a greater proportion of 'normal' results will appear to be members of the Down's syndrome group. This results in a greater number of false-positive cases and, therefore, a reduction in the apparent efficacy of uE$_3$. We must be extremely careful to ensure that the population parameters used in Down's syndrome screening are truly representative of reality. This is an important lesson because it demonstrates that procedures that appear to work in a simulated population should not be accepted unless they have been proved to work using 'real' data.

How many analytes should we use?

There are two considerations that must be taken into account when deciding how many analytes can be used in Down's syndrome screening. The first must be efficacy: using only one analyte (AFP) there is detection of Down's syndrome pregnancies but the efficiency is very low. Addition of a second analyte results in greatly enhanced detection and, therefore,

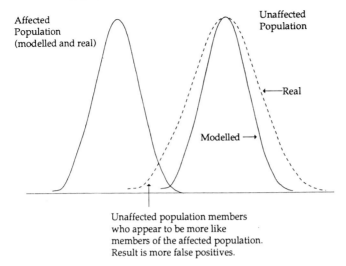

Fig. 4.7. Increased false-positive results occur if the population S.D. for the 'normal' cases is too small.

it can be taken that at least two analytes are required but is it necessary or beneficial to use more? The lack of improvement in detection due to adding uE_3 in Fig. 4.6 suggests that there may be no benefit from extra analytes but this is based on only a small number of cases. A second approach to determining the maximum number of analytes required is to examine how many analytes can be used before the result becomes too imprecise to be of any practical value. It may be argued that imprecision is immaterial since each extra analyte extends the range of possible risks that may result, thereby separating normal and affected groups more efficiently. For example, using AFP alone the range of possible risk lies from approximately 1:100 to 1:10 000 and the addition of hCG expands this range to approximately 1:30 to 1:100 000. This argument, however, is specious because the aim of biochemical investigation is to give the correct result to each patient. Therefore, imprecision must not become so great that confidence can no longer be placed in any individual result. The zone where precision is most important is close to the cut-off point between high- and low-risk decisions: poor precision here may be a cause of false-negative as well as false-positive results and even with a 'double test' significant variation has been reported (Selby *et al.*, 1993). Therefore, it must be concluded that if the addition of an extra analyte increases the uncertainty about the correct result beyond an acceptable limit then there is no point in adding the extra analyte to the screening test.

From the equations 4.2–4.4, it can be seen that as more analytes are added, the number of times each result is used in the risk calculation algorithm increases. Thus for one analyte screening, each value is used once in determination of the standard deviate for the unaffected population and once for the Down's syndrome population distribution. For two analyte screening, each analyte result is used four times (once for the standard deviate and once for the correction factor for both normal and Down's syndrome distributions). For triple analyte screening, each result is used nine times, etc. It is obvious that if there is an error in the result, then as more analytes are added this error may be multiplied. Since all laboratory results have errors inherent in their determination, there must be errors in the final Down's syndrome risk estimation. To determine these errors algebraically is extremely difficult and, therefore, it is better to measure them experimentally or by computer simulation (Reynolds, 1992).

Experimental imprecision may be assessed by repeatedly assaying a single sample. Using four different samples, AFP and hCG were each assayed in replicate ($n = 22$) and the results used to derive likelihood ratios (uE_3 is not assayed routinely in the laboratories in South Wales and, therefore, was not included in this process). Coefficients of variation (CV) were derived for all four cases and the mean CV was taken to give an assessment of the imprecision of screening. For AFP-only screening, the CV was 12.3% and for AFP + hCG screening, the mean was 24.7%. A computer simulation using representative individual assay CVs derived from a manufacturer's kit insert data was also performed. CVs used were: AFP, 5.8%; hCG, 5.1%; and uE_3, 8.7%. For AFP-only screening, the CV of likelihood ratios was 8.6%; for AFP + hCG screening the CV was 15.7%; and for triple testing the CV was 23.8%. The manufacturer's precision data reported smaller CVs than those found in practice and when the simulation was repeated using the slightly higher CVs found in the experimental study, the combined CV was shown to increase by 12% per analyte; this was similar to the experimental study. Thus, the probable experimental CV for the triple test would be approximately 36%. This is in the middle of the range of CVs reported for experimental triple test imprecision by Holding (1991) who found that for the triple test imprecision measured by CV lay in the range 21.4–47.8%.

Analytical imprecision has long been considered important in clinical chemistry and, therefore, many studies have been made into its effect on the utility of results in clinical practice. As early as 1963 it was proposed that a maximum CV of 10% should be allowable although this was later amended to 20% for certain analytes (Tonks, 1963, 1968). Furthermore, surveys of clinicians have shown that CVs greater than 20% are totally unacceptable for clinical use (Elion-Gerritzen, 1980; Skendzel *et al.*, 1985). A CV of 20% means that the 95% confidence limits for a result is approximately $\pm 40\%$. Thus if the CV becomes 50% the limit of confidence is approximately $\pm 100\%$ or, for any given estimation of risk (n), the confidence limit would lie from risk $= 1:0$ to $1:2n$. Thus even a risk of $1:10\,000$ could still conceivably be a high-risk result that was mis-classified purely due to analytical imprecision. Therefore, it is vital that we limit imprecision as far as possible and, in view of the 20% limit that is considered to be the limit of acceptability for other clinical chemistry results, it is reasonable to believe that Down's syndrome screening results should have a similar tolerance. This implies that the maximum number of analytes that is viable is two.

The importance of accurate gestation dating

The conversion of patient results to MoMs to remove the effect of the changes in analyte concentration with gestation has already been described. However, what has not been considered is the problem of deciding which median to use to determine the MoM. Gestation dating is a major problem: relying on the woman's dates may be acceptable as often even the date of conception can be accurately remembered, but there are many cases where this is not true. Menstrual cycles may be irregular and it is quite possible for the estimated date of conception to be out by as much as 4 weeks. Therefore, it is necessary to check by ultrasound that gestation dates are correct, preferably before screening takes place. It is totally wrong to check the gestation dates of those women who have a high-risk result from screening in order to remove them from the amniocentesis group. This can only result in a loss of detection since for each woman whose date reassignment results in a low-risk decision there is likely to be another for whom date reassignment would have indicated that the change should be from the low-risk to the high-risk group.

Once it is accepted that accurate gestation dating is crucial and that ultrasound assessment is necessary before screening takes place, a decision must be made about how gestation dates are to be expressed. It is common practice in many hospitals for dates to be expressed in integer weeks with the date derived from a table of biparietal diameters (BPD). This is undesirable because it can cause a very large variation in the calculated risk simply due to the imprecision of an ultrasound dating compared to

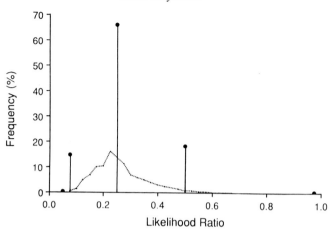

Fig. 4.8. The distribution of likelihood ratios produced when gestation dating is in integer weeks (solid line with circles) and using BDP-derived dates (dotted line).

the 'true' gestation date. Ultrasound measurement is as prone to 'assay' imprecision as any other measurement in biomedicine (Reynolds, 1992). However, because ultrasound produces a numerical value, it may either be used directly to derive medians instead of first converting it to a date (Reynolds *et al.*, 1992a) or used via a formula to convert to an 'exact' date (BMUS, 1990). Since the formula will always convert a given BPD to the same date this is effectively the same as using the BPD directly to derive medians. However, it has the advantage that if the scan is performed on a different day from the one on which the blood sample was collected, the difference may be added (or subtracted) as necessary.

Figure 4.8 shows a simulation of the effect of using integer week-derived medians and exact date-derived medians on likelihood ratios assuming no laboratory imprecision on 10 000 simulated gestation datings for a single sample. The most striking feature is the multi-modality when integer-week medians are used, but the wide range of possible likelihood ratios resulting from integer-week dating (range approximately from 0.1 to 1.0) is also significant. This occurs because of over- or under-estimation of BPD to such an extent that a different week of gestation is predicted and, in this simulation, over 30% of the simulated datings resulted in mis-classification. This multi-modal peak effect can be eliminated simply by changing the method of expressing the ultrasound dates. In the same figure, the distribution for 'exact' dating shows that a smaller range of likelihood ratios with a mono-modal pattern results.

is quite low. Nevertheless, the graph shows an approximately 5% increase in detection when weight correction is performed.

A further maternal factor that may influence analyte concentrations is maternal height. The increase in body fat in obesity results in a decrease in the proportional volume of body water (Lassiter and Gottschalck, 1974). Thus, for two women of equal weight but widely differing heights, the dilution effect may be different. In actuality, the effect is so small as to be negligible and maternal weight correction alone is sufficient (Reynolds *et al.*, 1992b).

The influence of the mathematics of screening on detection and false-positive rates for different maternal ages

In Down's syndrome screening, a standard risk cut-off is usually used to determine who should be offered amniocentesis. From the age-related risk profile shown in Fig. 4.1 and the description of how Down's syndrome risk estimates are derived, it is obvious that the likelihood ratio required to convert the age-related risk to a high risk will be dependent on maternal age. Since the likelihood ratio is dependent on the degree to which a serum analyte profile is atypical of normal and the AFP and hCG levels are independent of age, it follows that in younger women the degree of abnormality in the serum picture must be greater to identify them as being members of the high-risk group (Reynolds *et al.*, 1993a). By computer simulation of populations of 100 000 unaffected and 100 000 Down's syndrome-affected pregnancies, the proportion of women in each age group for both affected and unaffected populations whose serum results would be sufficient to cause them to have a high-risk result were estimated. This allows the detection rates, false-positive rates and the predictive value for each age group to be derived. Figures 4.13–4.15 show the age-related false-positive rates, detection rates and predictive values for AFP screening and for AFP + total hCG screening. The results for triple analyte screening have been left off the diagrams for clarity as they were similar to the results for the AFP + hCG combination.

The significant point to notice from these graphs is that in young women, who make up the majority of the pregnant population, the predicted detection rate is much lower (approximately 40%) than the aggregate detection rate of greater than 60% that is usually the rate that is discussed during prescreen counselling in antenatal clinics. However, it is also obvious that the false-positive rates in younger women are lower. Similarly in older women, the detection rate is far greater than 60% and

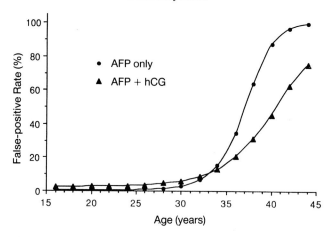

Fig. 4.13. Age-related false-positive rate for risk cut-off 1:300.

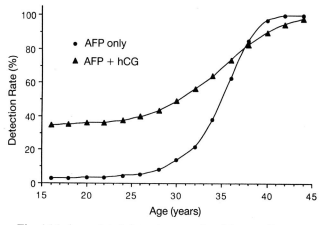

Fig. 4.14. Age-related detection rate for risk cut-off 1:300.

approaches 100% in the oldest age groups. However to achieve 100% detection, the false-positive rates are also increased, up to nearly 80% in 45-year-old women for the double test. These sigmoid characteristics are purely due to the shape of the maternal age and Down's syndrome incidence relationship and have many effects on the entire Down's syndrome screening process; for example, comparison of different studies is made more difficult because for effective comparison the population age structure must be the same. It would be possible to give a screening programme the appearance of being more successful purely by restricting

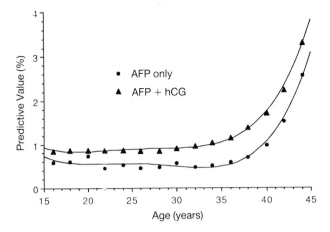

Fig. 4.15. Age-related predictive value of a positive result for risk cut-off 1:300.

the screen to older women. Conversely, in countries where it is the practice to offer amniocentesis automatically to older women without first screening them, the screen may only be performed for young women and this would result in an apparently poor performance of a serum screening programme.

The age-related detection and false-positive rates may be of considerable value in pre-test counselling because they can be used to explain that the test is not 100% effective but that it will pick up a significant proportion of cases of Down's syndrome. The predictive value of a positive result is also important because it may be used in secondary counselling after a high-risk result has been received. An explanation that there is only a 1% chance that the fetus has Down's syndrome may be beneficial in reducing the stress generated by a 'positive' result.

Other mathematical treatments for results

The likelihood ratio method for calculating Down's syndrome risk estimates is an effective way of determining whether a patient's serum profile is more typical of Down's syndrome than of the normal situation but has one major deficiency: if a result is atypical of normal but is even more atypical of Down's syndrome, the final risk estimate will be a very low risk of Down's syndrome. However, such a result indicates further investigation (Wright *et al.*, 1993). This problem arises because the question asked is very specific: are these data characteristic of a Down's syndrome pregnancy? For example, the case arrowed in Fig. 4.16 has a

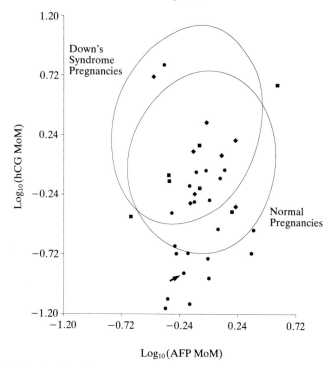

Fig. 4.16. Plot showing AFP and hCG results for trisomy 13 and 18 pregnancies reported in the literature. The ellipses represent the 99% confidence limits for unaffected and Down's syndrome pregnancies. The arrowed result has a Down's syndrome risk of 1:18 000 but is significantly atypical of normality (Wright *et al.*, 1993). Diagram reproduced by permission of the Editor of the *Annals of Clinical Biochemistry*.

calculated Down's syndrome risk of 1 in 18 000, but the fetus was affected by trisomy 18. In this case the 'incorrect' diagnosis could be avoided because the combination of AFP and hCG is so atypical of normal that it should be recognised as such. However, recognition of atypical results by eye is difficult, particularly when they are close to the borderlines of normality.

The two rings on the graph in Fig. 4.16 represent the 99% confidence contour such that a serum result profile that lies outside of the contour is only 1% likely to be typical of the parameters that define the distribution. These contours are defined by the Mahalanobis distance described at the beginning of this chapter. This value has the same distribution as the χ^2 distribution and, therefore, it is simple to determine whether a serum result profile is atypical of either the normal or the

Down's syndrome groups. The Mahalanobis distance has the same number of degrees of freedom as the number of analytes used to calculate it. Therefore for AFP + hCG screening, a 99% cut-off can be defined as any score greater than 9.210. However, since addition of an atypicality cut-off could result in an increased amniocentesis rate for little extra detection, it is probably advisable that amniocentesis is not the automatic result of a sample being flagged as atypical. An atypical result should be used as an indicator that something is amiss; this may even be simply that the gestation dating is incorrect.

Conclusions

In conclusion, it has been shown that although the underlying mathematical principles behind the derivation of Down's syndrome risk estimates are quite simple, the interactions between the prior odds derived from maternal age, the variation in the odds-modifying likelihood ratio due to analytical and gestation-dating imprecision and the uncertainty about the correct population parameters result in an extremely complex situation. However, there are some essential factors that should be considered in Down's syndrome risk screening programmes.

(1) Since MoMs cannot be avoided until a better alternative is found, derivation of correct medians is crucial: the mid-point of the population MoM distribution should be 1.0 (or 0.0 if a log distribution is examined) and there should be a linear plot on probability paper.

(2) Assays for use in Down's syndrome screening must be optimised to the concentrations expected and population parameters must be derived using optimised assays. If two methods give different results, they will probably also give different MoM distributions and, therefore, risk estimates may need to be derived using assay-specific population parameters.

(3) A set of population parameters may work very well in simulations but very poorly when tested on a real population. Therefore, any study that relies on simulations to determine the benefit of adding extra or different analytes should be examined with caution until population studies prove that the benefit is genuine.

(4) Clinical chemistry is about giving the correct result to each individual patient: we must therefore ensure that the results we produce are as precise as possible. It appears that imprecision imposes a maximum limit of two analytes if Down's syndrome risks are to be estimated by the likelihood ratio method.

(5) Accurate gestation dating is crucial.

(6) Inter-centre biases in dating may be significant and it is vital that each screening programme should derive its own medians: when a programme is initiated it may be possible to use manufacturer's medians but these should be replaced by locally derived medians as soon as practically possible.

(7) Some maternal factors may affect the concentrations of analytes and hence alter the risk estimate.

(8) Other mathematical treatments for the results are possible and must be examined to determine whether they may be superior to the likelihood ratio method.

References

BMUS (British Medical Ultrasound Society Working Party on Fetal Measurements) (1990). *Clinical aplications of ultrasonic fetal measurement.* London: British Medical Ultrasound Society.

Canick, J., Knight, G., Palomaki, G. *et al.* (1988). Low second trimester serum unconjugated oestriol in pregnancies with Down's syndrome. *Br. J. Obstet. Gynaecol.*, **95**, 330–3.

Conover, W. (1980). *Practical Non-parametric Statistics*, 2nd Edn. New York: John Wiley.

Cuckle, H., Wald, N. & Thompson, S. (1987). Estimating a woman's risk of having a pregnancy associated with Down's syndrome using her age and serum alpha-fetoprotein. *Br. J. Obstet. Gynaecol.*, **94**, 387–402.

Elion-Gerritzen, W. (1980). Analytic precision in clinical chemistry and medical decisions. *Am. J. Clin. Path.*, **73**, 183–95.

Holding, S. (1991). Biochemical screening for Down's syndrome. *Br. Med. J.*, **302**, 1275.

Lassiter, W., Gottschalck, C. (1974). Volume and composition of the body fluids. pp. 1049–64. In *Medical Physiology*, 13th edn, ed. V. Mountcastle, pp. 1049–64. St Louis: Mosby.

Nørgaard-Petersen, B., Larsen, S., Arends, J., Svenstrup, B. & Tabor, A. (1990). Maternal serum markers in screening for Down syndrome. *Clin. Genet.* **37**, 35–43.

Palomaki, G. & Haddow, J. (1987). Maternal, serum α-fetoprotein, age and Down syndrome risk. *Am. J. Obstet. Gynecol.*, **156**, 460–3.

Parvin, C., Gray, D. & Kessler, G. (1991). Influence of assay method differences on multiple of the median distributions: maternal serum alpha-fetoprotein as an example. *Clin. Chem.*, **37**, 637–42.

Reynolds, T. (1992). Practical problems in Down syndrome screening: what should we do about gestation dating? What is the effect of laboratory imprecision? *Commun. Lab. Med.*, **1**, 31–8.

Reynolds, T. & John, R. (1992). A comparison of unconjugated estriol assay kits shows that expression of results as multiples of the median causes unacceptable variation in calculated Down syndrome risk factors. *Clin. Chem.*, **38**, 1888–93.

Reynolds, T. & Penney, M. (1990). The mathematical basis of multivariate risk analysis: with special reference to screening for Down syndrome associated pregnancy. *Ann. Clin. Biochem.*, **27**, 452–8.

Reynolds, T., Penney, M., Hughes, H. & John, R. (1991). The effect of weight correction on risk calculation for Down syndrome. *Ann. Clin. Biochem.*, **28**, 245–9.

Reynolds, T., Penney, M. & Hughes, H. (1992a). Ultrasonic dating of pregnancy results in significant errors in Down syndrome screening which may be minimised by use of biparietal diameter based means. *Am. J. Obstet. Gynaecol.*, **166**, 872–7.

Reynolds, T., Hughes, H. & Penney, M. (1992b). Weight correction revisited: does maternal height affect serum AFP and hCG levels. *Commun. Lab. Med.* **1**, 103–5.

Reynolds, T., Nix, B., Dunstan, F. & Dawson, A. (1993a). Age related detection rates in Down syndrome screening: an aid to counselling. *Obstet. Gynecol.*, **81**, 447–50.

Reynolds, T., John, R. & Spencer, K. (1993b). The utility of unconjugated estriol in Down syndrome screening is not proven. *Clin. Chem.*, **39**, 2023–5.

Selby, C., Stirland, B., Meakin, J., Powditch, S. & Marenah, C. (1993). Within and between batch variability of the estimation of Down's syndrome risks. *Proceedings of the ACB National Meeting*, Vol. 37, p. 37. London: Association of Clinical Biochemists.

Skendzel, L., Barnett, R. & Platt, R. (1985). Medically useful criteria for analytical performance of laboratory tests. *Am. J. Clin. Path.*, **83**, 200–5.

Tonks, D. (1963). A study of the accuracy and precision of clinical chemistry determinations in 170 Canadian laboratories. *Clin. Chem.*, **9**, 271–303.

Tonks, D. (1968). A quality control program for quantitative clinical chemistry. *Can. J. Med. Technol.*, **30**, 38–54.

Wald, N., Cuckle, H., Densem, J. *et al.* (1988a). Maternal serum screening for Down's syndrome in early pregnancy. *Br. Med. J.*, **297**, 883–8.

Wald, N., Cuckle, H., Densem, J. *et al.* (1988b). Maternal serum oestriol as an antenatal screening test for Down's syndrome. *Br. J. Obstet. Gynaecol.*, **95**, 334–41.

Wald, N., Cuckle, H., Demsem, J. *et al.* (1992). Maternal serum screening for Down's syndrome: the effect of routine ultrasound scan determination of gestational age and adjustment for maternal weight. *Br. J. Obstet. Gynaecol.*, **99**, 144–9.

Wright, D., Reynolds, T. & Donovan, C. (1993). Assessment of atypicality: an adjunct to screening for Down syndrome that facilitates detection of other chromosomal defects. *Ann. Clin. Biochem.*, **30**, 578–83.

5

Measurement of human chorionic gonadotrophin (hCG) as a screening test for Down's syndrome

T. CHARD AND R. ILES

Low levels of maternal serum α-fetoprotein (AFP) in association with a chromosomally abnormal fetus were first documented by Merkatz and colleagues (1984). This finding led to the suggestion that other biochemical products of the fetoplacental unit, including human chorionic gonado-trophin might also show characteristic abnormalities (Chard et al., 1984). In 1987 the reality of this concept was shown by Bogart and colleagues, with the demonstration of elevated levels of hCG in maternal blood in the presence of a Down's syndrome fetus. The phenomenon has now been confirmed by numerous authors. It is also apparent that maternal serum hCG is probably the single most efficient index of Down's syndrome risk, and its measurement is included as part of almost all screening programmes for this condition.

Biochemistry of human chorionic gonadotrophin

Human chorionic gonadotrophin (hCG) is a member of a family of four glycoprotein hormones, the other members being luteinising hormone (LH), follicle-stimulating hormone (FSH), and thyrotrophin-stimulating hormone (TSH). Each of these consists of two subunits: an α-subunit (92 amino acid residues), which is almost identical in all four hormones, and a β-subunit that is characteristic of the individual hormone (Bahl et al., 1972; Morgan et al., 1975). The β-subunit of hCG is a single chain of 145 amino acid residues. Of the first 121 N-terminal amino acid residues, 80% are identical with those in β-LH. The C-terminus of β-hCG has a 24 amino acid residue extension not present in β-LH. Both subunits of the molecule must be combined for biological activity but the β-subunit determines the specificity of the action (Strickland and Puett, 1981). The α-subunit is coded by a single gene on chromosome 6 and the β-subunit by a family of six genes on chromosome 19 (Graham *et al.*, 1987); only two of the latter genes are believed to contribute to synthesis of placental hCG (Talmadge *et al.*, 1984). However, recent studies suggest that at least five are transcriptionally functional (Bo and Boime, 1992). Once dimerisation of the two subunits has occurred, the hormone is very rapidly released, almost none being stored within the cell: in contrast to the pituitary gland there is no evidence for calcium-dependent exocytosis of secretory granules (Hussa, 1981).

Chorionic gonadotrophin is produced by the placental syncytiotrophoblast (and possibly also the cytotrophoblast; Kurman *et al.*, 1984). The syncytiotrophoblast is a continuous layer of cells which forms the surface of the chorionic villi. It is thus in direct contact with the maternal bloodstream but is separated from fetal blood by a basement membrane, connective tissue and fetal vascular endothelium.

Throughout most of pregnancy the α-subunit is synthesised in greater quantities than the β-subunit (Boothby *et al.*, 1983). Small amounts of free α-subunit appear in maternal blood, where the pattern is a progressive increase to a plateau at 36 weeks (i.e. similar to other placental products such as hPL) (Cole *et al.*, 1984; Nagy *et al.*, 1994). The pattern of hCG levels in fetal blood is similar to that in the mother but at 2–3% of the concentration (Clements *et al.*, 1976). At term, the levels in the female fetus are substantially higher than those in the male (Obiekwe and Chard, 1982). The levels and pattern of hCG in amniotic fluid do not mirror maternal blood (Iles *et al.*, 1992). The half-life of hCG shows multiple components with an initial fast phase of 6 hours (Wehman *et al.*, 1984). For the free subunits the clearance rates are much faster, with fast components of 0.2 hours for free α-subunits and 0.68 hours for free β-subunits (Wehman and Nisula, 1980). In urine some hCG is in the form of intact hormone (10–25%) while the remainder consists of free β-subunit and, in particular, a fragment known as 'β-core' which is synthesised from hCG in the kidney (Wehman *et al.*, 1990).

The mechanisms which control the levels of hCG in maternal blood are unknown. The other proteins of the placenta, and the steroid hormones, all show a progressive rise throughout pregnancy which closely parallels the growth of the fetus and placenta. Many factors can affect the release of hCG from placental tissues *in vitro*. Numerous studies have been performed on the possible role of gonadotrophin-releasing hormone (GnRH), which undoubtedly is present in the placenta (Gibbons *et al.*, 1975; Lee *et al.*, 1981). However, although there appears to be extensive evidence for a role of GnRH *in vitro*, little or no effect has been shown with *in vivo* studies (Perez-Lopez *et al.*, 1984; Kim *et al.*, 1987). In addition, many of the studies have employed concentrations of materials which would generally be regarded as pharmacological rather than physiological. It is also difficult to perceive any anatomical or physiological basis for suggesting that the types of feedback mechanism which operate in the hypothalamic–pituitary–gonadal axis might also apply to the placenta. The general conclusion is that the trophoblast is effectively a free-running tissue, in which the major factors determining synthesis and secretion are the mass of the trophoblast and uteroplacental bloodflow.

It has been shown that β-hCG synthesised by bladder tumour cells *in vitro* can be stimulated by interferon-alpha (IFN-α) (Iles and Chard, 1989). This is of particular interest in the light of the fact that the receptors for IFN-α are coded on chromosome 21, and that hCG levels are elevated in pregnancies with a trisomy 21 fetus.

In the early weeks of pregnancy, hCG may be the major luteotrophic signal from the implanting embryo. It has been postulated that, in the second trimester, hCG is the principal stimulus to synthesis of testosterone by the fetal testis, but there is now clear experimental evidence against this suggestion (Word *et al.*, 1989). Another fetal role proposed for hCG is an adrenocorticotrophic action. However, the pattern of hCG secretion (if this is the same in the fetus as in the mother) shows no obvious correlation with the development of fetal adrenal function.

Factors affecting circulating levels of hCG

Gestation

This is the major factor determining the circulating levels of hCG. Chorionic gonadotrophin is secreted by the blastocyst. It appears in maternal blood shortly after implantation and then increases rapidly until 8 weeks of gestation. The levels show little change at 8–12 weeks, decline to 18 weeks and thereafter remain fairly constant until term. The change in hCG concentrations is relatively small over the critical 16–18 week period, so that interpretation of hCG levels is less affected than that of the other analytes by inaccuracies in gestational dating.

Diurnal variation

Over a 24-hour period, there is some short-term random variation in blood hCG levels but no circadian rhythm (Houghton *et al.*, 1982).

Fetal sex

From approximately 18 weeks until term the levels of hCG are higher in mothers carrying a female fetus (Obiekwe and Chard, 1982; Leporrier *et al.*, 1992). At earlier stages there is no variation with fetal sex (Muller *et al.*, 1993).

Fetal weight

There is a clear relationship between maternal hCG levels and fetal weight at term (Obiekwe and Chard, 1982) but not in mid-pregnancy. In twin pregnancies, the multiple of median (MoM) of hCG levels at 15–22 weeks has been estimated at 1.84 (Word *et al.*, 1989) and 2.4 (Muller *et al.*, 1993).

Race

Median hCG levels are higher in blacks than in whites (Muller and Boue, 1990; Simpson *et al.*, 1990; Kulch *et al.*, 1993). Some have not been able to confirm this observation (Petrocik *et al.*, 1989; Bogart *et al.*, 1991), though Bogart was able to show a 9.8% difference after correction for maternal weight. Bogart and colleagues (1991) also showed that levels in orientals were 16% higher than those in white women.

Smoking

Levels of hCG are lower in smokers than in non-smokers (Bernstein *et al.*, 1989; Cuckle *et al.*, 1990; Bartels *et al.*, 1993).

IVF pregnancies

Levels of hCG in this group do not differ from normal pregnancies (Muller *et al.*, 1993).

Fetal abdominal wall defects

Levels of hCG in this group appear to be elevated (mean MoM 1.82 in 16 pregnancies) (T. Chard, unpublished data).

Maternal weight

There is an inverse relationship between maternal weight and circulating hCG levels (Suchy and Yeager, 1990; Bogart *et al.*, 1991; Bartels *et al.*, 1993)

Other complications of pregnancy

Low levels of hCG are associated with threatened and incomplete abortion (Salem *et al.*, 1984; Mason *et al.*, 1993). High levels of hCG in the second trimester are associated with complications later in the pregnancy including intrauterine growth retardation, proteinuric hypertension and fetal death (Bewley *et al.*, 1992; Lieppman *et al.*, 1993; Muller *et al.*, 1993; Tanaka *et al.*, 1993). Levels are normal or slightly reduced in women with insulin-dependent diabetes mellitus (Wald *et al.*, 1992a; Palomaki *et al.*, 1994). The potential clinical value of mid-trimester biochemistry in predicting third trimester complications is considered in more detail in Chapter 24.

Factors affecting assays for hCG

The design of assays for Down's screening is considered in detail in other chapters. The assays for hCG are generally robust, but with some variation in absolute levels as recorded by different sets of reagents, even using common standards. This problem is easily overcome by the development of normal ranges for a given set of reagents (e.g. a commercial kit) together with meticulous ongoing quality control. Failure to use reliable reference ranges probably explains why early data from the UK Quality Assurance Scheme revealed marked between-laboratory, within-analyte group differences in calculated risks (Ellis, 1993). The results of assays for intact hCG do not seem to be affected by the type of sample (serum or plasma) or conditions of sample storage (fresh, stored frozen, etc.) (Petrocik *et al.*, 1989). A potentially serious problem affecting assays for free β-subunit arises from the fact that intact hCG may fragment into subunits, especially after storage or at high temperatures (Fig. 5.1; Gau *et al.*, 1984). For example, if blood is stored unseparated at room temperature, the free β-subunit concentration increases by 14% at 24 hours and 43% at 4 days (Stevenson *et al.*, 1993). Generation of free β-subunits on storage might explain the apparent superior detection of Down's syndrome achieved with assays for free β-subunit; most studies have been performed retrospectively on samples which may have been stored for many years. Because the normal proportion of free β-subunit in the circulation is relatively small (3%), a 1% breakdown of intact hCG could increase measured free β-subunit by 30%. However, Spencer and colleagues (1993) have presented evidence that the instability of intact hCG is unlikely to be a serious problem in routine clinical practice.

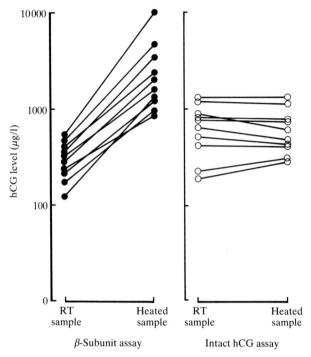

Fig. 5.1. Ten samples of pregnancy serum (11–14 weeks) were heated at 56°C for 6 hours. hCG levels were measured in the β-subunit assay and in the intact hCG assay (modified from Gau *et al.*, 1984). Heat dissociation has been used in the immunoassay of individual subunits (Nagy *et al.* 1994).

Levels of hCG in pregnancies with a chromosomally abnormal fetus

Maternal levels of intact hCG in pregnancies with a Down's syndrome fetus are generally higher than those in a normal pregnancy (Table 5.1). Analysis of the mid-trimester results shown in Table 5.1, with weighting according to the number of cases of Down's syndrome in each study, reveals an overall MoM of 2.09. This phenomenon is much more striking at 15–21 weeks than at 7–14 weeks of gestation. In combination with maternal age and AFP, measurement of hCG (intact or free β-subunit) would lead to the ascertainment of 60–70% of cases of Down's syndrome (Wald *et al.*, 1988, 1992b). In the first trimester, intact hCG levels have little or no predictive value, unlike free β-subunit (Brock *et al.*, 1990; Aitken *et al.*, 1993). Some authors (e.g. Muller and Bouc, 1990; Muller *et al.*, 1993) advocate the use of hCG alone as a screening test.

Table 5.1. *Studies on levels of intact hCG in relation to*
Down's syndrome[a]

Author	Stage of gestation (weeks)	No. of controls (normals)	No. of Down's syndrome	hCG levels in Down's syndrome (MoM)
Bogart *et al.*, 1987	18–25	74	17	2.77
Wald *et al.*, 1988	13–27	385	77	2.04
Osathanondh *et al.*, 1989	16–22		26	2.59
Brock *et al.*, 1990	7–14	63	21	1.43
Nørgaard-Pedersen *et al.*, 1990	14–18	328	42	1.57
Suchy and Yeager, 1990	15–22	614	16	2.4
Mancini *et al.*, 1991	15–18	831	9	2.33
Bogart *et al.*, 1991	15–21	3173	6	2.135
Crossley *et al.*, 1991	15–20	410	49	2.18
Phillips *et al.*, 1992	15–20	600	7	2.7
Ryall *et al.*, 1992	15–21	171	57	2.12
Spencer *et al.*, 1992	14–21	2862	90	2.13
van Lith *et al.*, 1992	13–27	1348	24	1.19
Herrou *et al.*, 1992	15–19	10 000	24	2.96
Crandall *et al.*, 1993	11–15	836	11	1.73

[a] Studies in which MoM values are not given for individual analytes
have not been included and studies on subunits of hCG are dealt with
in later chapters.

In contrast to Down's syndrome, trisomy 18 is associated with low
levels of maternal hCG (Muller and Boue, 1990; Nørgaard-Pedersen
et al., 1990; Crossley *et al.*, 1991), though there is some evidence for a
bimodal distribution with some very low levels and some high levels
(Muller *et al.*, 1993). This finding has been incorporated as a predictive
factor in some screening programmes (e.g. Palomaki *et al.*, 1992). Levels
of hCG are also lower in triploidy (Kohn *et al.*, 1991; Mason *et al.*, 1992)
though again there is some evidence of a bimodal distribution (Muller
et al., 1993). Therefore, it has been proposed that low levels are found in
digynic triploids and high levels in diandric triploids (Haig, 1993; Goshen,
1994). In trisomy 13, levels of hCG are normal (Crossley *et al.*, 1991), or
high (Muller *et al.*, 1993). High levels of hCG have also been reported in
cases of monoparental disomy of chromosome 16 (Vaughan *et al.*, 1994)
and in sex chromosome aneuploidies (Barnes-Kedar *et al.*, 1993) including
Turner's syndrome (Wenstrom *et al.*, 1994).

Conclusions

Measurement of hCG, whether of the intact molecule or the free β-subunit, is the single best marker of Down's syndrome pregnancy. There are few confounding factors, though both high and low levels may be found in association with other complications of pregnancy. Measurement of the free β-subunit is probably superior in predictive efficiency to that of the dimer though not all workers agree with this (e.g. Milunsky *et al.*, 1993). There are also residual concerns about the stability of these molecules which need to be addressed in the design of a screening programme.

References

Aitken, D.A., McCaw, G., Crossley, J.A. *et al.* (1993). First trimester biochemical screening for fetal chromosome abnormalities and neural tube defects. *Prenatal Diagn.*, **13**, 681–9.

Bahl, O.P., Carlson, R.B., Bellisario, R. & Swaminathan, N. (1972). Human chorionic gonadotropin amino acid sequence of the alpha and beta subunits. *Biochem. Biophys. Res. Commun.*, **48**, 416–22.

Barnes-Kedar, A., Amiel, A., Maor, O. & Fejgin, M. (1993). Elevated human chorionic gonadotropin levels in pregnancies with sex chromosome abnormalities. *Am. J. Med. Genet.*, **45**, 356–7.

Bartels, I., Hoppe-Sievert, B., Bockel, B., Herold, S. & Caesar, J. (1993). Adjustment formulae for maternal serum alpha-fetoprotein, human chorionic gonadotropin, and unconjugated oestriol to maternal weight and smoking. *Prenatal Diagn.*, **13**, 123–30.

Bernstein, L., Pike, M.C., Lobo, R.A., Depue, R.H., Ross, R.K. & Henderson, B.E. (1989). Cigarette smoking in pregnancy results in marked decrease in maternal hCG and oestradiol levels. *Br. J. Obstet. Gynaecol.*, **96**, 92–6.

Bewley, S., Chard, T., Grudzinskas, G., Cooper, D. & Campbell, S. (1992). Early prediction of uteroplacental complications of pregnancy using Doppler ultrasound, placental function tests and combination testing. *Ultrasound Obstet. Gynaecol.*, **2**, 333–7.

Bo, M. & Boime, I. (1992). Identification of the transcriptionally active genes of the chorionic gonadotropin β gene in vivo. *J. Biol. Chem.*, **267**, 3179–84.

Bogart, M.H., Panadian, M.R. & Jones, O.W. (1987). Abnormal maternal serum chorionic gonadotropin levels in pregnancies with fetal chromosome abnormalities. *Prenatal Diagn.*, **7**, 623–30.

Bogart, M.H., Jones, O.W., Felder, R.A. *et al.* (1991). Prospective evaluation of maternal serum human chorionic gonadotropin levels in 3428 pregnancies. *Am. J. Obstet. Gynecol.*, **165**, 663–7.

Boothby, M., Kukowska, J. & Boime, I. (1983). Imbalanced synthesis of human choriogonadotropin alpha and beta subunits reflects the steady state levels of the corresponding mRNAs. *J. Biol. Chem.*, **258**, 9250–3.

Brock, D.J., Barron, L., Holloway, S., Liston, W.A., Hillier, S.G. & Seppala, M. (1990). First trimester maternal serum biochemical indicators in Down syndrome. *Prenatal Diagn.*, **10**, 245–51.

Chard, T., Lowings, C. & Kitau, M.J. (1984). Alphafetoprotein and chorionic gonadotropin levels in relation to Downs syndrome. *Lancet*, **ii**, 750.

Clements, J.A., Reyes, F.I., Winter, J.S.D. & Faiman, C. (1976). Studies on human sexual development. III. Fetal pituitary and serum and amniotic fluid concentrations of LH, CG and FSH. *J. Endocrinol. Metab.*, **42**, 9–19.

Cole, L.A., Kroll, T.G., Ruddon, R.W. & Hussa, R.O. (1984). Differential occurrence of free beta and free alpha subunits of human chorionic gonadotropin (hCG) in pregnancy sera. *J. Clin. Endocrinol. Metab.*, **58**, 1200–2.

Crandall, B.F., Hanson, F.W., Keener, M.S., Matsumoto, B.S. & Miller, W. (1993). Maternal serum screening for alpha-fetoprotein, unconjugated estriol, and human chorionic gonadotropin between 11 and 15 weeks of pregnancy to detect fetal chromosome abnormalities. *Am. J. Obstet. Gynecol.*, **168**, 1864–9.

Crossley, J.A., Aitken, D.A. & Connor, J.M. (1991). Prenatal screening for chromosome abnormalities using maternal serum chorionic gonadotrophin, alpha fetoprotein, and age. *Prenatal Diagn.*, **11**, 83–101.

Cuckle, H.S., Wald, N.J., Densem, P. *et al.* (1990). The effect of smoking in pregnancy on maternal serum alpha-fetoprotein, unconjugated oestriol, human chorionic gonadotrophin, progesterone and dehydroepiandrosterone sulphate levels. *Br. J. Obstet. Gynaecol.*, **97**, 272–6.

Ellis, A.R. (1993). Antenatal screening for Down's syndrome – can we do better? *Ann. Clin. Biochem.*, **30**, 421–4.

Gau, G., Rice, A. & Chard, T. (1984). Increase of hCG levels following heating of serum. *J. Obstet. Gynaecol.*, **5**, 21–3.

Gibbons, J.M., Mitnick, M. & Chieffo, V. (1975). In vitro biosynthesis of TSH- and LH-releasing factors by the human placenta. *Am. J. Obstet. Gynecol.*, **121**, 127–33.

Goshen, R. (1994). The genomic basis of the beta-subunit of human chorionic gonadotropin diversity in triploidy. *Am. J. Obstet. Gynecol.*, **170**, 700.

Graham, M.Y., Otani, T., Boime, I., Olson, M.V., Carle, G.F. & Chapline, D.D. (1987). Cosmid mapping of the human chorionic gonadotrophin beta-subunit genes by field-inversion gel electrophoresis. *Nucl. Acids Res.*, **15**, 4437–48.

Haig, D. (1993). Genomic imprinting, human chorionic gonadotropin, and triploidy. *Prenatal Diagn.*, **13**, 151.

Herrou, M., Leporrier, N. & Leymarie, P. (1992). Screening for fetal Down syndrome with maternal serum hCG and oestriol: a prospective study. *Prenatal Diagn.*, **12**, 887–92.

Houghton, D.J., Newnham, J.P., Lo, K., Rice, A. & Chard, T. (1982). Circadian variation of circulating levels of four placental proteins. *Br. J. Obstet. Gynaecol.*, **89**, 831–5.

Hussa, R.O. (1981). Human chorionic gonadotropin, a clinical marker: review of its biosynthesis. *Ligand Rev.*, **3**, 6–43.

Iles, R.K. & Chard, T. (1989). Enhancement of ectopic beta-human chorionic gonadotrophin expression by interferon. *J. Endocrinol.*, **123**, 501–7.

Iles, R.K., Wathen, N.C., Campbell, D.J. & Chard, T. (1992). Human chorionic gonadotrophin and subunit composition of maternal serum and coelomic and amniotic fluids in the first trimester of pregnancy. *J. Endocrinol.*, **135**, 563–9.

Kim, S.J., Nam Koong, S.E., Lee, J.W., Jung, J.K., Kang, B.C. & Park, J.S.

(1987). Response of human chorionic gonadotrophin to luteinising hormone-releasing hormone stimulation in the culture media of normal human placenta, choriocarcinoma cell lines and in the serum of patients with gestational trophoblastic disease. *Placenta*, **8**, 257–64.

Kohn, G., Zamir, R., Zer, T., Amiel, A. & Fejgin, M. (1991). Significance of very low maternal serum human chorionic gonadotropin in prenatal diagnosis of Triploidy. *Prenatal Diagn.*, **11**, 277.

Kulch, P., Keener, S., Matsumoto, M. & Crandall, B.F. (1993). Racial differences in maternal serum human chorionic gonadotropin and unconjugated oestriol levels. *Prenatal Diagn.*, **13**, 191–5.

Kurman, R.J., Young, R.H., Norris, H.J., Main, C.S., Lawrence, W.D. & Scully, R.E. (1984). Immunocytochemical localisation of placental lactogen and chorionic gonadotropin in the normal placenta and trophoblast tumours, with emphasis on intermediate trophoblast and the placental site trophoblastic tumour. *Int. J. Gynecol. Pathol.*, **3**, 101–21.

Lee, J.N., Seppala, M. & Chard, T. (1981). Characterization of placental luteinizing hormone releasing factor-like material. *Acta Endocrinol.*, **96**, 394–7.

Leporrier, N., Herrou, M. & Leymarie, P. (1992). Shift of the fetal sex ratio in hCG selected pregnancies at risk for Down syndrome. *Prenatal Diagn.*, **12**, 703–4.

Lieppman, R.E., Williams, M.A., Cheng, E.Y. *et al.* (1993). An association between elevated levels of human chorionic gonadotropin in the midtrimester and adverse pregnancy outcome. *Am. J. Obstet. Gynecol.*, **168**, 1852–7.

Mancini, G., Perono, M., Dall'Amico, D. *et al.*, (1991). Screening for fetal Down's syndrome with maternal serum markers – an experience in Italy. *Prenatal Diagn.*, **11**, 345–52.

Mason, G., Linton, G., Cuckle, H. & Holding, S. (1992). Low maternal serum human chorionic gonadotrophin and unconjugated oestriol in a triploidy pregnancy. *Prenatal Diagn.*, **12**, 545–47.

Mason, G., Lindow, S., Ramsden, C., Cuckle, H. & Holding, S. (1993). Low maternal serum oestriol and chorionic gonadotropin in the prediction of adverse pregnancy outcome. *Prenatal Diagn.*, **13**, 223–5.

Merkatz, J.R., Nitowsky, H.M., Macri, J.N. & Johnson, W.E. (1984). An association between low maternal serum alpha-fetoprotein and fetal chromosomal abnormalities. *Am. J. Obstet. Gynecol.*, **14**, 886–94.

Milunsky, A., Nebiolo, L.M. & Bellet, D. (1993). Maternal serum screening for chromosome defects: human chorionic gonadotropin versus its free-beta subunit. *Fetal Diagn. Ther.*, **8**, 221.

Morgan, F.J., Birken, S. & Canfield, R.E. (1975). The amino acid sequence of human chorionic gonadotropin. The alpha subunit and beta subunit. *J. Biol. Chem.*, **250**, 5247–58.

Muller, F. & Boue, A. (1990). A single chorionic gonadotropin assay for maternal screening for Down's syndrome. *Prenatal Diagn.*, **10**, 389–98.

Muller, F. Aegertier, P. & Boue, A. (1993). Prospective maternal serum human chorionic gonadotropin screening for the risk of fetal chromosome anomalies and of subsequent fetal and neonatal deaths. *Prenatal Diagn.*, **13**, 29–43.

Nagy, A.M., Glinoer, D., Picelli, G. *et al.* (1994). Total amounts of circulating human chorionic gonadotrophin alpha and beta subunits can be assessed throughout human pregnancy using immunoradiometric assays calibrated with the unaltered and thermally dissociated heterodimer. *J. Endocrinol.,* **140**, 513.

Nørgaard-Pedersen, B., Larsen, S.O., Arends, J., Svenstrup, B. & Tabor, A. (1990). Maternal serum markers in screening for Down syndrome. *Clin. Genet.,* **37**, 35–43.

Obiekwe, B.C. & Chard, T. (1982). Human chorionic gonadotrophin levels in maternal blood in late pregnancy: relation to birthweight, sex and condition of the infant at birth. *Br. J. Obstet Gynaecol.,* **89**, 543–6.

Osathanondh, R., Canick, J.A., Abell, K.B. *et al.* (1989). Second trimester screening for trisomy 21. *Lancet,* **ii**, 52.

Palomaki, G.E., Knight, G.J., Haddow, J.E., Canick, J.A., Saller, D.N. & Panizza, D.S. (1992). Prospective intervention trial of a screening protocol to identify fetal trisomy 18 using maternal serum alpha-fetoprotein, unconjugated oestriol, and human chorionic gonadotropin. *Prenatal Diagn.,* **19**, 925–30.

Palomaki, G.E., Knight, G.J. & Haddow, J.E. (1994). Human chorionic gonadotropin and unconjugated oestriol measurements in insulin-dependent diabetic pregnant women being screened for fetal Down syndrome pregnancy. *Prenatal Diagn.,* **14**, 65.

Perez Lopez, L.R., Robert, J. & Teigeiro, J. (1984). Prl, TSH, FSH, beta-hCG and oestriol response to repetitive (triple) LRH/TRH administration in the third trimester of human pregnancy. *Acta Endocrinol.,* **106**, 400–4.

Petrocik, E., Wassman, E.R. & Kelly, J.C. (1989). Prenatal screening for Down syndrome with maternal serum human chorionic gonadotropin levels. *Am. J. Obstet. Gynecol.,* **161**, 1168–73.

Phillips, O.P., Elias, S., Shulman, L.P., Anderson, R.N., Morgan, C.D. & Leigh Simpson, J. (1992). Maternal serum screening for fetal Down syndrome in women less than 35 years of age using alpha-fetoprotein, hCG, and unconjugated estriol: a prospective 2-year study. *Obstet. Gynecol.,* **80**, 353–8.

Ryall, R.G., Staples, A.J., Robertson, E.F. & Pollard, A.C. (1992). Improved performance in a prenatal screening programme for Down's syndrome incorporating serum-free hCG subunit analyses. *Prenatal Diagn.,* **12**, 251–61.

Salem, H.T., Ghaneimah, S.A., Shaaban, M.M. & Chard, T. (1984). Prognostic value of biochemical tests in the assessment of fetal outcome in threatened abortion. *Br. J. Obstet. Gynaecol.,* **91**, 382–85.

Simpson, J.L., Elias, S., Morgan, C.D., Shulman, L., Umstot, E. & Anderson, R.N. (1990). Second trimester maternal serum human chorionic gonadotrophin and unconjugated oestriol levels in blacks and whites. *Lancet,* **335**, 1459–60.

Spencer, K., Coombes, E.J., Mallard, A.S. & Milford Ward, A. (1992). Free beta human choriogonadotropin in Down's syndrome screening: a multicentre study of its role compared with other biochemical markers. *Ann. Clin. Biochem.,* **29**, 506–18.

Spencer, K., Macri, J.N., Carpenter, P., Anderson, R. & Krantz, D.A. (1993). Stability of intact chorionic gonadotropin (hCG) in serum, liquid whole blood and dried whole blood filter paper spots: impact on screening for Down syndrome by measurement of free beta-hCG subunit. *Clin. Chem.,* **39**, 1064–8.

Stevenson, H.P., Leslie, H. & Sheridan, B. (1993). Serum free beta-human chorionic gonadotropin concentrations increase in unseparated blood specimens. *Ann. Clin. Biochem.*, **30**, 99–100.

Strickland, T.W. & Puett, D. (1981). Contribution of subunits to the function of luteinizing hormone/human chorionic gonadotropin recombinants. *Endocrinology*, **109**, 1933–42.

Suchy, S.F. & Yeager, M.T. (1990). Down syndrome screening in women under 35 with maternal serum hCG. *Obstet. Gynecol.*, **76**, 20–4.

Talmadge, K., Boorstein, W.R., Vamvakopoulos, N.C., Gething, M.J. & Fiddes, J.C. (1984). Only three of the seven human chorionic gonadotrophin β-subunit genes can be expressed in the placenta. *Nucl. Acids Res.*, **12**, 8415–36.

Tanaka, M., Natori, M., Kohno, H., Ishimoto, H., Kobayashi, T. & Nozawa, S. (1993). Fetal growth in patients with elevated maternal serum hCG levels. *Obstet. Gynecol.*, **81**, 341–3.

van Lith, J.M. (1992). First trimester maternal serum human chorionic gonadotrophin as a marker for fetal chromosomal disorders. The Dutch Working Party on Prenatal Diagnosis. *Prenatal Diagn.*, **12**, 495–504.

Wald, N.J., Cuckle, H.S., Densem, J.W. et al. (1988). Maternal serum screening for Down's syndrome in early pregnancy. *Br. Med. J.*, **297**, 883–7.

Wald, N.J., Cuckle, H.S., Densem, J.W. & Stone, R.B. (1992a). Maternal serum unconjugated oestriol and human chorionic gonadotrophin levels in pregnancies with insulin-dependent diabetes: implications for screening for Down's syndrome. *Br. J. Obstet. Gynaecol.*, **99**, 51–3.

Wald, N.J., Kennard, A., Densem, J.W., Cuckle, H.S., Chard, T. & Butler, L. (1992b). Antenatal maternal serum screening for Down's syndrome: results of a demonstration project. *Br. Med. J.*, **305**, 391–4.

Wehman, R.E. & Nisula, B.C. (1980). Characterization of a discrete degradation product of human chorionic gonadotropin β-subunit in humans. *J. Endocrinol.*, **51**, 101–5.

Wehman, R.E., Amer, S., Rosa, C. & Nisula, B.C. (1984). Metabolism, distribution and excretion of purified human chorionic gonadotropin and its subunits in man. *Ann. Endocrinol.*, **45**, 291–5.

Wehman, R.E., Blithe, D.L., Akar, A.H. & Nisula, B.C. (1990). Disparity between β-core levels in pregnancy urine and serum: implications for the origin of urinary β-core. *J. Clin. Endocrinol. Metab.*, **70**, 371–8.

Wenstrom, K.D., Williamson, R.A. & Grant, S.S. (1994). Detection of Turner syndrome with multiple-marker screening. *Am. J. Obstet. Gynecol.*, **170**, 570.

Word, R.A., George, F.W., Wilson, J.D. & Carr, B.R. (1989). Testosterone synthesis and adenylate cyclase activity in the early human fetal testis appear to be independent of human chorionic gonadotropin control. *J. Clin. Endocrinol. Metab.*, **69**, 204–8.

Vaughan, J., Ali, Z., Bower, S., Bennett, P., Chard, T. & Moore, G. (1994). Human maternal uniparental disomy for chromosome 16 and Fetal development, in press.

6

The measurement of hCG subunits in screening for Down's syndrome

K. SPENCER

Human chorionic gonadotrophin (hCG) is a 39.5 kDa dimeric glycoprotein composed of two non-identical subunits: the α-subunit (15 kDa) and the β-subunit (23 kDa). The α-subunit is composed of 92 amino acid residues and is virtually identical to that of the other pituitary glycoprotein hormones LH, FSH and TSH. The β-subunits on the other hand are hormone specific and it is this that confers specific biological activity when the two subunits (α and β) are non-covalently linked together. Much of the details of the synthesis, secretion and control of hCG production is poorly understood. Only one gene is known to code for the α-subunit (located on chromosome 6) and this is expressed within the placenta and the pituitary, whilst at least six (possibly seven) genes are known to code for the β-subunit (all clustered on chromosome 19). Of the β genes, only two are transcribed and expressed in the placenta. Control of secretion of β-subunits is thought to be the rate-limiting step to the production of intact hCG and this is influenced in a positive way by cyclic AMP, insulin, calcium, interleukin-1, fibroblast growth factor, placental-derived gonadotrophin-releasing hormone and epidermal growth factor. Inhibitory influences include prolactin, progesterone and inhibin (Ren and Braunstein, 1992).

Following the identification by Merkatz et al. (1984) of an association between low levels of maternal serum α-fetoprotein (AFP) and pregnancies affected by fetal chromosomal abnormalities, Chard et al. (1984) suggested that levels of other fetal placental markers (particularly hCG) might be abnormal in Down's syndrome pregnancies. It was three years later however that Bogart et al. (1987) showed that maternal serum levels of total hCG were elevated in Down's syndrome pregnancies and that in some cases α-hCG was also increased. Confirmation of Bogart's findings and the incorporation of AFP and total hCG measurements with measurements of maternal serum unconjugated oestriol (uE_3), by Wald *et al.* (1988), led to a proposed screening programme for Down's syndrome for which it was predicted that detection rates of 60% could be achieved at a false-positive rate of 5%.

More recently, studies looking specifically at the free subunits of hCG (Macri *et al.*, 1990; Spencer, 1991; Spencer and Macri, 1992; Ryall *et al.*, 1992; Spencer *et al.*, 1992a, 1993a) have indicated that the specific measurement of these free subunits may offer a further improvement in Down's syndrome detection rate both in the second trimester and the first trimester (Spencer *et al.*, 1992b; Aitken *et al.*, 1993b; Macri *et al.*, 1993b).

Free α-hCG

The early studies of Bogart *et al.* (1987, 1989) identified a possible role for free α-hCG in maternal serum in the detection of pregnancies at risk of fetal chromosomal anomalies. In both studies, Bogart found median levels of free α-hCG in second trimester pregnancies complicated by fetal Down's syndrome to be approximately twice that of unaffected pregnancies. Using a cut-off of 2.0 Multiples of the median (MoM), Bogart *et al.* (1987) claimed an 88% detection rate for Down's syndrome with a 6.8% false-positive rate. It is surprising, therefore, that Bogart's subsequent study concentrated on the measurement of total hCG alone (Bogart *et al.*, 1991).

Bogart *et al.* (1989) demonstrated that neither intact hCG nor free α-hCG levels in the first trimester were useful for the detection of Down's syndrome pregnancies. Ozturk *et al.* (1990), on the other hand, have shown that free β-free α-hCG ratios are low in the first trimester of trisomy 18 cases and yet are normal in cases of trisomy 21. Data from Kratzner *et al.* (1991) indicate that free α-hCG levels are lower in first trimester cases of Down's syndrome and confirm that in the second trimester its median levels in Down's syndrome were twice that of controls. Ryall *et al.* (1992) have also shown that, in the second trimester, levels of free α-subunits are higher in Down's syndrome, with a median level of 1.39 MoM. However our own studies (Spencer, 1993a) using a commercial free α-glycoprotein subunit assay have been unable to confirm the elevation of free α-subunits in the second trimester in 36 cases of Down's syndrome (median MoM = 0.99). Furthermore, our unpublished study of 48 cases of Down's syndrome, using the Bioclone assay as employed by Ryall *et al.* (1992), has confirmed that free α-hCG levels in Down's syndrome pregnancies are not significantly elevated (median MoM = 1.15).

These data suggest that a case for the use of free α-hCG subunits in screening for Down's syndrome has not yet been made.

Free β-hCG

Second trimester retrospective studies

In recent years two groups independently showed that free β-hCG levels in maternal serum are elevated in Down's syndrome pregnancies (Macri *et al.*, 1990; Spencer, 1991). This has subsequently been confirmed by Crossley *et al.* (1991) and Ryall *et al.* (1992). Macri's study showed that free β-subunits combined with AFP measurement and maternal age yielded an overall detection rate of 72.4% at a 5% false-positive rate. He also noted an increased detection rate at 14–16 weeks of gestation compared with cases later in gestation. Spencer (1991) was the first to show directly the advantage of measuring free β-hCG rather than total hCG; his study found a 66% detection rate using free β-hCG compared with only 52% using total hCG. Because of the small number of Down's cases in the study (29) this difference was not statistically significant.

A further study, looking at a group of Down's cases in the 16th week of gestation compared with a group in the 17th week (Spencer and Macri, 1992), confirmed that higher detection rates were achieved earlier in gestation, largely as a result of the higher median MoM free β-hCG found in pregnancies in early gestation (2.32 compared with 2.045). However, the difference in detection rates between the 16th (78%) and 17th week (57%) was not statistically significant because of the small number of cases studied.

A large multicentre study by Spencer *et al.* (1992a) comprising 90 Down's cases and 2862 controls is perhaps the most definitive study with respect to the use of maternal serum markers in biochemical screening for Down's syndrome. This study showed that the median free β-hCG in cases of Down's syndrome was 2.41, compared with 2.03 for total hCG, 0.70 for AFP and 0.74 for uE$_3$. The study showed that free β-hCG was the marker with the best discriminatory power (Fig. 6.1). When analytes were combined with maternal age, the best results were achieved using a combination of AFP and free β-hCG, with a detection rate of 66% at a 5.9% false-positive rate. When total hCG was used, a detection rate of 55.3% was achieved at the same false-positive rate. This difference was statistically significant. The improvement in detection using free β-hCG has been supported by Cuckle and Lilford (1992) who used mathematical modelling techniques to show that the population parameters from the

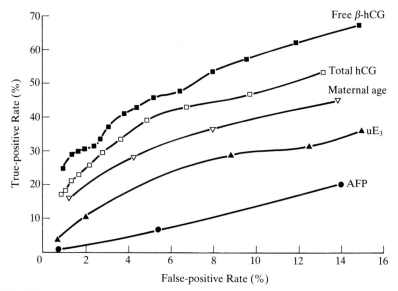

Fig. 6.1. Receiver Operator Characteristic curves depicting variation of false-positive rate with true-positive rate for markers of Down's syndrome analysed independently. (Spencer *et al.*, 1992a, reproduced with permission.)

Spencer *et al.* (1992a) study could indeed lead to an 8 to 10% improvement in detection rate. The study by Spencer *et al.* (1992a) also showed that inclusion of uE_3 did not improve screening performance (Fig. 6.2) (see Chapter 9). In analysing the data by gestational age band we were able to confirm that detection rates in the 14–16 week gestational band were greater than those in the 17–21 week band (77% versus 54%); this difference was statistically significant. We have subsequently shown (Spencer *et al.*, 1993d) that since the maternal age and median AFP of the two groups were very similar, the additional detection rate achieved in the early gestation group was largely as a result of the higher median free β-hCG MoM in this group (2.52 versus 2.32). Spencer *et al.* (1992a) also showed that, in women under 30 years the free β-hCG protocol detected more than twice as many cases of Down's syndrome than the total hCG protocol.

In an editorial to the original paper by Spencer (1991), Knight and Cole (1991) felt that a case for free β-hCG measurement could not be justified for three reasons.

(1) The difference between total hCG and free β-hCG detection rates was not statistically significant.

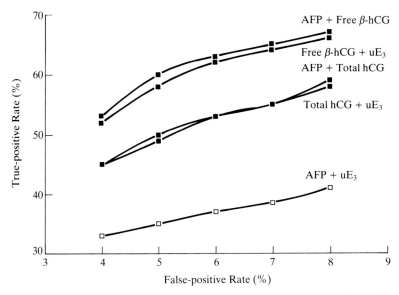

Fig. 6.2. Receiver Operator Characteristic curves depicting the variation of false-positive rate with true-positive rate for various combinations of biochemical markers of Down's syndrome analysed multivariately with maternal age. (Spencer *et al.*, 1992a, reproduced with permission.)

(2) Free β-hCG may be an unstable molecule and the concentration increases when samples are left at room temperature for more than 30 minutes.

(3) Great care would be needed in interpreting data from different assays because of different specificity.

The data from our recent large study (Spencer *et al.*, 1992a) has shown that the difference between total hCG and free β-hCG is statistically significant; this answers the first criticism of Knight and Cole. We have also shown (Spencer *et al.*, 1993b) that free β-hCG is stable for 70 hours at 20°C and for 35 hours as liquid whole blood; stability of filter paper blood spots can be assured for at least 7 days at 37°C. Furthermore, both the Macri assay (Macri *et al.*, 1993a) and the CIS assay used by our group, show insignificant cross-reactivity with intact hCG. The assays are highly comparable (Spencer and Macri, 1992; Spencer *et al.*, 1993a) and the CIS assay which uses the FBT11 monoclonal capture antibody should also measure the 'nicked' and 'non-nicked' forms of free β-hCG (Kardana and Cole, 1992).

A novel assay for the simultaneous measurement of AFP and free β-hCG has been developed (Macri *et al.*, 1992) and a six-centre UK trial of this assay has recently been published (Spencer *et al.*, 1993a). This included 168 Down's cases, 1457 controls, 66 cases of open spina bifida and 54 cases of anencephaly; the median AFP in the Down's group was 0.80 MoM and the median free β-hCG was 2.52 MoM. Detection rates for anencephaly and open spina bifida were similar to those in the combined UK Collaborative Study (1977). The study confirmed that detection rates for Down's syndrome were enhanced in earlier gestation with detection rates in the 14–16 week group being 70.6% compared with 54.2% at the later periods. False-positive rates in these two groups were also unchanged and the increased detection was due to the higher median free β-subunit MoM in the earlier gestational period (2.71 MoM compared with 2.30 MoM). Detection rates by maternal age band were also similar to those reported in our earlier study (Spencer *et al.*, 1992a), with detection rates of 52.4% even in the 20 to 24 year age group (2.3% false-positive rate). Our groups have now accumulated data on more than 480 cases of Down's syndrome; the median MoM shows a significantly higher median (2.64 MoM) than that from a similar sized meta analysis of 559 cases using total hCG (2.05 MoM) (Wald and Cuckle, 1992).

Wald and Hackshaw (1993) have recently suggested that the potential benefits to the use of free β-hCG may not be achievable. They argue, with no substantiating data, that there is a significant deviation from linearity in the distribution of the probability density function of log free β-hCG MoM. Wald and Hackshaw's comments are at variance with our published data from the combined observations from six centres participating in the clinical trial of the Dual Analyte assay (Spencer *et al.*, 1993a), our own routine experience (Spencer, 1993b), experience in two other UK screening centres (Spencer *et al.*, 1993d) and preliminary data from Cuckle and Lilford (1993). As Fig. 6.3 clearly shows, no such deviation exists in either the unaffected or the affected populations; indeed it may be argued that free β-hCG follows Gaussian linearity more closely than does total hCG.

Prospective screening experiences

As pointed out by Cuckle and Lilford (1993), the relative merits of using free β-hCG versus intact or total hCG will ultimately be determined by large prospective studies. We have been screening prospectively using our AFP and free β-hCG protocol since April 1991. In the year to 31 March

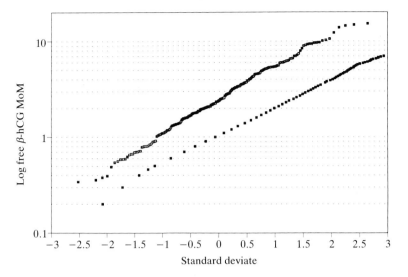

Fig. 6.3. The probability density distribution function of log free β-hCG (MoM) in cases of Down's syndrome (upper curve, $n = 246$) and in unaffected (lower curve, $n = 6557$) cases. (Spencer, 1993b, reproduced with permission.)

1992, we screened a total of 8317 pregnancies of which 8179 were singleton pregnancies. Our screening population is largely Caucasian (80%) with 10% of the population being Asian and only 3% of Afro/Caribbean origin. The median age of the population was 28 years with 10.6% of the population being 35 years or older. Gestational dating in our patients was by last menstrual period (LMP) in 57.5%, by ultrasound-confirmed LMP dates in 21.6% and dating by ultrasound in 20.9%. Weight correction was applied to AFP in 91% of the cases in which maternal weight information was available (median weight 64.0 kg), no correction was made to free β-hCG during this period. Assuming a birth incidence of 1.3 per thousand and allowing for a 25% fetal loss rate in Down's syndrome between the second and third trimester, in our population of 8179 pregnancies we would expect to observe 13.3 cases of Down's syndrome. By following outcome through our cytogenetic services, maternity services and birth outcome records we have ascertained 16 cases of Down's syndrome. Of these 16 cases, 12 (75%) were initially identified by the screening programme. In order to detect these cases, 6.8% of women had results identified as 'at increased risk'; after ultrasound revision of gestational dates this was reduced to 5.1%. This ultrasound revision of gestational dates also resulted in 1 case of Down's syndrome being re-classified as 'not at increased risk', leaving a final detection rate of 69%. Of the 5.1% of women identified as 'at increased risk', 89% accepted an offer of amniocentesis. Only 1 case of fetal loss within 28 days of the amniocentesis was identified (0.23%). Additionally the screening programme identified cases of Turner's syndrome (Laundon *et al.*, 1993), renal agenesis, hydronephrosis and cases of fetal death or impending fetal demise (Spencer and Carpenter, 1993).

In the screening period 1 April 1992 to 31 March 1993, for which preliminary data are available, the population screened was 8091 singleton pregnancies. We have ascertained 10 cases of Down's syndrome in the 5344 pregnancies that have gone to completion. Of these 10 cases we have identified 8 (80%), with 4.9% of pregnancies being identified as 'at increased risk' after gestational date revision.

The impact of free β-hCG screening in our Health District is best looked at in terms of the proportion of Down's syndrome cases avoided per year over the past decade (Fig. 6.4). At best, our experience using maternal age only (≥ 37) averaged a 10% avoidance; with AFP and maternal age this rose to just over 30%; but with free β-hCG, AFP and maternal age this has risen to 70%. Similar experience in other centres is summarised in Table 6.1 (Spencer *et al.*, 1993c).

First trimester screening

A small number of studies have reported on the measurement of biochemical markers in the first trimester of pregnancies affected by Down's syndrome. These studies have mainly been from samples collected from women prior to chorionic villus sampling (CVS) and as such they represent a pre-selected population. In such studies (Cuckle *et al.*, 1988; Brock *et al.*, 1990; Nebiolo *et al.*, 1990; Crandall *et al.*, 1991; Johnson *et al.*, 1991; Kratzner *et al.*, 1991; van Lith, 1992) AFP and uE$_3$ values have been shown to be low in cases of Down's syndrome (approximately 0.7 MoM), whilst studies with total hCG have shown this marker to be largely unaltered in first trimester Down's samples.

As a result of the foresight of our colleagues at the Duncan Guthrie Institute of Medical Genetics in Glasgow, we have had the opportunity to study biochemical markers in a unique set of first trimester samples collected from an unselected pregnant population. Consecutive maternal serum samples were collected between 6 and 14 weeks of gestation from 14 000 women attending antenatal clinics between January 1987 and April 1990 in the West of Scotland. Serum samples from these women were

β-hCG and AFP and cut-off criteria in both trimesters which would generate a 5% false-positive rate, we have demonstrated (Fig. 6.7) that the same cases would be identified in the first trimester as would have been identified using this protocol in the second trimester. Although these data are based on a small number of cases, it seems likely that the same case can be detected at a much earlier time window (8–12 weeks) than that used currently. PAPP-A or Schwangerschafts protein (SP1) which also show lower values in first trimester trisomies and normal or only marginally elevated values in second trimester trisomies, are unlikely to offer the same benefits as free β-hCG which is equally effective from 8 to 22 weeks of gestation (Aitken *et al.*, 1993a).

Conclusions

There is now a firm body of evidence that free β-hCG has better detection efficiency than total hCG and that this applies earlier in the second trimester (14–16 weeks). This earlier screening opportunity has obvious benefits for counselling, amniocentesis and the delays in obtaining results of karyotyping. Even taking the wider screening period of 14 to 22 weeks, detection efficiencies of 70% or greater are now being demonstrated using free β-hCG in prospective studies using two rather than three analytes. Finally we have demonstrated that free β-hCG and AFP can be used in the first trimester and this eventually may lead to screening programmes at this time.

References

Aitken, D.A., McKinnon, D., Crossley, J.A. *et al.* (1993a). Changes in the maternal serum concentrations of PAPP-A and SP-1 in Down's syndrome pregnancies between the first and second trimesters. In *Proceedings of the ACB National Meeting*, 1993, ed. S.M. Martin, S.P. Halloran & A.J.E. Green, p. 72. London: Association of Clinical Biochemists.

Aitken, D.A., McCaw, G., Crossley, J.A. *et al.* (1993b). First trimester biochemical screening for fetal chromosome abnormalities and neural tube defects. *Prenatal Diagn.*, **13**, 681–9.

Bogart, M.H., Pandian, M.R. & Jones, O.W. (1987). Abnormal maternal serum chorionic gonadotropin levels in pregnancies with fetal chromosome abnormalities. *Prenatal Diagn.*, **7**, 623–30.

Bogart, M.H., Globus, M.S., Sorg, N.D. & Jones, O.W. (1989). Human chorionic gonadotropin levels in pregnancies with aneuploid fetuses. *Prenatal Diagn.*, **9**, 379–84.

Bogart, M.H., Jones, O.W., Felder, R.A. *et al.* (1991). Prospective evaluation of maternal serum human chorionic gonadotropin levels in 3428 pregnancies. *Am. J. Obstet. Gynecol.*, **165**, 663–7.

Brambati, B., Lazani, A. & Tului, L. (1991). Ultrasound and biochemical assessment of first trimester pregnancy. In *The Embryo: Normal and Abnormal Development and Growth.* ed. M. Chapman, J.G. Grudzinskas & T. Chard, pp. 181–94. Berlin: Springer-Verlag.

Brambati, B., Macintosh, M.C.M., Teisner, B. *et al.* (1993). Low maternal serum levels of pregnancy associated plasma protein A (PAPP-A) in the first trimester in association with abnormal fetal karyotype. *Br. J. Obstet. Gynaecol.,* **100**, 324–6.

Brock, D.J.H., Barron, L., Holloway, S., Liston, W.A., Hillier, S.G. & Seppala, M. (1990). First trimester maternal serum biochemical indicators in Down's syndrome. *Prenatal Diagn.,* **10**, 242–51.

Chard, T., Lowings, C. & Kitau, M.J. (1984). Alpha fetoprotein and chorionic gonadotropin levels in relation to Down syndrome. *Lancet,* **ii**, 750.

Crandall, B.F., Golbus, M.S., Goldberg, J.D. & Matsumoto, M. (1991). First trimester maternal serum unconjugated oestriol and alpha fetoprotein in fetal Down's syndrome. *Prenatal Diagn.,* **11**, 377–80.

Crossley, J.A., Aitken, D.A. & Connor, J.M. (1991). Free beta hCG and prenatal screening for chromosome abnormalities. *J. Med. Genet.* **28**, 570.

Cuckle, H. & Lilford, R. (1992). Antenatal screening for Down's syndrome. *Br. Med. J.,* **305**, 1017.

Cuckle, H. & Lilford, R. (1993). Antenatal screening for Down's syndrome. *Br. Med. J.,* **306**, 1199.

Cuckle, H.S., Wald, N.J., Barkai, G. *et al.* (1988). First trimester biochemical screening for Down syndrome. *Lancet,* **ii**, 851–2.

Johnson, A., Cowchock, F.S., Darby, M., Wapner, R. & Jackson, L.G. (1991). First trimester maternal serum alpha fetoprotein and chorionic gonadotropin in aneuploid pregnancies. *Prenatal Diagn.,* **11**, 443–50.

Kardana, A. & Cole, L.A. (1992). Polypeptide nicks cause erroneous results in assays of human chorionic gonadotropin free beta subunit. *Clin. Chem.,* **38**, 26–33.

Knight, G.J. & Cole, L.A. (1991). Measurement of choriogonadotropin free beta subunit: an alternative to choriogonadotropin in screening for fetal Down's syndrome. *Clin. Chem.* **37**, 779–82.

Kratzner, P.G., Globus, M.S., Monroe, S.E., Finkelstein, D.E. & Taylor, R.N. (1991). First trimester aneuploidy screening using serum human chorionic gonadotropin (hCG), free alpha hCG, and progesterone. *Prenatal Diagn.,* **11**, 751–65.

Laundon, C., Spencer, K., Macri, J.N. & Buchanan, P. (1993). Turner's syndrome detection by MSAFP/free Beta (hCG) screening. *J. Med. Genet.,* **30**, 340–1.

Macri, J.N., Kasturi, R.V., Krantz, D.A. *et al.* (1990). Maternal serum Down syndrome screening: free beta protein is a more effective marker than human chorionic gonadotropin. *Am. J. Obstet. Gynecol.,* **163**, 1248–53.

Macri, J.N., Spencer, K. & Anderson, R. (1992). Dual analyte immunoassay in neutral tube defect and Down's syndrome screening. *Ann. Clin. Biochem.* **29**, 390–6.

Macri, J.N., Spencer, K., Anderson, R., Cook, E.J. (1993a). Free beta chorionic gonadotropin: a cross reactivity study of two immunometric assays used in prenatal maternal serum screening for Down syndrome. *Ann. Clin. Biochem.,* **30**, 94–8.

Macri, J.N., Spencer, K., Aitken, D.A. *et al.* (1993b). First trimester free beta Down syndrome screening. *Prenatal Diagn.,* **13**, 557–62.

Merkatz, I.R., Nitowsky, H.M., Macri, J.N. & Johnson, W.E. (1984). An association between low maternal serum alpha fetoprotein and fetal chromosomal abnormalities. *Am. J. Obstet. Gynecol.*, **148**, 886–94.

Nebiolo, L., Ozturk, M., Brambati, B., Miller, S., Wands, J. & Milunsky, A. (1990). First trimester maternal serum alpha fetoprotein and human chorionic gonadotropin screening for chromosome defects. *Prenatal Diagn.*, **10**, 575–81.

Ozturk, M., Milunsky, A., Brambati, B., Sachs, E.S., Miller, S.L. & Wands, J.R. (1990). Abnormal maternal serum levels of human chorionic gonadotropin free subunits in trisomy 18. *Am. J. Med. Genet.*, **36**, 480–3.

Ren, S.G. & Braunstein, G.D. (1992). Human chorionic gonadotropin. *Semin. Reprod. Endocrinol.*, **10**, 95–105.

Ryall, R.G., Staples, A.J., Robertson, E.F. & Pollard, A.C. (1992). Improved performance in a prenatal screening programme for Down's syndrome incorporating serum free hCG subunit analysis. *Prenatal Diagn.*, **12**, 251–61.

Spencer, K. (1991). Evaluation of an assay of the free beta subunit of choriogonadotropin and its potential value in screening for Down's syndrome. *Clin. Chem.*, **37**, 809–14.

Spencer, K. (1993a). Free alpha hCG in Down's syndrome. *Am. J. Obstet. Gynecol.*, **165**, 132–5.

Spencer, K. (1993b). Screening for Down's syndrome. The role of intact hCG and free subunit measurement. *Scand. J. Clin. Lab. Invest.*, **53** (Suppl. 216), 79–96.

Spencer, K. & Macri, J.N. (1992). Early detection of Down's syndrome using free beta human choriogonadotropin. *Ann. Clin. Biochem.*, **29**, 349–50.

Spencer, K. & Carpenter, P. (1993). Prospective study of prenatal screening for Down's syndrome with free beta human chorionic gonadotrophin. *Br. Med. J.*, **307**, 764–8.

Spencer, K., Coombes, E.J., Mallard, A.S. & Milford Ward, A. (1992a). Free beta human choriogonadotropin in Down's syndrome screening: a multicentre study of its role compared with other biochemical markers. *Ann. Clin. Biochem.*, **29**, 506–18.

Spencer, K., Macri, J.N., Aitken, D.A. & Connor, J.M. (1992b). Free beta hCG as first trimester marker for fetal trisomy. *Lancet*, **339**, 1480.

Spencer, K., Macri, J.N., Anderson, R.V. et al. (1993a). Dual analyte immunoassay in neural tube defect and Down's syndrome screening: results of a multicentre clinical trial. *Ann. Clin. Biochem.*, **30**, 394–401.

Spencer, K., Macri, J.N., Carpenter, P., Anderson, R. & Krantz, D.A. (1993b). Intact hCG stability in serum, liquid whole blood and dried whole blood filter paper spots and its impact on free beta hCG Down's syndrome screening. *Clin. Chem.* **39**, 1064–8.

Spencer, K., Macri, J.N., Coombes, E.J. & Milford Ward, A. (1993c). Antenatal screening for Down's syndrome. *Br. Med. J.*, **306**, 1616.

Spencer, K., Coombes, E.J., Mallard, A.S. & Milford Ward, A. (1993d). Use of free beta hCG in Down's syndrome screening. *Ann. Clin. Biochem.*, **30**, 515–8.

Spencer, K., Aitkin, D.A., Macri, J.N., Anderson, R. & Connor, J.M. (1993e). PAPP-A as a marker of trisomy 21 in the first trimester. *Clin. Biochem. Rev.*, **14**, 284.

UK Collaborative Study (1977). Report of the UK Collaborative Study on alpha fetoprotein in relation to neural tube defects. Maternal serum alpha fetoprotein measurements in antenatal screening for anencephaly and spina bifida in early pregnancy. *Lancet*, **i**, 1323–32.

van Lith, J.M.M. (1992). First trimester maternal serum human chorionic gonadotrophin as a marker for fetal chromosomal disorders. *Prenatal Diagn.*, **12**, 495–504.

Wald, N.J. & Cuckle, H.S. (1992). Biochemical screening. In *Prenatal Screening and Diagnosis*. ed. D.J.H. Brock, C.H. Rodeck & M.A. Ferguson-Smith. Edinburgh: Churchill Livingstone.

Wald, N.J. & Hackshaw, A. (1993). Antenatal screening for Down's syndrome. *Br. Med. J.*, **306**, 1198–9.

Wald, N.J., Cuckle, H.S., Densem, J.W. *et al.* (1988). Maternal serum screening for Down's syndrome in early pregnancy. *Br. Med. J.*, **297**, 883–7.

Wald, N.J., Stone, R., Cuckle, H.S. *et al.* (1992). First trimester concentrations of pregnancy plasma protein A and placental protein 14 in Down's syndrome. *Br. Med. J.*, **305**, 28.

7

The measurement of free β-hCG in screening for Down's syndrome

J.N. MACRI

Introduction

Prior to April of 1984 (Merkatz *et al.*, 1984), the only means of assessing a woman's risk of having a child with Down's syndrome was to determine her age. At age 35 years or over mothers are at sufficient risk for chromosomal anomalies (primarily Down's syndrome) to warrant offering conventional genetic counseling followed by amniocentesis and fetal cell karyotyping. While this crude screening method is effective in older mothers, it will only detect some 20% of cases of Down's syndrome since the majority of such affected fetuses (approximately 80%) are born to younger mothers.

In 1983, in studying the association between maternal and fetal complications and low maternal serum α-fetoprotein (MSAFP), we observed a strong correlation between low MSAFP and ultimate fetal loss (Davenport and Macri, 1983). Any association between low MSAFP and fetal chromosomal malformations eluded this initial study because pregnancy outcome data were secured from delivery room records which were often deficient in their notation of Down's syndrome or other chromosomal anomalies. It was the chance finding of a below-sensitivity MSAFP in our screening of a mother carrying a fetus affected by Edward's syndrome (trisomy 18) which led to the recognition of the association between low MSAFP and chromosomal trisomy (Merkatz *et al.*, 1984). Following this initial observation, further work on larger data bases clearly demonstrated the association between low MSAFP and trisomy 21 (Macri, 1986). The implication of these results, namely being able to screen maternal serum of an unselected pregnant population to determine those at increased risk for Down's syndrome, was indeed an exciting prospect. In early work, however, it was recognized that detection efficiency for Down's syndrome within the framework of a maternal serum screening protocol using low MSAFP would be mediocre at best. Estimates of detection rates of approximately 20–25% in Down's syndrome screening of younger mothers (under the age of 35 years) with low MSAFP were predicted and reported results have proven these predictions accurate (Macri, 1986; Cuckle *et al.*, 1987; Palomaki, 1986). It is for this reason that additional markers to improve detection efficiency in screening a younger population were actively sought.

Initial observations on the utility of unconjugated estriol (uE$_3$) (Canick *et al.*, 1988) as a marker for Down's syndrome have been controversial and serious questions remain as to the benefit of the addition of this marker to a screening protocol (Macri *et al.*, 1990a,b,c, 1991; Spencer, 1991; Reynolds, 1992; Reynolds and John, 1992; Spencer *et al.*, 1992a,b; Crossley *et al.*, 1993). The addition of serum intact human chorionic gonadotropin (hCG) assay to MSAFP, however, improves detection efficiency for Down's syndrome to as high as 55–60% (Bogart *et al.*, 1987; Wald *et al.*, 1988).

Maternal serum screening for Down's syndrome has been evaluated in a variety of ways. In some centers, MSAFP evaluation directed primarily at neural tube defect screening was applied simultaneously to Down's syndrome. In other centers, maternal serum hCG was added to the AFP assessment in a double test procedure. In all others, in spite of controversy on uE$_3$ assays, a triple marker screening approach has been utilized. It is clear that the process of maternal serum screening for Down's syndrome is evolving rapidly; current markers continue to be validated and new ones are sought to improve upon the process.

Initial observations on the utility of the new marker: free β-hCG

Recognizing the significant contribution to Down's syndrome screening which can be made by the addition of hCG assessment to that of low MSAFP, our laboratory sought to determine which of the various approaches to measuring intact hCG would perform optimally. It is well understood that hCG is a heterodimer consisting of α- and β-chains, non-covalently bound together. Current conventional two-site sandwich immunoassays can capture and measure the intact hCG molecule by targeting epitopes on the α-subunit initially and the β-subunit subsequently (Fig. 7.1). Alternatively, in the so-called β-subunit assay, intact hCG can

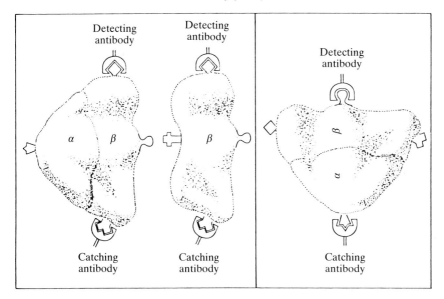

Fig. 7.1. Immunoassay methods in measuring intact hCG. Left panel illustrates the β-subunit assay while the right panel illustrates an α-β approach. (Reprinted from Macri *et al.* (1990d). *Am. J. Obstet. Gynecol.*, **163**, 1248–53.)

be assayed by targeting both the capture and the measurement epitopes on the β-subunit portion of the intact molecule. While this latter procedure indeed measures intact hCG (also capturing the relatively small number of free β-molecules present) it does so by virtue of antigenic sites on the β-chain only.

In initially assessing these two assay approaches to the measurement of intact hCG (Fig. 7.2), maternal sera taken from 26 documented Down's syndrome cases were used (Macri *et al.*, 1992a). It was observed that the α-β assay procedure did not yield the same detection efficiency as the β-subunit procedure for intact hCG. This observation remains unexplained in that both procedures are essentially capturing and measuring the same intact hCG molecule. However, the finding led us to the development of an immunoassay procedure which eliminated intact hCG from measurement. Instead, the assay targeted in a highly specific manner only unbound, free β-chains in the maternal circulation.

The development of a highly specific free β-subunit immunoassay took advantage of an antigenic site available at the interface of the α- and β-subunits. When α-chains and β-chains are combined (Fig. 7.3) to form the intact hCG molecule, the specific antigenic site used in the free β-hCG

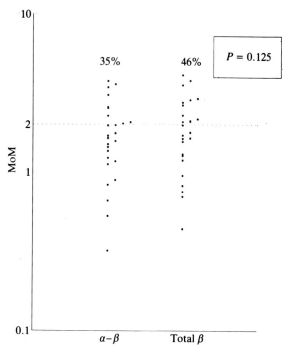

Fig. 7.2. Intact hCG levels in 26 cases of Down's syndrome using a β-subunit and an α-β immunoassay. The percentage values given are detection efficiency.

assay is not available. It is only when the free β-chain exists independently of the α-chain that the antigenic site becomes available for primary attachment to capture antibodies. Subsequently any available antigenic site on the β-subunit can be utilized as a secondary or measuring site for attachment of labeled antibody allowing for accurate quantification of free β-hCG.

   If such a free β-hCG assay system is to be effective, all cross-reactivity with the intact hCG molecule must be eliminated. Figure 7.4 demonstrates the relative levels of the free β-molecule compared to intact hCG during the second trimester of pregnancy. Free β-hCG represents less than 0.5% of intact hCG, therefore, any cross-reactivity with the intact molecule would result in a higher assay signal than that which would be expected from the free β-hCG molecule alone. Through a series of both competitive and non-competitive cross-reactivity studies, (Figs. 7.5, 7.6, Table 7.1) it was determined that our free β-hCG assay system possessed sufficiently little cross-reactivity to the intact hCG molecule to assure specific measurement of free β-hCG (Macri et al., 1992b).

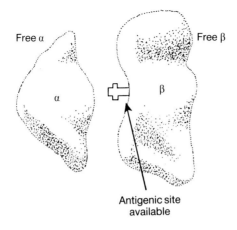

Free α

Free β

α

β

Antigenic site
available

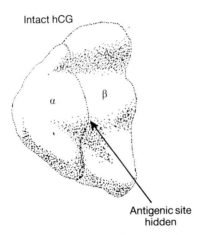

Intact hCG

α

β

Antigenic site
hidden

Fig. 7.3. Antigenic site employed in the development of a specific free β-subunit immunoassay. (Reprinted from Macri *et al.* (1990d). *Am. J. Obstet. Gynecol.*, **163**, 1248–53.)

Using the highly specific free β-hCG assay system on the same cases of Down's syndrome as shown in Fig. 7.2 revealed an even higher detection efficiency (Fig. 7.7). Selecting cases at less than 17 gestational weeks (13 cases, Fig. 7.8), the single analyte, free β-subunits showed levels at or above two multiples of the median (MoM) in 69% of cases. These early observations indicated that measurement of maternal serum free β-hCG might raise detection capability for Down's syndrome to levels higher than achieved with any marker previously reported.

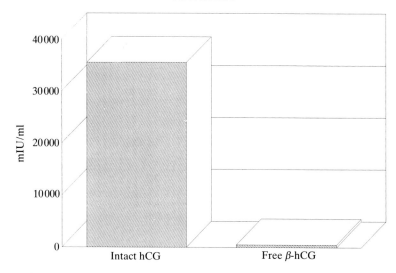

Fig. 7.4. Level of second trimester free β-subunits relative to intact hCG.

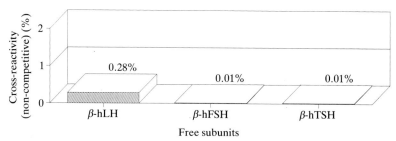

Fig. 7.5. Non-competitive cross-reactivity to free β-subunits.

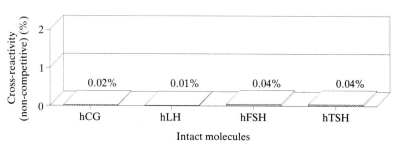

Fig. 7.6. Non-competitive cross-reactivity to intact molecules.

Table 7.1. *Competitive cross-reactivity of the free β-hCG assay with intact hCG*

Free β-hCG levels (ng/ml)	Apparent change in free β-hCG (ng/ml) at intact hCG levels of (IU/ml)			
	8	16	32	64
12.5	1.0	1.5	1.0	3.0
25.0	0.7	1.9	0.1	2.3
50.0	1.0	1.6	1.6	0.4

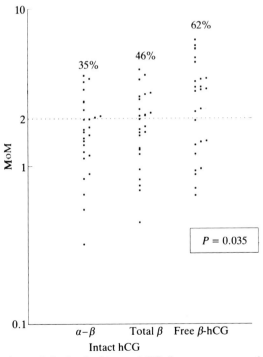

Fig. 7.7. Comparison of the level of intact hCG (by two assay methods) and free β-subunits in 26 cases of Down's syndrome. The percentage values given are the detection efficiency.

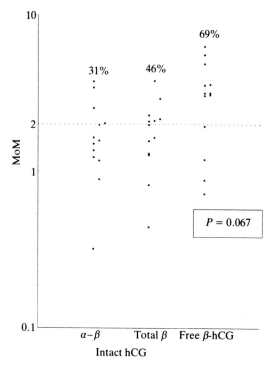

Fig. 7.8. Comparison of the level of intact hCG (by two assay methods) and free β-subunits in 26 cases of Down's syndrome prior to 17 gestational weeks.

Second trimester free β-hCG retrospective studies

Further evaluation of free β-hCG as a maternal serum marker for Down's syndrome initially included a direct comparison of free β-hCG and intact hCG in 242 controls and 101 patients carrying fetuses with trisomy 21. Figure 7.9a illustrates that, while the intact hCG level in maternal sera of affected cases is higher than that of controls, still higher levels of free β-hCG are seen in affected patients (Fig. 7.9b).

This comparison of two analytes provides information only on the relative level of each analyte in affected and unaffected states. To evaluate the effectiveness of free β-hCG assay as part of a protocol for assessing risk of Down's syndrome in the second trimester of pregnancy, the level of maternal serum free β-hCG must be combined in a multivariate discriminant analysis with maternal age and MSAFP.

Fig. 7.9. Level of second trimester intact hCG and free β-subunits in 242 unaffected and 101 Down's syndrome pregnancies: (a) intact hCG; (b) free β-subunits.

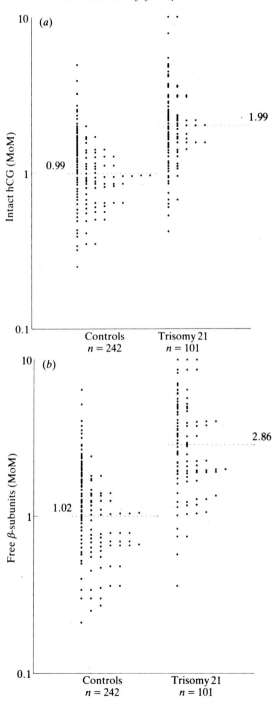

Table 7.2. *Down's syndrome screening results of free β-hCG, MSAFP and maternal age at 5% false-positive rate in initial study*

Gestational age (weeks)	Controls	Down's syndrome	Detection efficiency (%)
<17	240	15	80.0
≥17	210	14	64.3
14–22	450	29	72.4

In an initial study (Macri *et al.*, 1990d) of 450 controls and 29 documented cases of Down's syndrome in which maternal age, MSAFP and free β-hCG assessment were combined to produce patient risks for Down's syndrome, a detection efficiency (Table 7.2) as high as 80% in the early weeks of the second trimester was observed, with an efficiency of over 70% throughout the gestational testing range of 14 to 22 weeks. These encouraging findings were achieved while maintaining an initial false-positive rate of 5% or less.

Free β-hCG prospective screening protocol

In studies on prospective Down's syndrome screening, decisions must be made on the target population. In the USA, standards of care exist whereby mothers at or over the age of 35 years are considered at sufficient risk to warrant offering counseling and amniocentesis. This is theoretically capable of detecting 100% of cases of Down's syndrome in older mothers; therefore, the logical target population for screening is mothers under the age of 35 years. This younger population, while representing the vast majority of pregnancies (90–95%), is also the population which yields 80% or more of cases of Down's syndrome.

In view of the existing maternal age standard, younger mothers with maternal serum biochemical evaluations indicating increased risks would be similar to a 35-year-old, and this would trigger the offer of counseling and invasive diagnostic procedures. Hence, the protocol for prospective free β-hCG screening was restricted to mothers under the age of 35 years. Following biochemical screening, those patients demonstrating patient-specific risks equal to or greater than that of a 35-year-old were considered candidates for counseling and amniocentesis. Demographic data on maternal age, ethnicity and gestational age of this population are shown in Fig. 7.10.

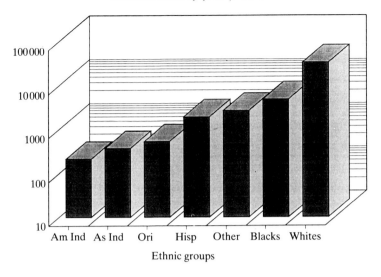

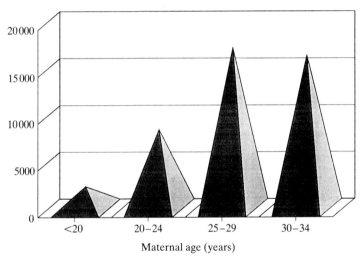

Fig. 7.10. Demographic data on 44 272 prospectively screened younger mothers. AM IND, American Indian; AS IND, Asian Indian; ORI, oriental; HISP, hispanic. (*continued*)

Results in screening younger mothers

In total, 44 272 women under the age of 35 years were screened (Table 7.3). Initial positive rates were acceptable and 29 of the 42 Down's syndrome cases (69%) were identified and confirmed at follow-up (Macri *et al.*, 1993a). This overall detection efficiency exceeds that using triple

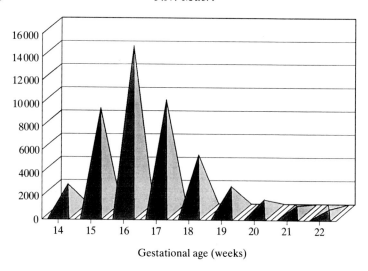

Gestational age (weeks)

Fig. 7.10 (*cont.*)

Table 7.3. *Results of a US prospective study of MSAFP/free β-hCG in women under 35 years*

Total number of patients screened	44 272
Patients initially found to be at increased risk	2465 (5.6%)
Patients offered amniocentesis after counseling and ultrasound	1688 (3.8%)
Down's syndrome cases ascertained by outcome gathering	42
Down's syndrome cases detected	29
Overall detection efficiency	69%
Detection at less than 17 weeks	73%
Detection at 17 weeks and after	63%

marker screening, and the enhanced detection in the earlier weeks of the second trimester (previously reported) exceeds any reported detection efficiency using intact hCG or uE_3 (Haddow *et al.*, 1992; Wald *et al.*, 1992) in either double or triple marker screening of younger mothers.

The observation of enhanced detection efficiency for Down's syndrome in earlier second trimester weeks has been assessed further by the addition of Down's syndrome cases retrospectively analyzed and added to our data base (Table 7.4). In 234 cases of Down's syndrome collected and evaluated either retrospectively or prospectively, an overall 12% improvement in detection efficiency (up to 82%) is seen when cases are evaluated earlier than 17 weeks of gestation (Macri *et al.*, 1993a). This level of free β-hCG

Table 7.4. *Down's syndrome detection efficiency in US studies*

	Gestational age < 17 weeks			Gestational age ≥ 17 weeks		
	No. DS cases	No. DS cases detected	(%)	No. DS cases	No. DS cases detected	(%)
Published retrospective study	26	21	80.8	34	21	61.8
Unpublished retrospective study[a]	98	83	84.7	34	28	82.4
US prospective study	26	19	73.1	16	10	62.5
Total	150	123	82.0	84	59	70.2

DS, Down's syndrome.
[a] 74% of unpublished retrospective Down's syndrome cases are from patients ≥ 35 years.

detection efficiency is more than 20% higher than that for either double or triple marker screening.

First trimester maternal serum screening

Second trimester maternal serum screening for open neural tube defects can achieve near 100% detection efficiency. However, attempts to move the testing window to the first trimester have not been successful. Maternal serum markers capable of detecting from 60% of Down's syndrome cases in the second trimester (Maternal Serum hCG combined with MSAFP) are similarly not effective in the first trimester (Cuckle *et al.*, 1988; Bogart *et al.*, 1989; Brock *et al.*, 1990). However, our recent report on 13 cases of first trimester Down's syndrome and 280 randomly selected first trimester control sera reveals that, unlike intact hCG, free β-hCG is elevated (1.9 MoM) in the first trimester and could serve as a screening marker (Spencer *et al.*, 1992c).

A more recent expansion of this earlier experience (Macri *et al.*, 1993b) with first trimester free β-hCG reveals that the median level of the analyte is even higher (2.2 MoM) than previously reported (Fig. 7.11). Thus

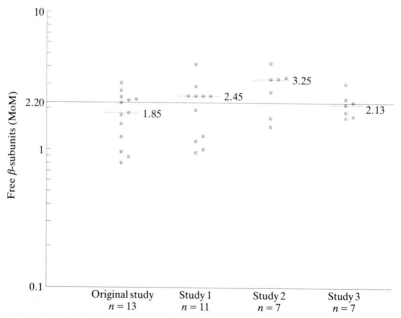

Fig. 7.11. Median first trimester free β-subunit levels in 38 Down's syndrome cases from four studies.

patients could be provided with the earliest possible alert (8 to 13 weeks) for chromosomal trisomy. The performance characteristics of free β-assay, however, in a prospective screening protocol in the first trimester remain to be defined, as does the place of other maternal serum markers. Not all samples in our initial studies were of sufficient volume to allow for evaluation of MSAFP and other markers; therefore, the calculation of risks was not possible.

Discussion

Maternal age-related invasive Down's syndrome testing has historically been applied to a small segment of the pregnant population (5–8%) with a theoretical 100% detection capability. This established protocol can only result in the detection of at most 20% of all cases of Down's syndrome. The application of non-invasive low MSAFP screening to mothers under the age of 35 years to identify an additional 5% of pregnancies at increased risk has provided us with the ability to identify an additional 25% of Down's syndrome. Comparison of the detection efficiency in these two groups, justifies the initiation of low MSAFP screening for Down's syndrome in younger mothers as being as effective as age-related Down's syndrome testing. The once unprecedented concept of non-invasive maternal serum screening for genetic malformations (neural tube defects being the first) is now expanding to other conditions and malformations. In doing so, the highest possible detection capability with the fewest possible false-positive results have been central to the acceptance of the process.

Newer Down's syndrome maternal serum screening markers now hold the promise of raising detection capability to a level approximating the efficiency of MSAFP screening for neural tube defects. The latest marker, maternal serum free β-hCG, has been used primarily in a double-analyte protocol with MSAFP. This marker has undergone extensive second trimester trials in Europe (mainly in the UK) and in our laboratory in the USA (Macri *et al.*, 1990d, 1992a, c, 1993a; Spencer, 1991; Larsen *et al.*, 1992; Spencer and Carpenter, 1992; Spencer and Macri, 1992; Spencer *et al.*, 1992a, b, d). Free β-assay has demonstrated, in retrospective and prospective evaluations, the highest detection capability of all previously reported markers.

Finally, the use of maternal serum free β-assay in the first trimester of pregnancy is a significant advantage. The detection efficiency of free β-hCG when used in combination with other markers remains to be assessed in the first trimester. Preliminary data suggest that first trimester MSAFP will contribute only marginally to Down's syndrome detection. With suitable MSAFP assays, and the possibility that additional and as yet unproven markers may prove effective, the contribution of free β-hCG in a multi-marker first trimester approach can be defined. Final acceptance of first trimester Down's syndrome screening will have to take into account the fact that first trimester maternal serum biochemical screening for neural tube defects (MSAFP) is not effective. The advantages, however, of a first trimester alert for chromosomal trisomy will, in all likelihood, outweigh other factors.

References

Bogart, M.H., Pandian, M.R. & Jones, O.W. (1987). Abnormal maternal serum chorionic gonadotropin levels in pregnancies with fetal chromosome abnormalities. *Prenatal Diagn.*, 7, 623–30.

Bogart, M.H., Golbus, M.S., Sorg, N.D. & Jones, O.W. (1989). Human chorionic gonadotropin levels in pregnancies with aneuploid fetuses. *Prenatal Diagn.*, 9, 379–84.

Brock, D.J.H., Barron, L., Holloway, S., Liston, W.A., Hillier, S.G. & Seppala, M. (1990). First trimester maternal serum biochemical indicators in Down syndrome. *Prenatal Diagn.*, 10, 245–51.

Canick, J.A., Knight, G.J., Palomaki, G.E., Haddow, J.E., Cuckle, H.S. & Wald, N.J. (1988). Low second trimester maternal serum unconjugated estriol in pregnancies with Down syndrome. *Br. J. Obstet. Gynaecol.*, 95, 330–3.

Crossley, J.A., Aitken, D.A. & Connor, J.M. (1993). Second trimester unconjugated estriol levels in maternal serum from chromosomally abnormal pregnancies using an optimized assay. *Prenatal Diagn.*, 13, 271–80.

Cuckle, H.S., Wald, N.J. & Thompson, S.G. (1987). Estimating a woman's risk of having a pregnancy associated with Down's syndrome using her age and serum alpha-fetoprotein level. *Br. J. Obstet. Gynaecol.*, 94, 387–402.

Cuckle, H.S., Wald, N.J., Barkai, G., Fuhrman, W., Altland, K. & Brambati, B. (1988). First trimester maternal serum biochemical indicators in Down syndrome. *Lancet*, ii, 851–52.

Davenport, D.M. & Macri, J.N. (1983). The clinical significance of low maternal serum alpha-fetoprotein. *Am. J. Obstet. Gynecol.*, 146, 657–61.

Haddow, J.E., Palomaki, G.E., Knight, G.J. et al. (1992). Prenatal screening for Down's syndrome with use of maternal serum markers. *N. Engl. J. Med.*, 327, 588–93.

Larsen, J., Garver, K., Frank, S. & Macri, J. (1992). Free beta hCG in Down syndrome screening. *Am. J. Obstet. Gynecol.*, 166, 350.

Macri, J.N. (1986). Critical issues in prenatal maternal serum alpha-fetoprotein screening for genetic abnormalities. *Am. J. Obstet. Gynecol.*, 155, 240–6.

Macri, J.N., Kasturi, R.V., Krantz, D.A., Cook, E.J., Sunderji, S.G. & Larsen, J.W. (1990a). Maternal serum Down syndrome screening: unconjugated estriol is not useful. *Am. J. Obstet. Gynecol.*, 162, 672–73.

Macri, J.N., Krantz, D.A., Kasturi, R.V. & Cook, E.J. (1990b). Measurement of unconjugated estriol by enzyme-linked immunosorbent assay fails to show an association with Down syndrome (letter). *Am. J. Obstet. Gynecol.*, **162**, 1634–35.

Macri, J.N., Kasturi, R.V., Krantz, D.A., Cook, E.J., Sunderji, S.G. & Larsen, J.W. (1990c). Maternal serum unconjugated estriol levels are lower in the presence of fetal Down syndrome (reply). *Am. J. Obstet. Gynecol.*, **163**, 1373–74.

Macri, J.N., Kasturi, R.V., Krantz, D.A. *et al.* (1990d). Maternal serum Down syndrome screening: free beta-protein is a more effective marker than human chorionic gonadotropin. *Am. J. Obstet. Gynecol.*, **163**, 1248–53.

Macri, J.N., Kasturi, R.V., Cook, E.J. & Krantz, D.A. (1991). Prenatal screening for Down's syndrome. *Br. Med. J.*, **303**, 468.

Macri, J.N., Anderson, R.W., Kasturi, R.V., Krantz, D.A. & Cook, E.J. (1992a). Enhanced Down syndrome detection with free beta (hCG). *Am. J. Hum. Genet.*, **51** (Suppl.), A418.

Macri, J.N., Spencer, K., Anderson, R.W. & Cook, E.J. (1992b). Free beta chorionic gonadotropin: a cross-reactivity study of two immunometric assays used in prenatal maternal serum screening for Down syndrome. *Ann. Clin. Biochem.*, **29**, 506–18.

Macri, J.N., Spencer, K. & Anderson, R. (1992c). Dual analyte immunoassay – a new approach to neural tube defect and Down syndrome screening. *Ann. Clin. Biochem.*, **29**, 390–6.

Macri, J.N., Spencer, K., Garver, K. *et al.* (1993a). Maternal serum free beta hCG screening; results of studies including 480 cases of Down syndrome. *Prenatal Diagn.*, in press.

Macri, J.N., Spencer, K., Aitken, D. *et al.* (1993b). First trimester free beta (hCG) screening for Down syndrome. *Prenatal Diagn.*, **13**, 557–62.

Merkatz, I.R., Nitkowski, H.M., Macri, J.N. & Johnson, W.E. (1984). An association between low maternal serum alpha-fetoprotein and fetal chromosome abnormalities. *Am. J. Obstet. Gynecol.*, **148**, 886–94.

Palomaki, G.E. (1986). Collaborative study of Down syndrome screening using maternal serum alpha-fetoprotein and maternal age. *Lancet*, **ii**, 1460.

Reynolds, T.M. (1992). Practical problems in Down syndrome screening: what should we do about gestational dating? What is the effect of assay precision on risk factors? *Commun. Lab. Med.*, **1**(2), 31–8.

Reynolds, T. & John, R. (1992). Comparison of assay kits for unconjugated estriol shows that expressing results as multiples of the median causes unacceptable variation in calculated risk factors for Down syndrome. *Clin. Chem.*, **38**, 1888–93.

Spencer, K. (1991). Evaluation of an assay of the free beta subunit of choriogonadotropin and its potential value in Down's syndrome. *Clin. Chem.*, **37**, 809–14.

Spencer, K. & Carpenter, P. (1992). Risk of Down syndrome and amniocentesis rate. *Br. Med. J.*, **304**, 640–1.

Spencer, K. & Macri, J.N. (1992). Early detection of Down's syndrome using free beta human choriogonadotropin. *Ann. Clin. Biochem.*, **29**, 349–50.

Spencer, K., Coombes, E.J., Selby, C., Mallard, A.S. & Ward, M.A. (1992a). Unconjugated oestriol has no place in second trimester Down's syndrome screening. *Clin. Chem.*, **38**, 952.

Spencer, K., Macri, J.N., Aitken, D. *et al.* (1992b). A clinical trial of a dual analyte immunoassay for free beta hCG and AFP and its application in NTD and Down's syndrome screening. *Clin. Chem.*, **38**, 952.

Spencer, K., Macri, J.N., Aitken, D.A. & Connor, J.M. (1992c). Free β-hCG as first trimester marker for fetal trisomy. *Lancet*, **339**, 1480.

Spencer, K., Coombes, J., Mallard, A.S. & Ward, A.F. (1992d). Free beta human choriogonadotropin in Down's syndrome screening: a multicentre study of its role compared with other biochemical markers. *Ann. Clin. Biochem.*, **29**, 506–18.

Wald, N.J., Cuckle, H.S., Densem, J.W. *et al.* (1988). Maternal serum screening for Down's syndrome in early pregnancy. *Br. Med. J.*, **297**, 883–7.

Wald, N.J., Kennard, A., Densem, J.W., Cuckle, H.S., Chard, T. & Butler, L. (1992). Antenatal maternal serum screening for Down's syndrome: results of a demonstration project. *Br. Med. J.*, **305**, 391–4.

8

Multiple hCG-related molecules

L.A. COLE

Occurrence of multiple hCG-related molecules

Human chorionic gonadotrophin (hCG) is a glycoprotein hormone produced by syncytiotrophoblast tissue in pregnancy and trophoblast disease. The hormone is composed of an α-subunit (92 amino acid residues) and a β-subunit (145 amino acid residues) held together by ionic and hydrophobic interactions. The α-subunit of hCG has the same peptide sequence as the α-subunits of the pituitary glycoprotein hormones. The β-subunit, however, is unique and distinguishes hCG from these other hormones. In early pregnancy, circulating hCG levels rise to a peak at 8 to 11 weeks after the last period. Levels diminish and reach approximately one fifth peak levels at 16 to 23 weeks, and remain close to this concentration until term (Fig. 8.1).

In addition to the hormone (intact hCG), a variety of uncombined or degraded molecules are produced with limited (less than 20%) or no biological activity (Fig. 8.2). These include nicked hCG, an hCG dimer severed between β-subunit residues 47 and 48 or, less commonly, between β-subunit residues 44 and 45. A portion of hCG molecules in all blood and urine samples and in WHO (1st IRP, 2nd and 3rd IS) and NIH (CR series) hCG standards, is severed or nicked at one or both of these sites (Bidart *et al.*, 1988; Nishimura *et al.*, 1988; Cole *et al.*, 1989, 1991; Puisieux *et al.*, 1990; Kardana *et al.*, 1991). Immunohistochemical studies (Kliman *et al.*, 1993), localized the nicked hCG to macrophages in the placenta. The proportion of nicked hCG molecules rises with advancing pregnancy (Cole *et al.*, 1993a). Averages of 9% (serum) and 8% (urine) nicked hCG molecules are present at 2 months of pregnancy, and 21%

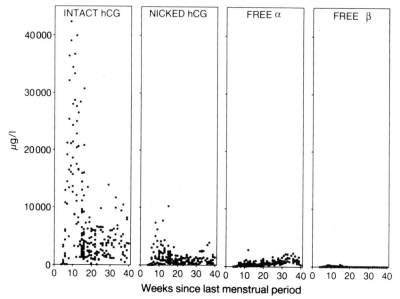

Fig. 8.1. Levels of intact hCG, nicked hCG and free subunits in 233 serum samples from different months of pregnancy. For comparison, all levels are plotted on the same scale (μg/l). Levels of intact (non-nicked) hCG were determined in the 'in house' B109 anti-hCG dimer (immobilized): enzyme-labeled anti-β antisera sandwich assay. Total hCG (nicked + non-nicked) was determined in a matched assay using 'in house' 2119 anti-α (immobilized): enzyme-labeled anti-β antisera, and the nicked hCG component deduced as total less intact. Free α was determined by the H7 anti-free α RIA and free β in the FBT11 anti-free β: enzyme-labeled anti-β antisera sandwich assay (Cole *et al.*, 1993a).

(serum) and 31% (urine) of nicked molecules are present by term (Figs. 8.1–3).

The β-subunit of hCG can be degraded in other ways (Fig. 8.2). hCG molecules missing the β-subunit C-terminal peptide (βCTP) have been isolated from urine samples in trophoblast disease (Kardana *et al.*, 1991). Recently, our laboratory tested 20 trophoblast disease serum samples. Values varied significantly in the β-hCG and βCTP antibody immuno-assays. In one sample values in the βCTP assay were as low as 2% of β-hCG assay levels, suggesting an almost complete absence of βCTP on this hCG (Cole and Kardana, 1992). Free α-subunit (free α) can also be detected in serum and urine (Figs. 8.1, 8.3). Like nicked hCG, the proportion of free α-subunit molecules rises with advancing pregnancy, from averages of 4.9% (serum) and 76% (urine) of hormone levels in the second month of pregnancy to 54% (serum) and 360% (urine) at term

cells and lower levels of hCG in the second or third trimesters from more differentiated or terminally differentiated syncytial tissues (Boime, 1991). Siler-Khodr and Khodr suggested a role for gonadotropin-releasing hormone (GnRH) in the regulation of hCG production (Khodr and Siler-Khodr 1978a,b; Siler-Khodr, 1988). hCG production is greatest in the first trimester when there is the largest number of cytotrophoblast or root cells and is least at term when these cells are sparse. Cytotrophoblast cells produce all the hypothalamic releasing hormones, including GnRH (Siler-Khodr, 1988). In cytotrophoblast monolayer cultures, GnRH can promote hCG production. In the placenta, GnRH may be produced by cytotrophoblast cells and act locally to promote hCG production by adjacent syncytiotrophoblast tissue (Khodr and Siler-Khodr 1978a,b). Work from Rao's laboratory has demonstrated hCG receptors on tropho-blast tissue, direct promotion of differentiation of trophoblast tissue by hCG, and autocrine or direct modulation of hCG levels by hCG itself (Lei and Rao, 1992; Lei *et al.*, 1992). All three mechanisms (differentiation, GnRH paracrine and hCG autocrine) may be needed to modulate hCG levels. Thus, GnRH may initially stimulate hCG production, and hCG itself amplify its own production by promoting differentiation of cytotro-phoblast cells, or inhibit it in later pregnancy by promoting terminal differentiation of syncytiotrophoblast cells.

Falling levels of hCG in the second and third trimesters of pregnancy may also be a reflection of nicking (Cole *et al.*, 1993a). hCG is increasingly nicked as pregnancy advances. Nicked hCG is unstable and dissociates into free α and nicked free β (dissociation half-life 22 ± 5.2 hours versus > 700 hours for intact hCG, Cole and Kardana, 1992). The 9% to 21% nicked hCG detected in pregnancy serum represents an equilibrium of continuously dissociating molecules. The true portion of nicked molecules produced by tissues may be much higher (Cole *et al.*, 1993a). A deactivation pathway has been proposed in which hCG is minimally nicked (and dissociated into free subunits) in the first 2 months of pregnancy (coinciding with the known 'purpose' of hCG to support the corpus luteum) and maximally nicked in the months thereafter. This pathway contributes to the decline of hCG levels and the parallel rise in urine free α and free β (free β + nicked free β + β-core) levels in the second and third trimesters of pregnancy. At this time we cannot say which is the principal pathway and can only suggest that differentiation, GnRH paracrine action, hCG autocrine effect, nicking/deactivation pathway, and possibly others all contribute to the modulation of hCG levels in the first, second and third trimesters of pregnancy.

The balance of α-subunit and β-subunit mRNAs in trophoblast cells changes as pregnancy advances. The cellular concentration of β-subunit mRNA is lower and of α-subunit mRNA is higher in term compared to first trimester tissues (Hoshina *et al.*, 1982). The change in the mRNA balance leads to an overproduction of α-subunit and possibly free α secretion (Boime, 1991; Hoshina *et al.*, 1982). Free α and nicked free β may also arise from dissociation of nicked hCG and the deactivation pathway. β-Core has been identified in placental explant cultures (Cole and Birken, 1988). While β-core could be of placental origin (trophoblast cells or associated macrophages), it also may arise in the circulation, liver or kidney from the degradation of nicked hCG (Wehmann and Nisula, 1980; Wehmann *et al.*, 1990; Cole *et al.*, 1993a). Nicked hCG dissociates releasing nicked free β. Leukocyte elastase can nick both hCG and free β. It can also degrade nicked free β (from free β or dissociation of nicked hCG) further by cleavage at β5–6, releasing peptide 1–5, and between β43 and 53 releasing residues 44–52, as might occur in β-core synthesis (Cole *et al.*, 1991, 1993a). This suggests that nicked hCG and nicked free β are the substrates for β-core synthesis.

The most obvious function for hCG in pregnancy is to maintain progesterone production by the corpus luteum. This function, however, is complete by 8 weeks of gestation, or before peak hCG levels are attained, making it unlikely that this is its only function. Other functions have been suggested, such as promotion of testosterone production in male fetuses. There may be additional physiologic roles for hCG that coincide with changing hCG levels. Nicked hCG, free β and β-core have minimal ($<20\%$ steroidogenic activity) or no corpus luteum-like activity (promotion of progesterone production). While they may simply be dissociation and degradation products that rapidly reduce hCG activity and clear hCG-related molecules from the circulation, they could have other yet-to-be-discovered physiologic functions.

Detection of multiple hCG-related molecules

Commercial kits employ a variety of methods to detect hCG. These include agglutination tests, radioimmunoassays, and multiple antibody sandwich tests. The agglutination test is either a latex or slide test and is strictly qualitative, giving a yes or no answer for pregnancy. In the β-hCG radioimmunoassay, a known amount of radioactive hCG competes with sample hCG to bind a limiting amount of β-hCG antibody. The amount of radioactivity bound is determined and from it the amount of sample hCG is deduced. The newer tests are multiple antibody sandwich type assays (Fig. 8.6). These are generally more specific and more sensitive than the single antibody tests. In this type of test one or more antibodies are attached to the inner surface of a tube or multititer plate, or on a glass bead or latex material. Sample is applied and the attached antibody captures and immobilizes the hCG in the sample. A further antibody raised against a distant site on hCG is added. This forms an antibody–hCG–antibody sandwich. The further antibody is labeled with a dye, with radioactivity or with an enzyme for spectrometric or fluorimetric detection. This labels and detects the amount of hCG in the sandwich.

If hCG was one molecule, rather than a group of related molecules, variations in kit results would be confined to cross-reactivities with luteinizing hormone, variances in detection level, and in choice of hCG standard (WHO 1st IRP versus 2nd IS). However, hCG is a group of related molecules, which causes additional or more serious problems. Agglutination tests and β-hCG radioimmunoassays use a single antibody to the hCG β-subunit. These kits usually detect intact (non-nicked) hCG, nicked hCG and all β-subunit-related molecules (free β, nicked free β and β-core) (Fig. 8.6). Multiple antibody sandwich assays using two different β-subunit antibodies (anti-β:labeled anti-β format assays) have similar specificities (Fig. 8.6). Sandwich assays using an anti-βCTP (immobilized): anti-β (labeled) antibody format have similar specificities, except that they do not detect molecules minus βCTP or β-core. Those using an anti-α (immobilized): anti-β (labeled) antibody format detect only hCG (intact hCG, nicked hCG and hCG missing βCTP); those using an anti-α (immobilized): anti-βCTP (labeled) format measure the same except that they do not detect hCG minus βCTP; and those using anti-hCG dimer (immobilized): anti-β (labeled) format only detect intact (or biologically active) hCG molecules (Cole *et al.*, 1991, 1993b; Cole and Kardana, 1992). These antibody formats are found today in quantitative and qualitative pregnancy test kits. in a survey of 29 hCG kits available in the USA, nine were βhCG radioimmunoassays or dye or agglutination tests, seven were anti-α:anti-β format, two were anti-βCTP:anti-α format, two were anti-βCTP:anti-β format, four were anti-β:anti-β format and five were anti-hCG dimer:anti-β format type immunoassays (Cole *et al.*, 1983).

Differences in the specificities of hCG immunoassays for intact hCG, nicked hCG, molecules missing βCTP, free β and β-core lead to conflicting results (Cole and Kardana, 1992; Cole *et al.*, 1993b). Kits give conflicting results with the same serum sample, and different doctor's office or home pregnancy tests give either true-positive or false-negative results with a

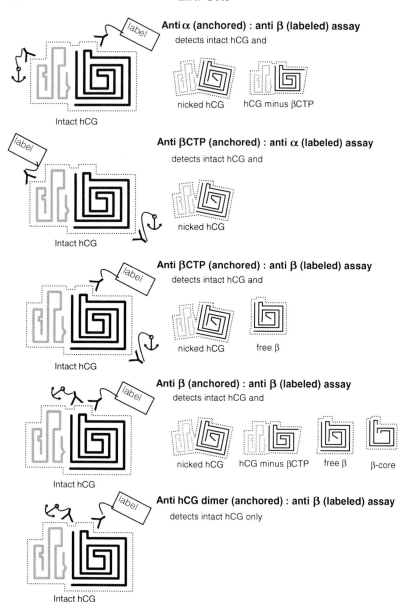

Fig. 8.6. Antibody configurations used in hCG sandwich-type immunoassays. Anchored means immobilized on a bead, tube, multititer plate or latex material; labeled means linked to enzyme, radioactive iodine, or colored dye. Structures are representations of intact hCG, nicked hCG, hCGs minus βCTP and free β as illustrated in Fig. 8.2. Specificities for intact hCG and other hCG-related molecules are those indicated in other publications (Cole and Kardana, 1992; Cole *et al.*, 1991).

single urine specimen. In our own laboratory we tested 20 pregnancy and 20 trophoblast disease serum samples with ten different hCG immuno-assays, two each of five formats (Table 8.1) and all calibrated with the same hCG standard. Major variation was apparent in the results from the ten assays with pregnancy (coefficient of variation 15.1%) and with trophoblast disease (coefficient of variation 28.2%) serum samples. Results with pregnancy samples ranged from 64 to 154% of mean value (2.4-fold difference), and with trophoblast disease samples ranged from 4.4 to 252% of mean value (57-fold difference). Two types of assay gave particularly aberrant results with trophoblast disease serum samples. The two anti-hCG dimer (immobilized): anti-β (labeled) sandwich assay kits, which detect intact hCG, gave consistently low results with trophoblast disease samples (67% and 80% of mean values, respectively). The two anti-βCTP (immobilized): anti-β (labeled) sandwich assays gave sporadic low and high results: in one case giving results 4.4% and 5.0% of mean values, respectively and in three others results over 130% of mean values. Variations were antibody-format dependent. If one type of kit gave low or high results so did other kits using the same antibody format. We conclude that hCG assay results are format dependent and may vary significantly when determined by a different antibody format assay. While we cannot say which measurement (intact hCG, intact plus nicked hCG, etc.) or which format of kit is the most correct, we can suggest that manufacturers mark kits appropriately so that the confusion caused by conflicting hCG values can be avoided. Results, cut-off levels and doubling rates from different format kits should be clearly distinguished.

Clinical applications of multiple hCG-related molecules

hCG determination is used for detecting intra- and extrauterine pregnancies, for predicting trophoblast disease, Down's syndrome fetuses, and in following the therapy of choriocarcinoma, testicular cancer and certain other malignancies. These are dealt with elsewhere. Here we focus on new applications and supporting roles for the hCG-related molecules, nicked hCG, hCG minus β-hCG, free α, free β and β-core. Papers describing clinical applications for hCG-related molecules are listed in Table 8.2.

Generation of multiple hCG-related molecules is an ongoing process in serum and urine samples. The nicked component of hCG is continuously dissociating releasing nicked free β. This can falsely elevate free β measurements. The effect of storage of nicked hCG on free measurements can be estimated. If one considers that hCG in serum from first trimester

Table 8.1. *Inter-assay discordance in hCG results: Sera from 20 pregnancies and 20 trophoblast disease samples tested in 10 immunoassay kits*

	hCG (ng/ml)									
	2119 'in house' anti $\alpha:\beta$	Hybritech Tandem anti $\alpha:\beta$	B109 'in house' anti hCG:β	Serono MAIAclone anti hCG:β	Abbott hCGβ15/15 anti $\beta:\beta$	Biomerica hCG anti $\beta:\beta$	DPC hCG β RIA	Amersham Amerlex-M β RIA	Organon NML anti bCTP:β	CC11 'in house' anti βCTP:β
Pregnancy samples										
1	100	98	89	119	70	108	103	107	115	68
2	111	102	102	123	76	99	103	113	119	72
3	132	110	113	134	95	115	118	117	138	73
4	192	163	142	205	136	178	167	174	206	169
5	285	254	259	315	257	273	294	302	371	238
6	659	521	537	648	572	586	533	556	706	666
7	796	672	687	796	737	845	672	701	990	699
8	1275	1114	1064	1301	976	1271	1109	1234	1120	887
9	1542	1400	1642	1416	1596	1354	1436	1480	1664	1840
10	1553	1029	1164	1088	983	1383	1011	1444	945	707
11	1568	1400	1716	1516	1598	2133	1378	1390	1676	1782
12	2006	2212	2484	2526	2572	2188	2080	2888	2438	2680
13	2042	1440	1944	1896	2116	1748	1514	1876	1944	2188
14	2696	2554	2412	3060	3290	2574	2594	3174	2920	2812
15	3590	3050	4080	3400	3650	2730	3080	3320	3440	4480
16	3680	2850	4080	3550	3510	2920	2750	3110	3380	4830
17	5550	5040	6390	5470	5730	4370	5220	5180	5520	7110
18	7420	6250	7010	6780	6950	5470	6140	6310	7630	7840
19	9160	8060	9460	10110	8670	8500	5940	8550	11020	9700
20	9160	6980	9620	8950	9380	7240	7990	8740	8490	10820

Table 8.1 (cont.)

hCG (ng/ml)

	2119 'in house' anti α:β	Hybritech Tandem anti α:β	B109 'in house' anti hCG:β	Serono MAIAclone anti hCG:β	Abbott hCGβ15/15 anti β:β	Biomerica hCG anti β:β	DPC hCG β RIA	Amersham Amerlex-M β RIA	Organon NML anti bCTP:β	CC11 'in house' anti βCTP:β
	42	61	30	69	86	59	70	72	76	53

Trophoblast disease samples

	2119 'in house' anti α:β	Hybritech Tandem anti α:β	B109 'in house' anti hCG:β	Serono MAIAclone anti hCG:β	Abbott hCGβ15/15 anti β:β	Biomerica hCG anti β:β	DPC hCG β RIA	Amersham Amerlex-M β RIA	Organon NML anti bCTP:β	CC11 'in house' anti βCTP:β
1	876	954	1081	1124	2374	1161	1147	1562	1742	1160
2	2830	3680	4500	4400	4700	3540	3930	4460	3940	2790
3	3220	3280	4150	4050	4730	3250	3730	4160	3940	3380
4	3420	3870	4740	4520	5990	3910	4650	5080	5520	3970
5	4470	4900	5220	5330	5070	4540	5440	5710	5520	3220
6	7510	7700	7710	9640	8850	8130	7410	8810	8160	8400
7	11 200	10 460	4520	10 300	26 680	11 200	12 120	19 240	18 220	15 220
8	14 380	14 540	16 020	14 700	36 000	14 780	17 820	24 700	24 320	17 340
9	15 080	14 600	17 140	14 560	13 240	13 880	14 960	14 920	14 700	8900
10	29 600	40 320	37 800	43 440	48 080	38 160	62 760	33 880	40 280	32 680
11	35 400	32 000	43 000	32 200	63 600	32 100	37 900	46 200	47 600	47 400
12	46 400	44 100	48 000	42 200	57 400	42 900	50 900	57 500	42 800	48 000
13	51 900	55 100	57 100	64 600	67 500	57 800	54 500	54 100	61 300	72 500
14	57 000	62 100	62 500	69 900	75 600	62 500	73 700	66 800	73 800	67 900
15	58 800	59 300	69 900	65 800	76 900	62 900	57 400	60 500	64 900	74 300
16	96 100	111 900	116 100	123 700	134 000	108 200	97 900	129 600	112 100	111 100
17	104 300	115 200	122 900	110 700	134 100	112 700	103 900	130 900	117 900	140 800
18	136 400	150 800	221 500	178 200	218 900	154 700	134 700	196 200	182 800	153 000
19	152 400	82 600	96 300	90 500	97 700	92 100	81 200	201 600	3990	3468

Table 8.2. *Publications describing clinical applications for hCG-related molecules*

Carbohydrate variants of hCG as a marker of trophoblast disease
Mizuochi *et al.*, 1983, 1985
Cole, 1987
Amano *et al.*, 1988
Imamura *et al.*, 1987

Nicked hCG as a marker of trophoblast disease
Nishimura *et al.*, 1988
Puisieux *et al.*, 1990
Cole *et al.*, 1991

Free β as a marker of Down's syndrome and other trisomies
Ozturk *et al.*, 1990
Macri *et al.*, 1990
Spencer, 1991, 1992
Knight and Cole, 1991

Free β as a marker of testicular cancer
Madersbacher *et al.*, 1990, 1992
Blumsohn and Morris, 1990

Free β as a marker of trophoblast disease
Cole *et al.*, 1983
Khazaeli *et al.*, 1986, 1989
Ozturk *et al.*, 1987, 1988
Fan *et al.*, 1987
Berkowitz *et al.*, 1989
Kardana and Cole, 1992

Free β as a marker of ectopic pregnancy or spontaneous abortion
Cole *et al.*, 1987
Letterie and Hay, 1991

Free β as a marker of non-trophoblastic cancers
Weintraub and Rosen, 1973
Hagen *et al.*, 1976
Kahn *et al.*, 1977
Nagelberg *et al.*, 1985, 1989
Iles *et al.*, 1989
Marcillac *et al.*, 1992
Alfhan *et al.*, 1992

Urine β-core as a marker of non-trophoblastic cancers
Masure *et al.*, 1981
Cole *et al.*, 1982, 1988a,b, 1990
Papapetrou and Nicopoulou, 1986
Kardana *et al.*, 1988

Table 8.2 (*cont.*)

Wong *et al.*, 1988
Cole and Nam, 1989
Nam *et al.*, 1990a,b,c
Norman *et al.*, 1990
McGill *et al.*, 1990
Schwartz *et al.*, 1991
Lee *et al.*, 1991
Maruo *et al.*, 1991
Mochizuki *et al.*, 1991
Kinugasa *et al.*, 1992
D'Agostino *et al.*, 1992
Alfhan *et al.*, 1992

Free α as a marker of trophoblast disease
Elegbe *et al.*, 1984
Ozturk *et al.*, 1988

Free α as a marker of non-trophoblastic cancers
Kourides *et al.*, 1976
Franchimont *et al.*, 1978
Huang *et al.*, 1989
Marcillac *et al.*, 1992

While we have tried to make this list complete, it is possible we may have missed some papers. We apologise to the authors of any manuscript we have missed.

pregnancy is 9% nicked and contains 0.91% free β (mass percentage of hCG level; Cole *et al.*, 1993a), then storage for 22 hours at 37°C would amplify free β measurements by 290%. Dissociation of hCG is governed by the Law of Mass Action. Therefore, storage for a certain time at room temperature (20°C) may elevate free β measurement 70%, while storage in a refrigerator (4°C) would elevate it 16%. Care must be taken to refrigerate or freeze samples, preferably within 30 minutes of collection.

Measurements of free β levels have proven useful in the diagnosis of trophoblast disease. Numerous publications (Cole *et al.*, 1983; Khazaeli *et al.*, 1986, 1989; Fan *et al.*, 1987; Ozturk *et al.*, 1987, 1988; Berkowitz *et al.*, 1989; Kardana and Cole, 1992; and others) show higher free β-subunit to hCG ratios in sera from patients with persistent trophoblast disease than in those from patients with hydatidiform mole, with the latter being higher than in normal first trimester pregnancies. In our own experience, using samples frozen within 30 minutes of collection, 0 of 12 women with first trimester pregnancy, 11 of 12 with hydatidiform mole and 6 of 6 with persistent trophoblast disease had free β levels exceeding

1.0% of hCG concentration. Free β levels averaged $0.53 \pm 0.18\%$ (S.D.) in pregnancy, $5.2 \pm 5.6\%$ in hydatidiform mole and $11.6 \pm 8.0\%$ of hCG levels in persistent trophoblast disease samples (Kardana and Cole, 1992). The results were improved by measuring nicked free β instead of total (all) free β (Kardana and Cole, 1992). Ozturk and colleagues used free β measurement in the differential diagnosis of pregnancy and complete mole, complete mole and choriocarcinoma, and in the early prediction of recurrence in patients with choriocarcinoma (Ozturk et al., 1988).

Recent reports also indicate higher concentrations of free β in patients with Down's syndrome and other trisomy pregnancies (Macri et al., 1990; Ozturk et al., 1990; Spencer, 1991, 1992). There are now commercial kits for measuring free β (Sys Corporation, Bioclone Australia and Wallac DELFIA) and free β assays have been introduced at some testing centers. hCG levels are approximately 2-fold higher than normal in Down's syndrome pregnancies (Bogart et al., 1987). Elevated hCG levels and unduly low α-fetoprotein and unconjugated estriol levels are all suggestive of Down's syndrome and are now used together as a 'triple test' for pre-screening for Down's syndrome fetuses (Cranick, 1990). Research by Macri et al. (Chapter 7) and Spencer et al. (Chapter 6) indicate that free β measurement offers an improvement over hCG determination, and they suggest the use of free β alone or of the free β and α-fetoprotein combination for screening for Down's syndrome. In our experience, using samples frozen within 30 minutes of collection, hCG levels were 1.8-fold higher in Down's syndrome ($n = 9$, 8552 ± 2525 ng/ml, mean $\pm$ S.D.) than in control serum samples ($n = 48$, 4690 ± 3133 ng/ml). Free β levels were 2.3-fold different: 34 ± 32 ng/ml in Down's syndrome versus 15 ± 11 ng/ml in control serum samples. Most of the differences between levels of free β in control and Down's syndrome sera was due to nicked free β molecules (Rotmensch et al., 1992). Calculated nicked free β (total minus intact free β) levels were 21 ± 26 ng/ml in the Down's syndrome and 4.0 ± 4.9 ng/ml in the control group, or approximately 5-fold different. In this small test series, nicked free β was a better marker than total (all) free β or hCG. Larger studies are needed with many more Down's syndrome samples to evaluate nicked free β as a marker of Down's syndrome.

Low levels of free β have been associated with ectopic pregnancy and spontaneous abortion (Cole et al., 1987; Letterie and Hay, 1991). Overall, unduly high or very low free β, or nicked free β, levels are indicative of problems in pregnancy; high serum free β levels (>0.1 ng/ml) or high urine β-core levels (>3 fmol/mol) in non-pregnant subjects are indicative of cancer.

Acknowledgements

Some of the research described in this review was supported by National Institute of Health grants CA44131 and CA46828 to Laurence A. Cole. Antibody 2119-12 used in the 'in house' total hCG was donated to our laboratory by Unipath, Inc., Bedford, England. Antibody B204 and B109 used in the 'in house' β-core and intact hCG assays were gifts from Drs O'Connor, Krichevsky and Canfield at Colombia University, New York, and antibody FBT11 from Drs Bellet and Bidart of Institute Gustave Roussy in Paris, France. We also wish to thank Dr Glenn Braunstein at Cedars-Sinai Medical Center in Los Angles who collected the serial pregnancy serum samples for hCG determination (Fig. 7.1).

References

Alfhan, H., Haglund, C., Roberts, P. & Stenman, U.H. (1992). Elevation of free β-subunit of human choriogonadotropin and core β fragment of choriogonadotropin in serum and urine of patients with malignant pancreatic and biliary disease. *Cancer Res.*, **52**, 4628–33.

Amano, J., Nishimura, R., Mochizuki, M. & Kobata, A. (1988). Comparative study of the mucin-type sugar chains of human chorionic gonadotropin present in the urine of patients with trophoblastic diseases and healthy pregnant women. *J. Biol. Chem.*, **263**, 1157–65.

Berkowitz, R., Ozturk, M., Goldstein, D., Bernstein, M., Hill, L. & Wands, J.R. (1989). Human chorionic gonadotropin and free subunits' serum levels in patients with partial and complete hydatidiform moles. *Obstet. Gynecol.*, **74**, 212–16.

Bidart, J.-M., Puisieux, A., Troalen, F., Foglietti, M.J., Bohuon, C. & Bellet, D. (1988). Characterization of the cleavage product in the human choriogonadotropin β-subunit. *Biochem. Biophys. Res. Comm.*, **154**, 626–32.

Birken, S., Agosto, G., Amr, S. *et al.* (1988a). Characterization of antisera distinguishing carbohydrate structures in the β-carboxyl-terminal region of human chorionic gonadotropin. *Endocrinology*, **122**, 2054–63.

Birken, S., Armstrong, E.G., Kolks, M.A.G. *et al.* (1988b). Structure of human chorionic gonadotropin β-subunit core fragment from pregnancy urine. *Endocrinology*, **123**, 572–83.

Blumsohn, A. & Morris, B.W. (1990). Measurement of free choriogonadotropin beta-subunit in patients with testicular tumors. *Clin. Chem.*, **36**, 2009–15.

Bogart, M.H., Pandian, M.R. & Jones, O.W. (1987). Abnormal maternal serum chorionic gonadotropin levels in pregnancies with fetal chromosome abnormalities. *Prenatal Diagn.*, **7**, 623–30.

Boime, I. (1991). Human placental hormone production is linked to the stage of trophoblast differentiation. *Trophoblast Res.*, **5**, 57–60.

Cole, L.A. (1987). The O-linked oligosaccharides are strikingly different on pregnancy and choriocarcinoma hCG. *J. Clin. Endocrinol. Metab.*, **65**, 811–13.

Cole, L.A. & Birken, S. (1988). Origin and occurrence of human chorionic gonadotropin β-subunit core fragment. *Mol. Endocrinol.*, **2**, 825–30.

Cole, L.A. & Kardana, A. (1992). Discordant results in human chorionic gonadotropin assays. *Clin. Chem.*, **38**, 263–70.

Cole, L.A. & Nam, J.H. (1989). Urinary gonadotropin fragment measurements in the diagnosis and management of ovarian cancer. *Yale J. Med. Biol.*, **62**, 367–78.

Cole, L.A., Birken, S., Sutphen, S., Hussa, R.O. & Pattillo, R.A. (1982). Absence of the COOH-terminal peptide on ectopic human chorionic gonadotropin beta subunit (hCG beta). *Endocrinology*, **110**, 2198–2200.

Cole, L.A., Hartle, R.J., Laferla, J.J. & Ruddon, R.W. (1983). Detection of the free beta subunit of human chorionic gonadotropin (hCG) in cultures of normal and malignant trophoblast cells, pregnancy sera, and sera of patients with choriocarcinoma, *Endocrinology*, **113**, 1176–8.

Cole, L.A., Kroll, T.D. & Ruddon, R.W. (1984). Differential occurrence of free α and free β subunits of human chorionic gonadotropin (hCG) from pregnancy sera. *J. Clin. Endocrinol. Metab.*, **50**, 1200–2.

Cole, L.A., Restrepo-Cand, H., Lavy, G. & DeCherney, A. (1987). hCG free beta-subunit an early marker of outcome of *in vitro* fertilization clinical pregnancies. *J. Clin. Endocrinol. Metab.*, **64**, 1328–30.

Cole, L.A., Wang, Y., Elliott, M. *et al.* (1988a). Urinary human chorionic gonadotropin free beta-subunit and core fragment: a new marker of gynecologic cancers, *Cancer Res.*, **48**, 1356-60.

Cole, L.A., Schwartz, P.E. & Wong, Y. (1988b). Urinary gonadotropin fragments (UGF) in cancers of the female reproductive system: I. Sensitivity and specificity, comparison with other markers. *Gynecol. Oncol.*, **31**, 82–90.

Cole, L.A., Kardana, A. & Birken, S. (1989). The isomers, subunits and fragments of hCG. *Serono Symposia Publ.*, **65**, 59–79.

Cole, L.A., Nam, J.H., Chang, K.C., Chambers, J.T. & Schwartz, P.E. (1990). Urinary gonadotropin fragment, a new tumor marker: II. For differentiating a benign from a malignant pelvic mass. *Gynecol. Oncol.*, **36**, 391–4.

Cole, L.A., Kardana, A., Andrade-Gordon, P. *et al.* (1991). The heterogeneity of hCG: III. The occurrence, biological and immunological activities of nicked hCG. *Endocrinology*, **129**, 1559–67.

Cole, L.A., Kardana, A., Park, S.-Y. & Braunstein, G.D. (1993a). The deactivation of hCG by nicking and dissociation. *J. Clin. Endocrinol. Metab.*, **76**, 704–710.

Cole, L.A., Seifer, D.B., Kardana, A. & Braunstein, G.D. (1993b). Selecting human chorionic gonadotropin immunoassays: consideration of cross-reacting molecules in first-trimester serum and urine. *Am. J. Obstet. Gynecol.*, in press.

Cranick, J.A. (1990). Screening for Down syndrome using maternal serum alpha-fetoprotein, unconjugated estriol and hCG. *J. Clin. Immunoassay*, **13**, 30–3.

D'Agostino, R.S., Cole, L.A., Ponn, R.B., Stern, H. & Schwartz, P.E. (1992). Urinary gonadotropin fragment in patients with lung and esophageal disease. *J. Surg. Oncol.*, **49**, 147–50.

Elegbe, R.A., Pattillo, R.A., Hussa, R.O., Hoffmann, R.G., Damole, I.O. & Finlayson, W.E. (1984). Alpha subunit and human chorionic gonadotropin in normal pregnancy and gestational trophoblastic disease. *Obstet. Gynecol.*, **63**, 335–41.

Fan, C., Goto, S., Furuhashi, Y. & Tomoda, Y. (1987). Radioimmunoassay of the serum free beta-subunit of human chorionic gonadotropin in trophoblastic disease. *J. Clin. Endocrinol. Metab.,* **64**, 313–18.

Franchimont, P., Reuter, A. & Gaspard, U. (1978). Ectopic production of hCG and its α- and β-subunits. In *Current Topics In Experimental Endocrinology*, Vol. 3. ed. L. Martini & V.H.T. James, pp. 202–16. New York: Academic Press.

Hagen, C., Gilby, E.D., McNeilly, A.S., Olgaard, K., Bondy, P.K. Rees, L.H. (1976). Comparison of circulating glycoprotein hormones and their subunits in patients with oat cell carcinoma of the lung and uraemic patients on chronic dialysis. *Acta Endocrinol. (Copenh.)* **83**, 26–32.

Hoshina, M., Boothby, M. & Boime, I. (1982). Cytological localization of chorionic gonadotropin α and placental lactogen mRNAs during development of the human placenta. *J. Cell. Biol.,* **93**, 190–8.

Huang, S.C., Hsieh, C.Y., Hwang, J.L., Ouyang, P.C. & Chen, H.C. (1989). Free alpha subunit of human chorionic gonadotropin in women with non-trophoblastic tumors. *Taiwan I Hsueh Hui Tsa Chih,* **88**, 215–18.

Iles, R.K., Jenkins, B.J., Oliver, R.T.D., Blandy, J.P. & Chard, T. (1989). Beta human chorionic gonadotropin in serum and urine. A marker for metastatic urothelial cancer. *Br. J. Urol.,* **64**, 241–4.

Imamura, S., Armstrong, G.A. Birken, S., Cole, L.A. & Canfield, R.E. (1987). Highly specific and sensitive measurements of desialylated forms of human chorionic gonadotropin with lectin immunoradiometric assays. *Clin. Chim. Acta,* **163**, 339–49.

Johansson, E.N.B. (1979). Plasma levels of progesterone in pregnancy measured by a rapid competitive protein binding technique. *Acta Endocrinol. (Copenh.),* **61**, 607–17.

Kahn, C.R., Rosen, S.W., Weintraub, B.D., Fajans, S.S. & Gorden, P. (1977). Ectopic production of chorionic gonadotropin and its subunits by islet-cell tumors. *N. Engl. J. Med.,* **297**, 565–7.

Kardana, A. & Cole, L.A. (1990). Serum hCG beta-core fragment is masked by associated macromolecules. *J. Clin. Endocrinol. Metab.,* **71**, 1393–5.

Kardana, A. & Cole, L.A. (1992). Polypeptide nicks cause erroneous results in human chorionic gonadotropin free β-subunit assays. *Clin. Chem.,* **38**, 26–33.

Kardana, A., Taylor, M.E., Southall, P.J., Boxer, G.M., Rowan, A.J. & Bagshawe, K.D. (1988). Urinary gonadotropin peptide isolation and purification, and its immunohistochemical distribution in normal and neoplastic tissues. *Br. J. Cancer,* **58**, 281–6.

Kardana, A. Elliott, M.E., Gawinowicz, M.A., Birken, S. & Cole, L.A. (1991). The heterogeneity of hCG: I. Characterization of peptide variations in 13 individual preparations of hCG. *Endocrinology,* **129**, 1541–50.

Khazaeli, M.B., Hedayat, M.M., Hatch, K.D. *et al.* (1986). Radioimmunoassay of free beta subunit of human chorionic gonadotropin as a prognostic test for persistent trophoblastic disease in molar pregnancy. *Am. J. Obstet. Gynecol.,* **155**, 320–5.

Khazaeli, M.B., Buchina, E.S., Pattillo, R.A., Soong, S.J. & Hatch, K.D. (1989). Radioimmunoassay of free beta-subunit of human chorionic gonadotropin in diagnosis of high-risk and low-risk gestational trophoblastic disease. *Am. J. Obstet. Gynecol.,* **160**, 444–9.

Khodr, G.S. & Siler-Khodr, T.M. (1978a). The effect of luteinizing hormone-releasing factor on human chorionic gonadotropin secretion. *Fertil. Steril.,* **30**, 301–4.

Khodr, G.S. & Siler-Khodr, T.M. (1978b). Localization of luteinizing hormone-releasing factor in the human placenta. *Fertil. Steril.*, **29**, 523–6.

Kinugasa, M., Nishimura, R., Hasegawa, K., Okamura, M., Kimura, A. & Ohtsu, F. (1992). Assessment of urinary β-core fragment of hCG as a tumor marker of cervical cancer. *Acta Obstet. Gynecol. Japan*, **44**, 188–94.

Kliman, H.J., Less, K.S., Meaddough, E.L. & Cole, L.A. (1993). hCG degradation in the human chorionic villous core (abstract). *Serono Symposium on Glycoprotein Hormones*, Santa Barbara, CA: Raven Press.

Knight, G.J. & Cole, L.A. (1991). Measurement of choriogonadotropin free beta-subunit: an alternative to choriogonadotropin in screening for fetal Down's syndrome? *Clin. Chem.*, **37**, 779–82.

Kourides, I.A., Weintraub, B.D., Rosen, S.W., Ridgway, E.C., Kliman, B. & Maloof, F. (1976). Secretion of alpha subunit of glycoprotein hormones by pituitary adenomas. *J. Clin. Endocrinol. Metab.*, **43**, 97–102.

Lee, C.L., Iles, R.K., Shepherd, J.H., Hudson, C.N. & Chard, T. (1991). The purification and development of a radioimmunoassay for beta-core fragment of human chorionic gonadotrophin in urine: application as a marker of gynaecological cancer in premenopausal and postmenopausal women. *J. Endocrinol.*, **130**, 481–9.

Lei, Z.M. & Rao, Ch. V. (1992). Gonadotropin receptors in human fetoplacental unit: implications for hCG as an intracrine, paracrine and endocrine regulator of human fetoplacental function. *Trophoblast Res.*, **6**, 213–24.

Lei, Z.M., Rao, Ch.V., Acherman, D.M. & Day, T.G. (1992). The expression of human chorionic gonadotropin/human luteinizing hormone receptors in human gestational trophoblastic neoplasms. *J. Clin. Endocrinol. Metab.*, **74**, 1236–41.

Letterie, G.S. & Hay, D.L. (1991). Serial monitoring of human chorionic gonadotropin and free beta subunit secretion in ectopic pregnancy. *Clin. Exp. Obstet. Gynecol.*, **18**, 221–5.

Macri, J.N., Kasturi, R.V., Krantz, D.A. *et al.* (1990). Maternal serum Down syndrome screening: free beta-protein is a more effective marker than human chorionic gonadotropin. *Am. J. Obstet. Gynecol.*, **163**, 1248–53.

Madersbacher, S., Berger, P., Mann, K., Kuzmists, R. & Wick, G. (1990). Diagnostic value of free subunits of serum chorionic gonadotropin in testicular cancer. *Lancet*, **336**, 630–1.

Madersbacher, S., Klieber, R., Mann, K. *et al.* (1992). Free alpha-subunit, free beta-subunit of human chorionic gonadrotropin (hCG), and intact hCG in sera of healthy individuals and testicular cancer patients. *Clin. Chem.*, **38**, 370–6.

Marcillac, I., Troalen, F., Bidart, J.-M. *et al.* (1992). Free human chorionic gonadotropin beta subunit in gonadal and nongonadal neoplasms. *Cancer Res.*, **52**, 3901–7.

Maruo, T., Kitajima, T., Otani, T., Mochizuki, M., Nishimura, R. & Hasegawa, K. (1991). Clinical significance of the measurement of urinary hCG β-core fragment in patients with gynecologic malignant tumors. *Obstet. Gynecol. Japan*, **7**, 1197–1202.

Masure, H.R., Jaffe, W.L., Sickel, M.A., Birken, S., Canfield, R.E. & Vaitukaitis, J.L. (1981). Characterization of a small molecular size urinary immunoreactive human chorionic gonadotropin-like substance produced by the normal placenta and by hCG secreting neoplasms. *J. Clin. Endocrinol. Metab.*, **53**, 1014–20.

McGill, J., Cole, L.A., Nam, J. *et al.* (1990). Urinary gonadotropin fragment (UGF): a potential 'marker' of colorectal cancer. *J. Tumor Marker Oncol.,* **5**, 175–7.

Mise, T. & Bahl, O.P. (1980). Assignment of disulfide bonds in the α-subunit of human chorionic gonadotropin. *J. Biol. Chem.,* **255**, 8516–22.

Mise, T. & Bahl, O.P. (1981). Assignment of disulfide bonds in the β-subunit of human chorionic gonadotropin. *J. Biol. Chem.,* **256**, 6587–92.

Mizuochi, T., Nishimura, R., Derappe, C. *et al.* (1983). Structures of the asparagine-linked sugar chains of human chorionic gonadotropin produced in choriocarcinoma. Appearance of triantennary sugar chains and unique biantennary sugar chains. *J. Biol. Chem.,* **258**, 14126–9.

Mizuochi, T., Nishimura, R., Taniguchi, T. *et al.* (1985). Comparison of carbohydrate structure between human chorionic gonadotropin present in urine of patients with trophoblastic diseases and healthy individuals. *Japan J. Cancer Res.,* **76**, 752–9.

Mochizuki, M. *et al.* (1991). Clinical significance of the measurement of urinary hCG beta core fragment in patients with gynecologic malignant tumors (in Japanese). *Obstet. Gynecol. Japan,* **7**, 1197–1205.

Nagelberg, S.B., Cole, L.A. & Rosen, S.W. (1985). A novel form of ectopic human chorionic gonadotrophin beta subunit in the serum of a woman with epidermoid cancer. *J. Endocrinol.,* **107**, 403–8.

Nagelberg, S.B., Marmorstein, B., Khazaeli, M.B. & Rosen, S.W. (1989). Isolated ectopic production of the free beta subunit of chorionic gonadrotropin by an epidermoid carcinoma of unknown primary site. *Cancer,* **55**, 1924–30.

Nam, J.H., Cole, L.A., Chambers, J.T. & Schwartz, P.E. (1990a). Urinary gonadotropin fragment, a new tumor marker: I. Assay development and cancer specificity. *Gynecol. Oncol.,* **36**, 383–90.

Nam, J.H., Chang, K.C., Chambers, J.T., Schwartz, P.E. & Cole, L.A. (1990b). Urinary gonadotropin fragment, a new tumor marker: III. Use in cervical and vulvar cancers. *Gynecol. Oncol.,* **38**, 66–70.

Nam, J.H., Chambers, J.T., Schwartz, P.E. & Cole, L.A. (1990c). Urinary gonadotropin fragment, a new tumor marker: IV. Use in endometrial and uterine cancers. *Gynecol. Oncol.,* **39**, 353–7.

Nishimura, R., Ide, K., Utsunomiya, T., Kitajima, T., Yuki, Y. & Mochizuki, M. (1988). Fragmentation of the β-subunit of human chorionic gonadotropin produced by choriocarcinoma. *Endocrinology,* **123**, 420–5.

Norman, R.J., Buck, R.H., Aktar, B., Mayet, N. & Moodley, J. (1990). Dectection of a small molecular species of human chorionic gonadotropin in the urine of patients with carcinoma of the cervix and cervical intraepithelial neoplasia: comparison with other assays for human chorionic gonadotropin and its fragments. *Gynecol. Oncol.,* **37**, 254–9.

Ozturk, M., Bellet, D., Manil, L., Hennen, G., Frydman, R. & Wands, J. (1987). Physiological studies of human chorionic gonadotropin (hCG), αhCG, and βhCG as measured by specific monoclonal immunoradiometric assays. *Endocrinology,* **120**, 549–55.

Ozturk, M., Berkowitz, R., Goldstein, D., Bellet, D. & Wands, J. (1988). Differential production of human chorionic gonadotropin and free subunits in gestational trophoblast disease. *Am. J. Obstet. Gynecol.,* **158**, 193–9.

Ozturk, M., Milunsky, A., Brambati, B., Sachs, E.S., Miller, S.L. & Wands, J.R. (1990). Abnormal maternal serum levels of human chorionic gonadotropin free subunits in trisomy 18. *Am. J. Med. Genet.,* **36**, 480–3.

Papapetrou, P.D. & Nicopoulou, S.C. (1986). The origin of a human chorionic gonadotropin beta-fragment in the urine of patients with cancer. *Acta Endocrinol.*, **112**, 415–22.

Puisieux, A., Bellet, D., Troalen, F. *et al.* (1990). Occurrence of fragmentation of free and combined forms of the β-subunit of human chorionic gonadotropin. *Endocrinology*, **126**, 687–94.

Rosa, C., Amr, S., Birken, S., Wehmann, R. & Nisula, B. (1984). Effect of desialylation of human chorionic gonadotropin on its metabolic clearance rate in humans. *J. Clin. Endocrinol. Metab.*, **59**, 1215–19.

Rotmensch, S., Liberati, M., Kardana, A., Mahoney, M., Hobbins, J.C. & Cole, L.A. (1992). Peptide heterogeneity of human chorionic gonadotropin (hCG) and its β-subunit in Down syndrome pregnancies (abstract). *Annual Meeting of Society of Perinatal Obstetricians.*

Schwartz, P.E., Chambers, J.T., Taylor, K. *et al.* (1991). Early detection of ovarian cancer: preliminary results of the Yale Early Detection Program. *Yale J. Biol. Med.*, **64**, 573–82.

Siler-Khodr, T.M. (1988). Chorionic peptides. In *Cellular and Integrative Mechanisms in the Onset of Labor*, ed. D. McNellis, J.R.G. Challis, P.C. MacDonald, P. Nathanielsz & J. Roberts, pp. 213–32. Ithaca, New York: Perinatology Press.

Spencer, K. (1991). Evaluation of an assay of the free beta-subunit of choriogonadotropin and its potential value in screening for Down's syndrome. *Clin. Chem.*, **37**, 809–14.

Spencer, K. (1992). Free beta-hCG as first-trimester marker for fetal trisomy. *Lancet*, **339**, 1480.

Wehmann, R.E. & Nisula, B.C. (1980). Characterisation of a discrete degradation product of human chorionic gonadotrophin β-subunit in humans. *J. Clin. Endocrinol. Metab.*, **51**, 101–5.

Wehmann, R., Blithe, D., Akar, H. & Nisula, B. (1990). Disparity between β-core levels in pregnancy urine and serum: implications for the origin of urinary β-core. *J. Clin. Endocrinol. Metab.*, **70**, 371–8.

Weintraub, B.D. & Rosen, S.W. (1973). Ectopic production of the isolated beta subunit of human chorionic gonadotropin. *J. Clin. Invest.*, **52**, 3135–51.

Wong, Y., Schwartz, P.E., Chambers, J.T. & Cole, L.A. (1988). Urinary gonadotropin fragments (UGF) in cancers of the female reproductive system: II. Initial serial studies. *Gynecol. Oncol.*, **31**, 91–100.

Table 9.1. *Distribution of uE$_3$ by MoM using the Canick modification of the IM2 method and the specifically targeted second trimester assay (IM4)*

	MoM	
Percentile	IM2 kit	IM4 kit
2.5	0.71	0.35
5.0	0.78	0.47
10.0	0.83	0.58
25.0	0.89	0.75
50.0	1.00	1.00
75.0	1.15	1.36
90.0	1.27	1.70
95.0	1.35	1.86
97.5	1.45	2.11

Data from Reynolds and John (1992).

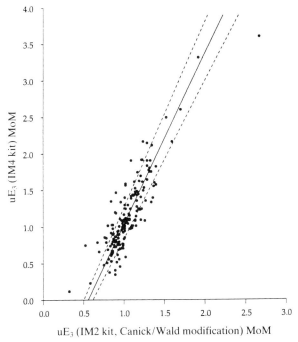

Fig. 9.2. Scatter plot comparing uE$_3$ MoMs for patient results using the IM2 modified method of Canick *et al.* (1988) and the IM4 assay. Solid line is the regression line, the dashed lines are the 95% confidence limits. (Reynolds and John (1992), reproduced with permission.)

Table 9.2. *Meta analysis of study reports of median or mean uE$_3$ levels in Down's syndrome pregnancies*

Study	Source	No. pregnancies	Median or mean
Fischer *et al.*, 1989	USA	26	0.52
Osanthanondh *et al.*, 1989	USA	26	0.62
Herrou *et al.*, 1992	France	24	0.64
Kellner *et al.*, 1991	USA	10	0.65
Del Junco *et al.*, 1989	USA	22	0.70
Ryall *et al.*, 1992	Australia	57	0.70
MacDonald *et al.*, 1991	USA	54	0.71
Haddow *et al.*, 1992	USA	35	0.72
Wald *et al.*, 1988a	UK	77	0.73
Mancini *et al.*, 1992	Italy	12	0.73
Mancini *et al.*, 1991	Italy	9	0.73
Spencer, 1991a	UK	29	0.73
Spencer *et al.*, 1992	UK	90	0.74
Reynolds *et al.*, 1993	UK	52	0.74
Nørgaard-Pedersen *et al.*, 1990	Denmark	42	0.74
Cheng *et al.*, 1993	USA	22	0.75
Davies *et al.*, 1991	UK/Germany	126	0.76
Heyl *et al.*, 1990	USA	16	0.77
Phillips *et al.*, 1992	USA	7	0.77
Canick *et al.*, 1988	USA	22	0.79
Crossley *et al.*, 1993	UK	49	0.79
Macri *et al.*, 1990a	USA	41	0.99
Macri *et al.*, 1990b	USA	27	1.09
Total No. cases		875	0.749

of 0.749. As seen in Table 9.2 there is a concentration of studies with a median between 0.7 and 0.8, with a few studies at the extremes of this distribution. Only the studies from Macri's group (Macri *et al.*, 1990a,b) have shown no difference in the median uE$_3$ between a Down's group and a control group.

Is oestriol a better predictor of Down's syndrome than other markers?

Data from our published study (Spencer *et al.*, 1992) of the use of four different markers in 90 cases of Down's syndrome and 2862 controls are summarised in Fig. 9.3. This figure shows the detection rate (% true positive) and the false-positive rate when each analyte is used independently and without combination with maternal age. On this basis both

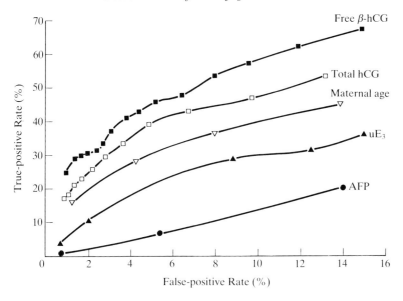

Fig. 9.3. Receiver Operator Characteristic (ROC) curves depicting variation of false-positive rate with true-positive rate for markers of Down's syndrome analysed independently. (Spencer *et al.*, 1992, reproduced with permission.)

AFP and uE_3 are seen to be less efficient predictors of Down's syndrome than maternal age, but total hCG and especially free β-hCG are considerably better at predicting Down's syndrome.

Can we describe the affected and unaffected populations statistically?

The original population paper of Wald *et al.* (1988a) suggested that, unlike AFP, uE_3 fitted a Gaussian frequency distribution without the need for log transformation of the data, yet the data as shown in Fig. 3 of that paper clearly showed Gaussian linearity only between a very narrow range of MoM values (0.4–1.4). Other studies have shown that uE_3 distributions only follow a Gaussian frequency distribution after log transformation (Nørgaard-Pedersen *et al.*, 1990; Spencer, 1991a; Reynolds *et al.*, 1991; Spencer *et al.*, 1992). Figures 9.4 and 9.5 show data from over 5000 sets of uE_3 data analysed with the IM4 kit and clearly demonstrate that log transformation is needed to make the data fit a Gaussian distribution. Recently Wald *et al.* (1992) have agreed that the data for uE_3 require log transformation in order to fit the Gaussian model.

K. Spencer

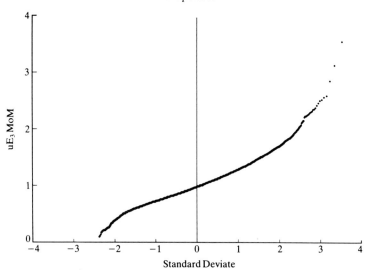

Fig. 9.4. Cumulative frequency distribution for uE_3 MoM from 5000 unaffected control cases.

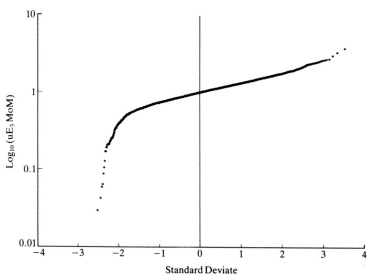

Fig. 9.5. Cumulative frequency distribution for Log_{10} uE_3 MoM from 5000 unaffected control cases.

Do we have the correct values for the statistical description of the populations?

The population parameters for use in Down's syndrome screening algorithms put forward by Wald *et al.* (1988b) have been considered by many to be the 'Gold Standard'. In Table VI of the Wald paper the population parameters for uE_3 and for AFP are said to be derived from data in the paper by Wald *et al.* (1988a). Table 9.3 shows the data specific to uE_3. On close examination it is difficult to reconcile the statement in the Wald *et al.* (1988a) paper that 'the correlation between uE_3 and log AFP is statistically significant ($r = 0.21$; $p < 0.05$ for Down's syndrome pregnancies and $r = 0.20$; $p < 0.001$ for unaffected pregnancies)' with the figures of 0.14 and 0.13 quoted in the appendix to the paper and used in the subsequent paper (Wald *et al.*, 1988b). Also it would appear that although AFP was measured on the samples in the Wald *et al.* (1988a) study using a modern sensitive IRMA assay, the actual statistics quoted are from the Cuckle *et al.* (1987) paper who used AFP values measured at the time the sample was taken, i.e. some 4 to 14 years earlier.

Table 9.4 shows the consensus picture for estimates of the width (standard deviation, S.D.) of the distribution of uE_3 in both the Down's and unaffected populations in a variety of studies. From this table it is clear that for studies using data that are not log transformed the consensus estimate of S.D. in the Down's group is closer to 0.29 rather than the 0.26 quoted by Wald *et al.* (1988a). Similarly for the unaffected group the estimate of Wald is again an under-estimate.

Wald *et al.* (1992) revised the estimates of the population parameters based on the use of ultrasound or last menstrual period (LMP) dates.

Table 9.3. *The 'Gold Standard' uE_3 population parameters after Wald et al., 1988a*

	Affected[a]	Unaffected[b]
No. cases	77	385
Median	0.73	1.00
Distribution	Linear	Linear
S.D.	0.26	0.27
Correlation: $\log_{10}$ AFP (MoM) versus $\log_{10}$ uE_3 (MoM)	0.14	0.13

[a] Down's syndrome pregnancies.
[b] Normal pregnancies.

Table 9.4. *Summary of studies showing the width (S.D.) of the uE_3 distribution*

| | Affected pregnancies | | | Unaffected pregnancies | |
	No. cases	S.D.	Distribution	No. cases	S.D.
Wald *et al.*, 1988a	77	0.26	Linear	385	0.27
Canick *et al.*, 1988	22	0.24[a]	Linear		
Heyl *et al.*, 1990	16	0.33	Linear	85	0.26
MacDonald *et al.*, 1991	54	0.29	Linear		
Crossley *et al.*, 1993	49	0.29	Linear	390	0.29
Swanson *et al.*, 1989			Linear	529	0.37
Spencer, 1991a	29	0.21	Log_{10}	140	0.16
Spencer *et al.*, 1992	90	0.21	Log_{10}	2862	0.15
Macri *et al.*, 1990b	27	0.26[a]	Log_{10}		
Macri *et al.*, 1990c	41	0.21[a]	Log_{10}		
Mancini *et al.*, 1991	9	0.15[a]	Log_{10}		
Nørgaard-Pedersen *et al.*, 1990	42	0.20	Log_{10}	291	0.12
Reynolds *et al.*, 1993	52	0.20	Log_{10}	536	0.19
Davies *et al.*, 1991	126	0.37	Log e	2765	0.30
Ryall *et al.*, 1992	57	0.41	Log e	171	0.34
Revised (adjusted)					
Wald *et al.*, 1992		0.194(LMP)[b] 0.174(scan)[c]	Log_{10}	1872	0.146(LMP) 0.118(scan)[c]

[a] Calculated from data presented in the study.
[b] Gestational dating by last menstrual period.
[c] Gestational dating by ultrasound scan.

For uE_3, unaffected pregnancies were measured with the IM4 kit and log transformation of the data was used. For the Down's population the samples were not analysed again and the data for this group were derived by taking the differences between the means, variances and co-variances for the Down's group and the unaffected group in the previous studies (Cuckle *et al.*, 1987; Wald *et al.*, 1988a,b). These differences were then added to the respective measurements in the newly measured unaffected population to achieve a 'derived' estimate for the Down's group. Clearly in the light of the data published by Reynolds and John (1992) on uE_3, the procedure used by Wald *et al.* (1992) to estimate Down's syndrome population parameters from data generated with the IM2 assay must now be of very questionable validity, as pointed out by Reynolds *et al.* (1993).

From Table 9.4, studies using the IM4 kit and log-transformed data show that the consensus S.D. for the Down's group is approximately 0.21, higher than that estimated by Wald *et al.* (1988a) for LMP-dated pregnancies. The data of Reynolds *et al.* (1993) which are based solely on ultrasound-dated pregnancies show an even greater difference between the measured S.D. and the estimate of Wald *et al.* (1992). With the unaffected population, the measured S.D. of Wald *et al.* (1992) also appears to be on the low side of consensus estimates. The impact of incorrect estimates of population parameters on the projected detection rate and false-positive rate with various analyte combinations has been discussed in Chapter 4.

Is oestriol an independent marker?

Table 9.5 examines the various estimates of the degree of correlation of uE_3 with AFP. As can be seen, the consensus estimate for the Down's syndrome group is close to 0.40 which is a highly significant correlation and almost twice that of the estimate for LMP-dated pregnancies published by Wald *et al.* (1992). For unaffected pregnancies, the consensus estimate is 0.26 which is close to the figure published by Wald *et al.* (1992) for LMP-dated pregnancies and considerably higher than that for ultrasound-dated pregnancies. Since most of the published studies contain an approximate 50:50 mix of ultrasound and LMP dating, one would expect

Table 9.5. *Summary of studies showing the size of the correlation of uE_3 with AFP*

	Affected			Unaffected	
	No. cases	*r*	Distribution	No. cases	*r*
Wald *et al.*, 1988a	77	0.14	Linear	385	0.13
Heyl *et al.*, 1990	16	0.08	Linear	85	0.13
Crossley *et al.*, 1993	49	0.44	Linear	390	0.25
Spencer, 1991a	29	0.62	Log_{10}	140	0.19
Spencer *et al.*, 1992	90	0.37	Log_{10}	2862	0.31
Nørgaard-Pedersen *et al.*, 1990	42	0.36	Log_{10}	291	0.33
Davies *et al.*, 1991	126	0.45	Log e	2765	0.27
Ryall *et al.*, 1992	57	0.46	Log e	171	0.32
Revised (*adjusted*) Wald *et al.*, 1992		0.22(LMP)[a] 0.08(scan)[b]	Log_{10}	1872	0.28(LMP)[a] 0.10(scan)[b]

Gestational dating by last menstrual period.
Gestational dating by ultrasound scan.

the consensus estimate to lie midway between the two estimates published by Wald *et al.*, but clearly this is not the case.

What does analytical error contribute to the error in the risk estimate?

Since the early 1960s the discipline of Clinical Biochemistry has been at the forefront of laboratory medicine and diagnosis in attempts to define the 'quality' of its work. All measurements, whether they be biochemical, physical or some other entity, have associated with them an error. In medicine, measurements are often made more difficult because of the influence of biological variation (in both health and disease) on the parameter measured. Some have argued that this pursuit of analytical excellence in Clinical Biochemistry has diverted us from the real task of understanding the molecular biochemistry of disease processes. However, without analytical excellence, or at least a knowledge of how good (or bad) measurements really are, we cannot interpret our data or better understand the molecular biochemistry of disease.

In Down's syndrome screening, error in the estimate of risk is important. If we quote a risk of 1 in 200 do we really understand the size of the uncertainty in this result, i.e. does it range from 1 in 150 to 1 in 250 or is the confidence interval much wider (Spencer and Carpenter, 1991)? One of the components that contributes to the error in the estimate of risk is gestational dating error, either based on incorrect recording of LMP dates, errors in the ultrasound measurement of gestation (Reynolds *et al.*, 1992) or how gestational dates are treated mathematically (Reynolds, 1992). Other errors include imprecision in the measurement of the various analytes.

In order to look at the impact of analyte imprecision on risk, Table 9.6 shows the between-assay imprecision (at Down's-like analyte levels) calculated as the median performance of five laboratories using the AFP,

Table 9.6. *Between-assay imprecision at Down's syndrome-like analyte levels: median performance of five laboratories using the Kodak assays*

Analyte	Concen-tration	(MoM)	S.D.	(MoM)	+2 S.D. as MoM	−2 S.D. as MoM
AFP	21	(0.70)	0.7	(0.02)	0.74	0.66
Total hCG	49	(2.00)	2.7	(0.11)	2.22	1.78
uE$_3$	3.0	(0.70)	0.35	(0.08)	0.86	0.54

MoM calculated at 16 weeks of gestation.

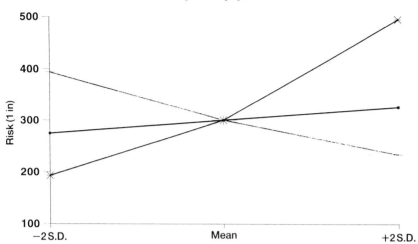

Fig. 9.6. Impact of analyte imprecision on risk calculated by varying one of the analytes by ±2 S.D. around its mean, whilst keeping the other two analytes fixed at their mean value. Risk calculated for a 25-year-old woman with a mean AFP of 0.70 MoM, total hCG mean of 2.00 MoM, uE_3 mean of 0.70 MoM and using the Wald *et al.* (1988b) algorithm. Analyte varied: AFP, ■; hCG, +; uE_3, *.

total hCG and uE_3 assays of Kodak Clinical Diagnostics. The table also shows the data expressed as MoM for a pregnancy of 16 weeks gestation and shows the MoM expressed as a ±2 S.D. range. If we then take these data and use them to calculate Down's syndrome risk using the Wald *et al.* (1988b) model, by keeping the maternal age fixed at 25 years and fixing two of the analytes at their mean MoM, we can show the effect of varying the third analyte from +2 S.D. to −2 S.D. and observe how this would influence risk. Figure 9.6 shows the results of such an experiment for each of the three analytes. It is clear that variation of uE_3 around its typical assay imprecision results in a variation of risk of some 300, which is twice that for total hCG (160) and 5-fold that for AFP (60). This obviously means that, of all analytes, variability in the measurement of uE_3 is likely to have the greatest influence on the variability of the risk. Spencer (1991b) and Reynolds (1992) have tried to simulate mathematically the impact of analytical error on the risk estimate when various analyte combinations were used. Reynolds has predicted that the use of two analytes is probably the optimum if the variability of the risk is to be kept below 20%, and that the addition of the third analyte (uE_3) adds significantly to the error in the risk, with coefficients of variation (CVs) of the order of 25–35%. Although Reynolds' data are based on computer simulation studies there

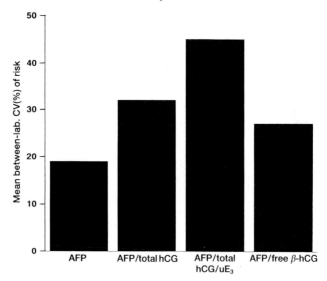

Fig. 9.7. UK EQAS scheme mean between-laboratory variation of risk estimate over the period April 1992–3, identified by analyte combination used.

is some evidence to support his model. For example, Fig. 9.7 shows data from the UKEQAS Scheme for Down's syndrome screening in which the mean between-laboratory variation in the estimate of risk is seen to increase almost linearly as further analytes are added such that with the triple-test combination an average between-laboratory CV of 45% is observed. Data from Holding (1991) also indicate that the CV of the risk is high in situations in which the triple test is used, but when dual combinations such as the AFP + free β-hCG protocol are used, variability of the risk is considerably less (10%) (Spencer and Carpenter, 1991). Clearly reporting a risk value which could have a within-laboratory between-assay CV as high as 20–30% is not acceptable.

How do oestriol estimates perform in practice?

The benchmark or 'Gold Standard' performance prediction for Down's syndrome screening is that based on the data published by Wald et al. (1988b). This study of 77 Down's syndrome cases and 385 unaffected cases predicted a 61% detection rate (CI: 49–72%) at a 5% false-positive rate when AFP, total hCG and uE_3 were used in combination. Using only AFP and total hCG, the predicted detection rate fell to 55% (CI: 43–66%) at the same false-positive rate. Clearly with overlapping confidence intervals the difference in the two detection rates cannot be considered statistically significant.

MacDonald *et al.* (1991) in a retrospective study of 54 Down's syndrome cases and 657 unaffected cases showed that using two analytes (AFP + total hCG) a 48% detection rate (CI: 34–62%) with a 6.2% false-positive rate was achieved. Using the same risk cut-off, they showed that when uE_3 was added, although the detection rate increased to 60% (CI: 45–72%) the false-positive rate also increased to 7.7%: almost certainly negating most of the benefit of the increased detection. This pattern of increased false-positive rate on the inclusion of uE_3 was also observed by Macri *et al.* (1991) when they incorporated uE_3 along with AFP and free β-hCG in a prospective evaluation of 1410 unaffected cases. They showed, at the same risk cut-off, that the false-positive rate increased from 5.3% to 7.5%, although the impact of this addition on detection rate was not investigated.

Our own published data (Spencer *et al.*, 1992) from a large retrospective study of 90 Down's syndrome cases and 2862 unaffected controls in which the performance of AFP + total hCG was compared with AFP + free β-hCG and both with and without uE_3, are summarised in the receiver operator characteristic (ROC) plot in Fig. 9.8. In this study, AFP and free β-hCG produced a 60% detection rate (CI: 49–70%) at a 5% false-positive rate; the inclusion of uE_3 made no change in either detection rate or false-positive rate. For AFP and total hCG, a 51% detection rate (CI: 40–62%) was achieved at a 5% false-positive rate; the inclusion of uE_3 resulted in a 1% fall in detection rate.

In a prospective study of 7718 women, Cheng *et al.* (1993) identified 19 out of 22 cases of Down's syndrome using the three marker approach, giving an 86% detection rate (CI: 65–97%) at a 5% false-positive rate. Excluding uE_3 would have resulted in the net loss of 1 case detected (detection rate 82%, CI: 60–95%) for the same false-positive rate. Haddow *et al.* (1992), in a similar prospective study that used the IM2 kit examined 25 207 women (36 Down's cases), observed a 64% detection rate (CI: 46–79%) with all three markers at an initial positive rate of 6.6%. Excluding uE_3 would have resulted in the net loss of 2 cases (1 gain, 3 losses) (detection rate 58%, CI: 41–75%). Also calculation from data presented in the prospective study of Phillips *et al.* (1992) shows that from a study of 9530 women (7 Down's cases) under 35 years of age, the inclusion of uE_3 resulted in no net increase in detection rate (57%, CI: 18–90%) since 1 case was gained by inclusion and 1 case was lost. Our own prospective evaluation of 5525 women (9 Down's cases) (K. Spencer,

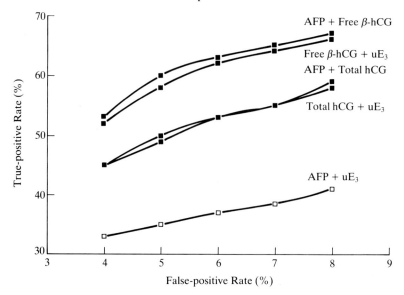

Fig. 9.8. ROC curves depicting variation of false-positive rate with true-positive rate for various combinations of biochemical markers of Down's syndrome analysed multivariately with maternal age (Spencer *et al.*, 1992; reproduced with permission).

unpublished observations) using the ALPHA software derived from the Wald *et al.* (1988b) algorithm and AFP/total hCG showed a 55% detection rate (CI: 21–86%) at a 5.4% false-positive rate. When uE_3 was included the detection rate remained the same but the false-positive rate rose to 6.6%. If the false-positive rate was fixed at 5.4%, 1 case of Down's syndrome was lost by the inclusion of uE_3, i.e. the detection rate fell to 44% (CI: 14–79%)   Data from a large retrospective clinical trial conducted by Kodak (Kodak, 1991), which included 126 Down's cases and 2765 controls, 70% of which were dated by ultrasound, also failed to demonstrate a conclusive benefit of uE_3. AFP and total hCG achieved a 55.4% detection rate at a 5% false-positive rate, adding uE_3 reduced this to 55.0% at the same false-positive rate. Therefore, even in very large studies, the benefits of including uE_3 cannot be demonstrated. Crossley *et al.* (1993) in a recently published retrospective study of 49 Down's cases and 390 controls have also shown that using AFP and total hCG a detection rate of 56% was achieved at a fixed 5% false-positive rate; this fell to 53% for the same false-positive rate when uE_3 was included. Furthermore, the data from Crossley *et al.* showed that uE_3 did not improve detection rate

Table 9.7. *The effect of ultrasound dating on* uE_3 *and AFP distribution in unaffected cases*

			S.D.	
	No. cases	Distribution	LMP^a	$Scan^b$
uE_3				
Wald *et al.*, 1992	1872	Log_{10}	0.146	0.118
Our data (unpublished)	1767	Log_{10}	0.166	0.132
AFP				
Wald *et al.*, 1992	1872	Log_{10}	0.202	0.191
Our date (unpublished)	1767	Log_{10}	0.158	0.147
Correlation r (AFP versus uE_3)			r (LMP)	r (Scan)
Wald *et al.*, 1992	1872		0.275	0.104
Our data (unpublished)	1767		0.361	0.236

[a] Gestational dating by last menstrual period.
[b] Gestational dating by ultrasound scan.

in younger women as was suggested by a short study of 18 Down's cases in women under 35 years of age by MacDonald *et al.* (1991).

Wald *et al.* (1992) revised the 'Gold Standard' population parameters based on the use of ultrasound or LMP dates, as previously described earlier. We have recently evaluated our own data (E.J. Coombes, M. Stroud and K. Spencer, unpublished data) with respect to the effect of ultrasound dating on both the width of the distribution of the unaffected populations and the influence of dating method on correlation with AFP. Our data, shown in Table 9.7, indicate a standard deviation of uE_3 for pregnancies dated by scan or LMP which is much wider than that found by Wald *et al.* Additionally, the correlation with AFP is still significant even in pregnancies dated by ultrasound. Of further note is our much tighter distribution for AFP; the effect of this would be to further reduce the influence of uE_3 in screening practice.

In a new study (Reynolds *et al.*, 1993), a set of 52 Down's syndrome cases prospectively collected in our screening programmes over the last 2 years are compared against 536 randomly selected unaffected controls. In this study, the new Wald parameters give a 5% fall in detection rate for a fixed 5% false-positive rate when uE_3 is added (Table 9.8).

Table 9.8. *Summary of detection rate and false-positive rate from the study by Reynolds* et al. *(1993) using the original (Wald* et al., *1988b) and new (Wald* et al., *1992) parameters in 52 Down's cases and 536 controls dated solely by ultrasound*

	Detection rate (%)	Confidence interval (%)	False-positive rate (%)
Original parameters			
AFP + total hCG	55	41–70	5.0
AFP + total hCG + uE_3	55	41–70	5.0
New parameters			
AFP + total hCG	55	41–70	5.0
AFP + total hCG + uE_3	50	34–64	5.0

Conclusion

The differences between the original non-optimised assay for uE_3 and a specifically optimised second-trimester assay for uE_3 have been well documented by Reynolds and John (1992). These data cast doubt on the data generated in the original studies using the IM2 kit. Certainly it is not appropriate to use population statistics derived from such an assay and then to apply these statistics to screening using the IM4 kit. Further it is inappropriate to take population statistics for the Down's group generated using the IM2 assay and then to 'adjust' the parameters for LMP dating and ultrasound dating on the basis of observations made in the unaffected population using the IM4 assay (as has been done by Wald *et al.*, 1992).

Undoubtedly levels of uE_3 are lowered in cases of fetal Down's syndrome. However, consensus estimates of the correlation with AFP have shown that the 'Gold Standard' estimate of Wald *et al.* (1988a,b) is probably an under-estimate, certainly for the Down's group and probably also for the unaffected population. Additionally, consensus estimates of the S.D. of uE_3 in both affected and unaffected populations would suggest that these were under-estimated by Wald's group.

The analytical error contributed by uE_3 is greater than the contribution from other analytes. Addition of uE_3 to screening programmes will result in a considerable widening of the error in the estimate of risk.

In practice small studies either show a positive or a negative contribution from uE_3. However the margins for error in these studies are great. This also applies to the larger studies, though in general they do not support the inclusion of uE_3.

On the basis of current evidence a case for the inclusion of uE_3 in Down's syndrome screening programmes has not and is unlikely to be proved.

References

Allen, E.J. & Lachelin, G.C.L. (1978). A comparison of plasma levels of progesterone, oestradiol, unconjugated oestriol and total oestriol with urinary total oestrogen levels in clinical practice. *Br. J. Obstet. Gynecol.,* **85**, 287–92.

Bishop, J.C., Dunstan, F.D.J., Nix, B.J., Reynolds, T.M. & Swift, A. (1993). All MoM's are not equal: some statistical properties associated with reporting results in the form of multiples of the median. *Am. J. Hum. Genet.,* **52**, 425–30.

Bogart, M.H., Pandian, M.R. & Jones, O.W. (1987). Abnormal maternal serum chorionic gondadotrophin levels in pregnancies with fetal chromosome abnormalities. *Prenatal Diagn.,* **7**, 623–30.

Canick, J.A. (1990). Screening for Down syndrome using maternal serum alpha-fetoprotein, unconjugated estriol and hCG. *J. Clin. Immunoassay,* **13**, 30–3.

Canick, J.A., Knight, G.J., Palomaki, G.E., Haddow, J.E., Cuckle, H.S. & Wald, N.J. (1988). Low second trimester maternal serum unconjugated oestriol in pregnancies with Down's syndrome. *Br. J. Obstet. Gynaecol.,* **95**, 330–3.

Cheng, E.Y., Luthy, D.A., Zebelman, A.M., Williams, M.A., Lieppman, R.E. & Hickok, D.E. (1993). A prospective evaluation of a second trimester screening test for fetal Down syndrome using maternal serum alpha fetoprotein, hCG, and unconjugated estriol. *Obstet. Gynecol.,* **81**, 72–7.

Compton, A.A., Kirkish, L.S., Parra, J., Stoecklein, S., Barclay, M.L. & McCann, D.S. (1979). Diurnal variations in unconjugated and total plasma estriol levels in late normal pregnancy. *Obstet. Gynaecol.,* **53**, 623–6.

Crossley, J.A., Aitken, D.A. & Connor, J.M. (1993). Second trimester unconjugated oestriol levels in maternal serum from chromosomally abnormal pregnancies using an optimized assay. *Prenatal Diagn.,* **13**, 271–80.

Cuckle, H.S., Wald, N.J. & Thompson, S.G. (1987). Estimating a woman's risk of having a pregnancy associated with Down's syndrome using her age and serum alpha-fetoprotein. *Br. J. Obstet. Gynaecol.,* **94**, 387–402.

Davies, C.J., Selby, C., Spencer, K. *et al.* (1991). Multicentre retrospective clinical trial for the prenatal detection of Down syndrome. *Clin. Chem.,* **37**, 943.

Del Junco, D., Greenberg, F., Darnule, A. *et al.* (1989). Statistical analysis of maternal age, maternal serum alpha fetoprotein, beta human chorionic gonadotrophin and unconjugated estriol for Down syndrome screening in mid trimester. *Am. J. Hum. Genet.,* **45**, A257.

Fischer, R.A., Suppnik, C.K., Peabody, C.T. *et al.* (1989). Maternal serum chorionic gonadotrophin, unconjugated estriol, and alpha fetoprotein in Down syndrome pregnancies. *Am. J. Hum. Genet.,* **45**, A259.

Haddow, J.E., Palomaki, G.E., Knight, G.J. *et al.* (1992). Prenatal screening for Down's syndrome with use of maternal serum markers. *N. Engl. J. Med.,* **327**, 588–93.

Herroue, M., Leporrier, N. & Leymarie, P. (1992). Screening for fetal Down syndrome with maternal serum hCG and oestriol: a prospective study. *Prenatal Diagn.*, **12**, 887–92.

Heyl, P.S., Miller, W. & Canick, J.A. (1990). Maternal serum screening for aneuploid pregnancy by alpha fetoprotein, hCG and unconjugated estriol. *Obstet. Gynecol.*, **76**, 1025–31.

Holding, S. (1991). Biochemical screening for Down's syndrome. *Br. Med. J.*, **302**, 1275.

Jorgensen, P.I. & Trolle, D. (1972). Low urinary oestriol excretion during pregnancy in women giving birth to infants with Down's syndrome. *Lancet*, **ii**, 782–4.

Kellner, L.H., Weiss, R.R., Neuer, M. & Bock, J.L. (1991). Maternal serum screening using alpha fetoprotein, beta-human chorionic gonadotropin and unconjugated estriol (AFP⁺) in the second trimester. *Am. J. Obstet. Gynecol.*, **164**, A636.

Kodak (1991). Trial results manual: a retrospective study. Down's syndrome and neural tube defect risk assessment. Amersham, UK: Kodak Clinical Diagnostics.

MacDonald, M.L., Wagner, R.M. & Slotrick, R.N. (1991). Sensitivity and specificity of screening for Down syndrome with alpha fetoprotein, hCG, unconjugated oestriol and maternal age. *Obstet. Gynecol.*, **77**, 63–8.

Macri, J.N., Kasturi, R.V., Krantz, D.A., Cook, E.J. & Larsen, J.W. (1990a). Maternal serum alpha fetoprotein (MS-AFP) patient specific risk reporting: its use and misuse. *Am. J. Hum. Genet.*, **46**, 587–90.

Macri, J.N., Krantz, D.A., Kasturi, R.V., Cook, E.J. & Larsen, J.W. (1990b). Measurement of unconjugated estriol by enzyme linked immunosorbent assay fails to show an association with Down syndrome. *Am. J. Obstet. Gynecol.*, **162**, 1634–5.

Macri, J.N., Kasturi, R.V., Krantz, D.A., Cook, E.J., Sunderji, S.G. & Larsen, J.W. (1990c). Maternal serum Down syndrome screening: unconjugated estriol is not useful. *Am. J. Obstet. Gynecol.*, **162**, 672–3.

Macri, J.N., Kasturi, R.V., Cook, E.J. & Krantz, D.A. (1991). Prenatal screening for Down's syndrome. *Br. Med. J.*, **303**, 468.

Mancini, G., Perona, M., Dall'aminco, D. *et al.* (1991). Screening for fetal Down's syndrome with maternal serum markers – an experience in Italy. *Prenatal Diagn.*, **11**, 245–52.

Mancini, G., Perona, M., Dall'aminco, C.D., Bollati, C., Fulvia, A. & Carbonara, A.O. (1992). hCG, AFP and uE₃ patterns in the 14–20th weeks of Down's syndrome pregnancies. *Prenatal Diagn.*, **12**, 619–24.

Nørgaard-Pedersen, B., Larsen, S.O., Arends, J., Svenstrup, B. & Tabor, A. (1990). Maternal serum markers in screening for Down syndrome. *Clin. Genet.*, **37**, 35–43.

Osathanondh, R., Canick, J., Abell, K.B. *et al.* (1989). Second trimester screening for trisomy 21. *Lancet*, **ii**, 52.

Parvin, C.A., Gray, D.L. & Kessler, G. (1991). Influence of assay method differences on multiple of the median distributions: maternal serum alpha fetoprotein as an example. *Clin. Chem.*, **37**, 637–42.

Phillips, O.P., Elias, S., Shulman, L.P., Andersen, R.N., Morgan, C.D. & Simpson, J.L. (1992). Maternal serum screening for fetal Down syndrome in women less than 35 years of age using alpha fetoprotein, hCG and unconjugated oestriol: a prospective 2-year study. *Obstet. Gynecol.*, **80**, 353–8.

Reynolds, T.M. (1992). Practical problems in Down syndrome screening: what should we do about gestation dating? What is the effect of assay precision on risk factors? *Comm. Lab. Med.*, **1**, 31–8.

Reynolds, T. & John, R. (1992). Comparison of assay kits for unconjugated estriol shows that expressing results as multiples of the median causes unacceptable variation in calculated risk factors for Down syndrome. *Clin. Chem.*, **38**, 1888–93.

Reynolds, T.M., Penney, M.D., Hughes, H. & John, R. (1991). The effect of weight correction on risk calculations for Down's syndrome screening. *Ann. Clin. Biochem.*, **28**, 245–9.

Reynolds, T., Penney, M. & Hughes, H. (1992). Ultrasonic dating of pregnancy results in significant errors in Down syndrome risk assessment which may be minimised by the use of biparietal diameter based means. *Am. J. Obstet. Gynecol.*, **166**, 872–7.

Reynolds, T.M., John, R. & Spencer, K. (1993). The utility of unconjugated estriol in Down syndrome screening is not proven. *Clin. Chem.*, **39**, 2023–5.

Ryall, R.G., Staples, A.J., Robertson, E.F. & Pollard, A.C. (1992). Improved performance in a prenatal screening programme for Down's syndrome incorporating serum free hCG subunit analyses. *Prenatal Diagn.*, **12**, 251–61.

Spencer, K. (1991a). Evaluation of an assay of the free beta subunit of choriogonadotropin and its potential value in screening for Down syndrome. *Clin. Chem.*, **37**, 809–14.

Spencer, K. (1991b). Analytical error in the calculation of risk in Down's syndrome screening. *Proceedings of the Association of Clinical Biochemists National Meeting* 1991, p. 107. London: Association of Clinical Biochemists.

Spencer, K. & Carpenter, P. (1991). Estimating risk of Down's syndrome. *Br. Med. J.*, **302**, 1536–7.

Spencer, K., Coombes, E.J., Mallard, A.S. & Ward, A.M. (1992). Free beta human chorionic gonadotropin in Down's syndrome screening: a multicentre study of its role compared with other biochemical markers. *Ann. Clin. Biochem.*, **29**, 506–18.

Swanson, J.R., Kenny, T. & Bissonnette, J. (1989). Maternal serum estriol in screening for Down's syndrome: significance of a high SD for the population. *Clin. Chem.*, **35**, 1193–4.

Wald, N.J. (1976). The detection of neural tube defects by screening maternal blood. In *Prenatal Diagnosis*, ed. A. Boue. *INSERM*, **61**, 227–38.

Wald, N.J., Cuckle, H.S., Densem, J.W. *et al.* (1988a). Maternal serum unconjugated oestriol as an antenatal screening test for Down's syndrome. *Br. J. Obstet. Gynaecol.*, **95**, 334–41.

Wald, N.J., Cuckle, H.S., Densem, J.W. *et al.* (1988b). Maternal serum screening for Down's syndrome in early pregnancy. *Br. Med. J.*, **297**, 883–7.

Wald, N.J., Cuckle, H.S., Densem, J.W., Kennard, A. & Smith, D. (1992). Maternal serum screening for Down's syndrome: the effect of routine ultrasound scan determination of gestational age and adjustment for maternal weight. *Br. J. Obstet. Gynaecol.*, **99**, 144–9.

10

Inhibin and CA 125 in Down's syndrome screening

J.M.M. VAN LITH

Inhibin

Inhibin is a gonadal protein that suppresses the synthesis and release of follicle stimulating hormone (FSH) in the anterior pituitary gland (Ying, 1988). During the menstrual cycle, ovarian follicles and corpora lutea secrete inhibin (MacLachlan et al., 1987a; Yamoto et al., 1991). Two forms of inhibin have been isolated (Kretser and Robertson, 1989; Healy et al., 1990; Dye et al., 1992). Both are dimers and are composed of an identical α-subunit linked by disulfide bonds to either of two β-subunits, inhibin A (α/βA) and inhibin B (α/βB). Structurally related to inhibin are activins composed of two β-subunits, activin A (βA/βA), activin AB (βA/βB) and activin B (βB/βB). Activins stimulate the production of FSH.

In pregnant women, the serum levels of immunoactive and bioactive inhibin are elevated above those found in non-pregnant women (Abe et al., 1990; Kettel et al., 1991; Tabei et al., 1991; Tovanabutra et al., 1993). During pregnancy inhibin reaches an initial peak value in the first trimester, declines after weeks 7–10 to remain relatively low during mid-gestation and, thereafter, gradually increases towards delivery. Shortly after conception, immediately after the appearance of human chorionic gonadotropin (hCG), there is an initial rise in inhibin levels, possibly reflecting secretion by the corpus luteum in response to stimulation by hCG (Santoro et al., 1992; Norman et al., 1993). The placenta will be the main source of inhibin synthesis, especially after the luteo-placental shift. Minami et al. (1992) reported immunohistochemical staining of all three subunits of inhibin in the syncytiotrophoblast. Petraglia et al. (1991) reported the α-subunit to be localized in the cytotrophoblast. The discrepancy might be explained by the difficulty of distinguishing syncytio-trophoblast and cytotrophoblast on the basis of histologic appearance, especially in placentae at term (Minami et al., 1992). The role of inhibin in pregnancy remains obscure. Inhibin and activin might have a paracrine function within the fetoplacental unit. Inhibin reverses the stimulating effect of activin on hCG production and suppresses the effects of gonadotropin-releasing hormone (GnRH) on hCG secretion (Petraglia *et al.*, 1987, 1989). Mersol-Barg *et al.* (1990) showed, in an *in vitro* placental explant culture model, that inhibin suppresses hCG secretion in term but not in first trimester placentae. Another possible role for inhibin and activin is in embryogenesis, as similar proteins have been reported to play a role in the embryogenesis of *Drosophila* and inhibin and activin mRNAs have been found in the embryogenesis of the rat (MacLachlan *et al.*, 1987b; Padgett *et al.*, 1987).

Inhibin and Down's syndrome

Second trimester

Van Lith *et al.* (1992) reported significant elevated levels of maternal serum immunoreactive inhibin during the second trimester in Down's syndrome pregnancies. This report was confirmed by Spencer *et al.* (1993) and Cuckle *et al.* (1993) (Table 10.1). In the three studies, inhibin was assayed using an enzyme immunoassay specific for the α-peptide of human inhibin. Inhibin can discriminate between pregnancies with a chromosomally normal and a Down's syndrome fetus. In van Lith's and Spencer's report, approximately 50% of the Down's syndrome pregnancies were above the 90th percentile. However, in Cuckle's report only 25% were above this value.

Before incorporating inhibin in a second trimester screening programme for Down's syndrome, it is important to know the correlation with other factors, especially hCG. Spencer and Cuckle calculated the correlation between inhibin and free β-hCG and hCG, respectively, which is for both

Table 10.1. *Results of studies of maternal serum immunoreactive inhibin and fetal Down's syndrome*

Study	Normal	Down's syndrome	MoM	95% CI	Positive (%)	Detection (%)
van Lith *et al.*, 1992	80	10	1.9	1.3–2.8	10	50
Spencer *et al.*, 1993	75	15	3.6	1.8–7.5	10	73
Cuckle *et al.*, 1993	90	19	1.3	0.9–1.9	10	25

0.70 in the Down's syndrome group and 0.26 in the normal group. The clear correlation between inhibin and hCG in Down's syndrome pregnancies means that not much information will be gained by measuring both markers. Thus, the sensitivity will be more or less the same. The correlation in the normal group is low, meaning extra information could be gained by measuring inhibin. This could increase the specificity, thus decreasing the number of false positives. This could be of advantage for Down's syndrome screening. More data are needed to calculate more precisely the impact of inhibin on maternal serum screening.

First trimester

The Dutch Working Party on Prenatal Diagnosis has initiated a study of first trimester biochemical markers for Down's syndrome (van Lith, 1992). As part of that multicentre study, inhibin was measured in 284 chromosomally normal and 23 Down's syndrome pregnancies (van Lith *et al.*, 1994). The median MoM in the Down's syndrome pregnancies was 1.3 (95% CI: 0.8–2.1). There was no significant difference between normals and Down's syndrome pregnancies.

Amniotic fluid

We measured inhibin in amniotic fluid samples (van Lith *et al.*, 1993a) collected at the antenatal diagnosis unit of the University Hospital of Groningen and stored frozen at $-70°C$. From the amniotic fluid bank, 30 samples from Down's syndrome and 90 samples from normal pregnancies were identified. The median MoM in the Down's syndrome pregnancies was 0.9 (95% CI: 0.7–1.2). The distributions of amniotic fluid inhibin did not differ between the two groups. However, it was notable that the concentration of inhibin in amniotic fluid was 10 times higher than in maternal serum.

Conclusion

Immunoreactive inhibin is elevated in maternal serum from Down's syndrome pregnancies in the second trimester. However, the role in second trimester maternal serum screening is likely to be minor. Inhibin levels correlate with those of hCG; inclusion of inhibin would have little effect on detection but might decrease false positives. There is no relation between the level of inhibin in first-trimester maternal serum or second-trimester amniotic fluid samples from Down's syndrome or normal pregnancies.

Cancer antigen 125 (CA 125)

CA 125 is a tumor-associated antigen used in gynecologic oncology, mainly for disease monitoring in patients with ovarian cancer (Yedema, 1992).

In normal pregnancies, maternal serum levels of CA 125 (MS-CA 125) show an increase during the first trimester and then decrease to low levels in the second trimester, remaining low until delivery (Niloff *et al.*, 1984; Seki *et al.*, 1986; Kobayashi *et al.*, 1989; Jacobs and Bast, 1989). CA 125 is present in decidua in relatively high concentrations and this is the most likely source of MS-CA 125 during pregnancy (O'Brien *et al.*, 1986; Kobayashi *et al.*, 1989). CA 125 might reach the maternal circulation directly via disruption of decidua or indirectly via a 'tubal reflux' mechanism (Quirk *et al.*, 1988; Kobayashi *et al.*, 1989).

The elevation of MS-CA 125 in the first trimester could result from trophoblastic invasion of decidua. Kobayashi *et al.* (1989) demonstrated increased levels of MS-CA 125 during induction and delivery when the decidua will be traumatized. During early gestation, high levels of MS-CA 125 were found some time before miscarriage and could also result from disruption of the decidua (Check *et al.*, 1990a). An association between high levels of MS-CA 125 and placental abruption supports a decidual source for CA 125 (Witt *et al.*, 1991). It seems likely that any disturbance of the decidua leads to increased levels of MS-CA 125.

CA 125 and Down's syndrome

Maternal serum

Check *et al.* (1990b) reported high levels of MS-CA 125 in chromosomally abnormal pregnancies that subsequently spontaneously aborted. Van Lith *et al.* (1991) reported low levels of MS-CA 125 in first-trimester Down's syndrome pregnancies. In a larger study, including both the first and the second trimesters and using an improved automated enzyme immunoassay for CA 125, van Lith *et al.* (1993b) could not confirm their initial results. Other reports showed no relation between MS-CA 125 and Down's syndrome (Spencer, 1991; van Blerk *et al.*, 1992; Norton and Golbus, 1992). Only Hogdall *et al.* (1992) found differences in both the first and second trimesters (Table 10.2).

Table 10.2. *Results of studies of maternal serum CA 125 and fetal Down's syndrome*

Study	Trimester	Down's syndrome	Difference detected
van Lith *et al.*, 1991	1st	9	Yes
Norton and Golbus, 1992	1st	15	No
van Lith *et al.*, 1993b	1st + 2nd	29	No
Hogdall *et al.*, 1992	1st + 2nd	14	Yes
Spencer, 1991	2nd	25	No
van Blerk *et al.*, 1992	2nd	10	No

Amniotic fluid

Levels of CA 125 in amniotic fluid are clearly elevated compared to the CA 125 concentration in maternal serum. Van Lith *et al.* (1993a) measured the amniotic fluid CA 125 level in 90 normal and 30 Down's syndrome pregnancies. They found a median MoM in the Down's syndrome pregnancies of 0.75 (95% CI: 0.58–0.91). This was significantly different from normals (Kolmogorov–Smirnov test). However, because of the large spread of individual concentrations, there was a considerable overlap between the distributions of the two groups.

Conclusion

Most studies show no relation of maternal serum CA 125 levels with fetal Down's syndrome in early pregnancy. Some differences could be explained by impending abortion. The lower levels of CA 125 in amniotic fluid in Down's syndrome pregnancy cannot be explained but is of no great clinical relevance. CA 125 is not a useful marker for Down's syndrome pregnancies.

References

Abe, Y., Hasegawa, Y., Miyamoto, K. *et al.* (1990). High concentrations of plasma immunoreactive inhibin during normal pregnancy in women. *J. Clin. Endocrinol. Metab.*, **71**, 133–7.

Check, J.H., Nowroozi, K., Winkel, C.A., Johnson, T. & Seefried, L. (1990a). Serum CA 125 levels in early pregnancy and subsequent spontaneous abortion. *Obstet. Gynecol.*, **75**, 742–3.

Check, J.H., Nowroozi, K., Vaze, M., Wapner, R. Seefried, L. (1990b). Very high CA 125 levels during early first trimester in three cases of spontaneous abortion with chromosomal abnormalities. *Am. J. Obstet. Gynecol.*, **162**, 674–5.

Cuckle, H.S., Holding, S. & Jones, R. (1993). Maternal serum inhibin levels in second trimester Down's syndrome pregnancies. *Prenatal Diagn.*, in press.

Dye, R.B., Rabinovici, J. & Jaffe, R.B. (1992). Inhibin and activin in reproductive biology, *Obstet. Gynaecol. Surv.*, **47**, 173–85.

Healy, D.L., Polson, D., Yohkachiya, T. & De Kretser, D. (1990). Inhibin and related peptides in pregnancy. *Ballière's Clin. Endocrinol. Metab.*, **4**, 233–47.

Hogdall, C.K., Hogdall, E.V.S., Arends, J., Nørgaard-Pedersen, B., Smidt-Jensen, S. & Larsen, S.O. (1992). CA-125 as a maternal serum marker for Down's syndrome in the first and second trimesters. *Prenatal Diagn.*, **12**, 223–7.

Jacobs, I. & Bast, R.C. (1989). CA 125 tumor-associated antigen; a review of literature. *Hum. Reprod.*, **4**, 1–12.

Kettel, L.M., Roseff, S.J., Bangah, M.L., Burger, H.G. & Yen, S.S.C. (1991). Circulating levels of inhibin in pregnant women at term: simultaneous disappearance with oestradiol and progesterone after delivery. *Clin. Endocrinol.*, **34**, 19–23.

Kobayashi, F., Sagawa, N., Nakamura, K. *et al.* (1989). Mechanism and clinical significance of elevated CA 125 levels in the sera of pregnant women, *Am. J. Obstet. Gynecol.*, **169**, 563–6.

Kretser de, D.M. & Robertson, D.M. (1989). The isolation and physiology of inhibin and related proteins. *Biol. Reprod.*, **40**, 33–47.

MacLachlan, R.I., Robertson, D.M., Healy, D.L., Burger, H.G. & de Kretser, D.M. (1987a). Circulating immunoreactive inhibin levels during the normal menstrual cycle. *J. Clin. Endocrinol. Metab.*, **65**, 954–61.

MacLachlan, R.I., Burger, H.G., Healy, D.L., de Kretser, D.M. & Robertson, D.M. (1987b). Circulating immunoactive inhibin in the luteal phase and early gestation of women undergoing ovulation induction. *Fertil. Steril.*, **48**, 1001–5.

Minami, S., Yamoto, M., Nakano, R. (1992). Immunohistochemical localization of inhibin/activin subunits in human placenta. *Obstet. Gynecol.*, **80**, 410–14.

Mersol-Barg, M.S., Miller, K.F., Choi, C.M., Lee, A.C. & Kim, M.H. (1990). Inhibin suppresses human chorionic gonadotropin secretion in term, but not first trimester, placenta. *J. Clin. Endocrinol. Metab.*, **71**, 1294–8.

Niloff, J.M., Knapp, R.C., Schaetzl, E., Reynolds, C. & Bast, R.C. (1984). CA 125 antigen levels in obstetric and gynecologic patients. *Obstet. Gynecol.*, **64**, 703–7.

Norman, R.J., Matthews, C.D., McLoughlin, J.W. *et al.* (1993). Inhibin and relaxin concentrations in early singleton, multiple and failing pregnancy: relationship to gonadotropin and steroid profiles. *Fertil. Steril.*, **59**, 130–7.

Norton, M.E. & Golbus, M.S. (1992). Maternal serum CA 125 for aneuploidy detection in early pregnancy. *Prenatal Diagn.*, **12**, 779–81.

O'Brien, T.J., Hardin, J.W., Bannon, G.A., Norris, J.S. & Quirk, J.G. (1986). CA 125 antigen in human amniotic fluid and fetal membranes. *Am. J. Obstet. Gynecol.*, **155**, 50–5.

Padgett, R.W., St Johnston, R.D., Gelbart, W.M. (1987). A transcript from Drosophila pattern gene predicts a protein homologous to the transforming growth-factor-B family. *Nature*, **325**, 81.

Petraglia, F., Sawchenko, P., Lim, A.T.W., Rivier, J. & Vale, W. (1987). Localization, secretion and action of inhibin in human placenta. *Science*, **237**, 187–9.

Petraglia, F., Vaughan, J. & Vale, W. (1989). Inhibin and activin modulate the release of gonadotropin-releasing hormone, human chorionic gonadotropin and progesterone from cultured human placental cells. *Proc. Natl. Acad. Sci. USA*, **86**, 5114–17.

Petraglia, F., Garuti, G.C., Calza, L., Roberts, V., Giardino, L. & Genazzani, A.R. (1991). Inhibin subunits in human placenta: localization and messenger ribonucleic acid levels during pregnancy. *Am. J. Obstet. Gynecol.*, **165**, 750–8.

Quirk, J.G., Brunson, G.L., Long, C.A., Bannon, G.A., Sanders, M.M. & O'Brien, T.J. (1988). CA 125 in tissues and amniotic fluid during pregnancy. *Am. J. Obstet. Gynecol.*, **159**, 644–9.

Santoro, N., Schneyer, A.L., Ibrahim, J. & Schmidt, C.L. (1992). Gonadotropin and inhibin concentrations in early pregnancy in women with and without corpora lutea. *Obstet. Gynecol.*, **79**, 579–85.

Seki, K., Kikuchi, Y., Uesato, T. & Kato, K. (1986). Increased serum CA 125 levels during the first trimester of pregnancy. *Acta Obstet. Gynecol. Scand.*, **65**, 583–5.

Spencer, K. (1991). Maternal serum CA 125 is not a second trimester marker for Down's syndrome. *Ann. Clin. Biochem.*, **28**, 299–300.

Spencer, K., Wood, P.J. & Anthony, F.W. (1993). Elevated levels of maternal serum inhibin immunoreactivity in second trimester pregnancies affected by Down's syndrome. *Ann. Clin. Biochem.*, **30**, 219–20.

Tabei, T., Ochiai, K., Terashima, Y. & Takanashi, N. (1991). Serum levels of inhibin in maternal and umbilical blood during pregnancy. *Am. J. Obstet. Gynecol.*, **164**, 896–900.

Tovanabutra, S., Illingworth, P.J., Ledger, W.L., Glasier, A.F. & Baird, D.T. (1993). The relationship between peripheral immunoactive inhibin, human chorionic gonadotrophin, oestradiol and progesterone during human pregnancy. *Clin. Endocrinol.*, **38**, 101–7.

van Blerk, M., Smitz, J., De Catte, L., Kumps, C., Van Der Elst, J., Van Steirteghem, A.C. (1992). Second trimester cancer antigen 125 and Down's syndrome. *Prenatal Diagn.*, **12**, 1062–6.

van Lith, J.M.M. for the Dutch Working Party on Prenatal Diagnosis (1992). First trimester maternal serum human chorionic gonadotrophin as a marker for fetal chromosomal disorders. *Prenatal Diagn.*, **12**, 495–504.

van Lith, J.M.M., Mantingh, A., Beekhuis, J.R., De Bruijn, H.W.A. & Breed, A.S.P.M. (1991). First trimester CA 125 and Down's syndrome. *Br. J. Obstet. Gynaecol.*, **98**, 493–4.

van Lith, J.M.M., Pratt, J.J., Beekhuis, J.R. & Mantingh, A. (1992). Second trimester maternal serum immunoreactive inhibin as a marker for fetal Down's syndrome. *Prenatal Diagn.*, **12**, 801–6.

van Lith, J.M.M., Mantingh, A., Pratt, J.J. & De Bruijn, H.W.A. (1993a). Amniotic fluid levels of inhibin and CA 125 in Down's syndrome pregnancies. *Prenatal Diagn.*, in press.

van Lith, J.M.M., Mantingh, A. & de Bruijn, H.W.A. (1993b). Maternal serum CA 125 in chromosomally normal and abnormal pregnancies. *Prenatal Diagn.*, **13**, 1123–32.

van Lith, J.M.M., Mantingh, A. & Pratt, J.J. (1994). First trimester maternal serum inhibin levels in chromosomally normal and abnormal pregnancies. *Obstet. Gynecol.*, **83**, 661–4.

Witt, B.R., Miles, R., Wolf, G.C., Koulianos, G.T. & Thorneycroft, I.H. (1991). CA 125 levels in abruptio placentae, *Am. J. Obstet. Gynecol.*, **164**, 1225–8.

Yamoto, M., Minami, S. & Nakano, R. (1991). Immunohistochemical localization of inhibin subunits in human corpora lutea during menstrual cycle and pregnancy. *J. Clin. Endocrinol. Metab.*, **73**, 470–7.

Yedema, C.A. (1992). Serum tumor marker CA 125 in gynaecological practice. Thesis. Utrecht: Elinkwijk.

Ying, S. (1988). Inhibins, activins and follistatins: gonadal proteins modulating the secretion of follicle-stimulating hormone. *Endocrine Rev.*, **9**, 267–93.

11

Schwangerschafts protein 1 (SP1) and biochemical screening for Down's syndrome

M.C.M. MACINTOSH

Schwangerschafts protein 1 (SP1) (also known as pregnancy-specific β_1-glycoprotein) is one of a group of proteins initially described as 'specific' to the placenta (Table 11.1). SP1 was first isolated by Russian workers in 1970 (Tatarinov and Masyukevich, 1970) and then independently a year later by Bohn (1971). The German name is now the most widely used. Meanwhile a group in Miami (Lin *et al.*, 1974) described four pregnancy-associated plasma proteins (PAPP-A/B/C/D) of which PAPP-C proved to be SP1. As further properties of this protein were discovered it was also given the name of pregnancy-specific β_1-glycoprotein.

SP1 is a glycoprotein with a molecular weight (MW) of 90 000 and β-1 electrophoretic mobility. Initial studies found two isoelectric points (Lin *et al.*, 1974). Subsequently Teisner and colleagues (1978) described two proteins with the immunochemical properties of SP1 in the serum of pregnant women. The first was the original protein described by Bohn and the second was larger (MW 400 000) and had α-2 electrophoretic mobility. This led to the designations SP1-α and SP1-β. It has been suggested that the larger molecule is formed as a combination of SP1-β and a non-pregnancy serum protein (Bohn, 1979; Ahmed and Klopper, 1980). The earlier studies did not discriminate between the two proteins but the major component in the serum is SP1-β.

In the human placenta, the fetal and maternal blood streams are separated by two layers of cells: the trophoblast and the vascular endothelium of the fetal capillaries. The trophoblast includes the syncytiotrophoblast, which is a continuous layer on the surface of the villi, and the cytotrophoblast, isolated cells on the fetal side of the syncytiotrophoblast that are prominent in the early placenta but become sparse toward term. The origin of SP1, as with most placental proteins, is the

Table 11.1. *Placental proteins*

Protein	
Human chorionic gonadotrophin	hCG
Human placental lactogen	hPL
Human placental growth hormone	hPGH
Schwangerschafts protein 1	SP1
Pregnancy-associated plasma protein A	PAPP-A
Placental protein 5	PP5
Placental alkaline phosphatase	PLAP
Placental cystine aminopeptidase	CAP

syncytiotrophoblast. It is not absolutely specific to pregnancy, being found in high concentrations in seminal plasma in the male and in ovarian follicular fluid in the female. A similar distribution is found with other placental proteins.

SP1 in normal pregnancy

SP1 appears in the blood 14 days after implantation (Grudzinskas *et al.*, 1977) and then rises rapidly in the first 6 weeks with a doubling time of 2 to 3 days (Grudzinskas *et al.*, 1979; Lenton *et al.*, 1981), a similar profile to that of human chorionic gonadotrophin (hCG). The rate of increase then slows for the remainder of the first trimester, followed by a more rapid rise in mid-trimester to reach a plateau near term. The resulting sigmoid curve (Fig. 11.1) is similar to the pattern of human placental lactogen (hPL). It reflects the growth in size of the placenta and the mass of active trophoblast.

SP1 in complications of pregnancy

In early pregnancy, maternal SP1 levels are predictive of the outcome of threatened abortion (Gordon *et al.*, 1978; Jandial *et al.*, 1978; Schultz-Larsen and Herz, 1978; Jouppila *et al.*, 1980; Sterzik *et al.*, 1986). As with hCG, SP1 levels are raised in trophoblast disease. In late pregnancy, low levels are associated with intrauterine growth retardation (Wurz *et al.*, 1981) and low birth weight with and without dysmaturity (Westergaard *et al.*, 1985). However SP1 assays have not been introduced into routine clinical practice as they confer no advantage over hCG and ultrasound.

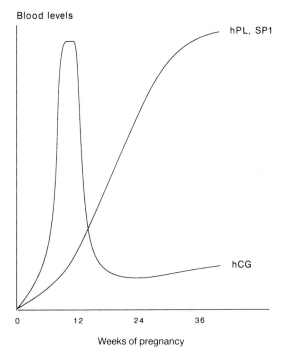

Fig. 11.1. Maternal blood levels of hCG, hPL and SP1 during pregnancy.

Maternal serum SP1 (MSSP1) levels and Down's syndrome pregnancies

The first biochemical marker to be associated with Down's syndrome was low levels of α-fetoprotein (Merkatz *et al.*, 1984). Subsequently other markers have been described, in particular hCG and unconjugated oestriol. A combination of these markers can identify some 60% of Down's syndrome pregnancies with a 5% screen-positive rate (Wald *et al.*, 1988). At least 12 other biochemical markers have been reported (Cuckle, 1992) including SP1. Current screening programmes address the second trimester (15–20 weeks). However with the advent of chorionic villus sampling (CVS) and early amniocentesis there are major efforts to identify first-trimester markers for Down's syndrome (reviewed by Macintosh and Chard, 1992, 1993).

Second trimester studies

Bartels and Lindemann (1988) were the first to report elevated levels of SP1 in Down's syndrome; the increase was similar to that of hCG.

Table 11.2. *Second trimester studies on maternal serum SP1 in chromosomally abnormal pregnancies*

Study	No. and type of abnormal pregnancy		MSSP1 (MoM)	Gestation (weeks)	Variation in normal median
Bartels and Lindemann, 1988	24	tr[a] 21	2.1 (mean of all samples)	16–19	26.9 mg/l throughout
	4	tr 18			
Wald et al., 1989	77	tr 21	1.2 (median of sample)		8% increase per week
Petrocik et al., 1990	46	tr 21	45/46: >1 MoM	15–20	
Bartels et al., 1990	43	tr 21	1.54 (median of all samples)	14–24	
	12	tr 18			
	2	tr 13			
	5	Others			
Spencer, 1991	18	tr 21	1.035 (median of sample)	16–18	16% increase per week
Graham et al., 1992	48	tr 21	1.17 (median)	15–20	8% increase per week
	9	tr 18	0.87 (median)		
	4	tr 13	1.01 (median)		
	9	SCA[a]	0.93 (median)		
	4	bal trans[b]	0.79 (median)		
	8	unbal trans[b]	0.52 (median)		

[a] Trisomy.
[b] Sex chromosome anomalies.
[c] Balanced and unbalanced translocations.

Subsequent studies (Table 11.2) have shown less striking elevations (Knight *et al.*, 1989; Wald *et al.*, 1989; Bartels *et al.*, 1990; Petrocik *et al.*, 1990; Graham *et al.*, 1992) or no association (Spencer, 1991). A possible reason for the disparity in findings is that in the original Bartel's study the maternal samples were taken after amniocentesis. However, a more likely explanation is the problem of determining stable normal medians with a limited sample size. All studies express data as multiples of the normal median (MoM). The normal median values for the second trimester (Table 11.2) in the studies vary from no change with gestational age (Bartels and Lindemann, 1988) to a 16% increase in value with each week (Spencer, 1991). Under- or overestimation of normal medians will yield a false increase or decrease in values expressed as MoM.

First trimester studies

Brock and colleagues (1990) published the first study on maternal levels of SP1 in the first trimester. They found reduced levels (0.79 MoM; 21 Down's syndrome pregnancies), although this was not statistically significant. A subsequent study (Macintosh *et al.*, 1993) found significantly reduced levels (0.4 MoM; 14 Down's syndrome pregnancies). There are two major differences between the studies. The Brock study used Down's syndrome cases diagnosed at birth and maternal samples were collected relatively late (only one was taken before 9 weeks). By contrast our own study comprised cases diagnosed at CVS and 13 of the 14 samples were collected before 9 weeks. When Down's syndrome cases are identified at CVS it is not known whether these would have survived to term. The low SP1 levels might therefore reflect the abortion process which is commonly associated with chromosomal abnormality. In addition, the reduction in SP1 may be greater in very early pregnancy.

Trisomy 18 and maternal serum biochemistry

Trisomy 18 pregnancies appear to be associated with very low maternal serum hCG in the second trimester (Table 11.3) although all studies are based on small numbers. There is also some evidence of a bimodal distribution of hCG levels with a few cases having very elevated levels (Bogart *et al.*, 1987; Blizer *et al.*, 1991; Greenberg *et al.*, 1992). Second-trimester MSSP1 levels are normal in trisomy 18 pregnancies when the corresponding levels of hCG are reduced (Bartels *et al.*, 1990; Graham *et al.*, 1992). In the first trimester, some but not all studies find either

Table 11.3. *Studies on hCG and SP1 levels in trisomy 18 pregnancies*

Study	Numbers	Gestation (weeks)		Analyte measured and findings
Second-trimester studies				
Bogart et al., 1987	3	19–20	hCG	2 very low, 1 very high
Bogart et al., 1989	2	18–21	hCG	Low
			αhCG	Normal
Bartels et al., 1990	12	14–24	hCG	7/12: <0.25 MoM; 1/12: >3.0 MoM
			SP1	Normal
Canick et al., 1990	10	15–21	hCG	Low (median 0.27 MoM)
Blizer et al., 1991	13	—	hCG	Low (median 0.27 MoM, range 0.05–2.29 MoM)
Crossley et al., 1991	4	15–20	hCG	All <0.4 MoM
Graham et al., 1992	9	15–20	hCG	Low (median 0.21 MoM)
			SP1	Normal (median 0.87 MoM)
Greenberg et al., 1992	14	15–18	hCG	9/14: <0.4 MoM; 3/4 very high
First trimester studies				
Ozturk et al., 1990	8	8–12	αhCG/hCG	High α-hCG/hCG
Nebiolo et al., 1990	6	8–12	αhCG/hCG	High α-hCG/hCG
Kratzer et al., 1991	7	9–12	hCG	High α-hCG/hCG
			αhCG/hCG	
van Lith, 1992	6	<13	hCG	Normal (median 0.8 MoM)
Macintosh et al., 1993	8	6–12	SP1	Normal (median 1.1 MoM)
Spencer et al., 1993	5	7–13	hCG	Low (median 0.17 MoM)

reduced hCG or raised αhCG/hCG ratios associated with trisomy 18. SP1 levels appear normal (Table 11.3).

Physiology of biochemical changes seen in chromosomally abnormal pregnancies

The mechanism of the biochemical changes observed in the serum of mothers with chromosomally abnormal pregnancies is unknown. In the second trimester in Down's syndrome there is an increase in most placental markers (hCG, hPL, SP1, progesterone) and a decrease in markers dependent on the presence of the fetus (oestriol, dehydro-epiandrosterone, AFP). In the first trimester the placental markers are not raised and in the case of SP1 may be reduced.

There have been two theories which might explain the biological phenomena. The combination of raised hCG levels and low AFP levels in the second trimester led to the hypothesis that the pregnancy was relatively immature. This was refuted by the observation of raised SP1 levels. Another explanation is that the placenta hypertrophies as a compensatory response to reduced fetal growth. The low levels of SP1 in the first trimester would imply that this compensation does not occur early on in the pregnancy.

The biochemical patterns depend on the type of chromosome abnormality. Thus low hCG levels in the second trimester in trisomy 18 pregnancies might be the result of a small placenta. However, SP1 levels (also a reflection of placental mass) in trisomy 18 appear to be normal in both the first and second trimesters. It is notable that a high proportion (70%) of Down's syndrome pregnancies in the second trimester survive to viability, as compared to the minority (30%) of trisomy 18 (Hook, 1983). The raised levels of placental proteins seen in the second trimester in Down's syndrome but not in other abnormalities may be the result of a process which maintains viability of these pregnancies.

Conclusions

In the second trimester, Down's syndrome is associated with raised MSSP1 levels. However, not all findings are consistent and some differences may be due to the lack of well established normal median values. It seems unlikely that measurement of SP1 in the second trimester would confer any advantage over the use of hCG. It also does not add significantly to detection rates when combined with the more commonly used markers (α-fetoprotein, hCG, oestriol). In the first trimester, preliminary findings show reduced levels associated with Down's syndrome but not to a degree which might suggest that it could be an efficient single marker. The changes seen in MSSP1 in Down's syndrome are not seen in trisomy 18. It is suggested that the increased levels of SP1 in the second trimester are secondary to a process maintaining viability in a Down's syndrome pregnancy.

References

Ahmed, A.G. & Klopper, A. (1980). Separation of two pregnancy associated plasma proteins with SP1 determinants and the conversion of SP1 beta to SP1 alpha. *Arch. Gynaecol.*, **230**, 95–108.

Bartels, I. & Lindemann, A. (1988). Maternal levels of pregnancy-specific β1-glycoprotein (SP-1) are elevated in pregnancies affected by Down's syndrome. *Hum. Genet.*, **80**, 46–8.

Bartels, I., Thiele, M. & Bogart, M.H. (1990). Maternal serum hCG and SP1 in pregnancies with fetal aneuploidy. *Am. J. Med. Genet.*, **37**, 261–4.

Blizer, M., Carmi, R., Blakemore, K., Andrews, N.J., Romem, I. & Schwarz, S. (1991). Low maternal serum human chorionic gonadotropin (MS-hCG) in the second trimester trisomy 18 pregnancies. *Am. J. Hum. Genet.*, **49**(Suppl.), 211.

Bogart, M.H., Pandian, M.R. & Jones, O.W. (1987). Abnormal maternal serum chorionic gonadotropin levels in pregnancies with fetal chromosome abnormalities. *Prenatal Diagn.*, **7**, 623–30.

Bogart, M.H., Golbus, M.S., Sorg, N.D. & Jones, O.W. (1989). Human chorionic gonadotropin levels in pregnancies with aneuploid fetuses. *Prenatal Diagn.*, **9**, 379–84.

Bohn, H. (1971). Nachweis und Charakteriserung von Schwangwerschaftsproteinen in der menschlichen Plazenta, sowie ihre quantitative immunologische Bestimmung im Serum schwangerer Frauen. *Arch. Gynakol.*, **210**, 440–57.

Bohn, H. (1979). Placental and pregnancy proteins. In *Carcino-embryonic Proteins*, ed. F.G. Lehmann, p. 279. Amsterdam: Elsevier.

Brock, D.J.H., Barron, L., Holloway, S., Liston, W.A., Hillier, S.G. & Seppala, M. (1990). First-trimester maternal serum biochemical indicators in Down syndrome. *Prenatal Diagn.*, **10**, 245–51.

Canick, J.A., Palomaki, G.E. & Osathanondh, R. (1990). Prenatal screening for trisomy 18 in the second trimester. *Prenatal Diagn.*, **10**, 546–8.

Crossley, J.A., Aitken, D.A. & Connor, J.M. (1991). Prenatal screening for chromosome abnormalities using maternal serum chorionic gonadotrophin, alpha-fetoprotein, and age. *Prenatal Diagn.*, **11**, 83–101.

Cuckle, H.S. (1992). Measuring unconjugated estriol in maternal serum to screen for fetal Down syndrome. *Clin. Chem.*, **38**, 1687–9.

Gordon, Y.B., Lewis, J.D., Pendlebury, D.J., Leighton, M. & Gold, J. (1978). Is measurement of placental function and maternal weight worthwhile? *Lancet* **1**, 1001–3.

Graham, G.W., Crossley, J.A., Aitken, D.A. & Connor, J.M. (1992). Variation in the levels of pregnancy specific β1-glycoprotein in maternal serum from chromosomally abnormal pregnancies. *Prenatal Diagn.*, **12**, 505–12.

Greenberg, F., Schmidt, D., Darnule, A.T., Weyland, B.R., Rose, E. & Alpert, E. (1992). Maternal serum α-fetoprotein, β-human chorionic gonadotropin, and unconjugated estriol levels in midtrimester trisomy 18 pregnancies. *Am. J. Obstet. Gynaecol.*, **166**, 1388–92.

Grudzinskas, J.G., Gordon, Y.B., Jeffrey, D. & Chard, T. (1977). Specific and sensitive determination of pregnancy-specific beta1-glycoprotein. *Lancet* **1**, 333–5.

Grudzinskas, J.G., Lenton, E.A. & Obiekwe, B.C. (1979). Studies on SP1 and PP5 in early pregnancy. In *Placental Proteins*, ed. A. Klopper & T. Chard, pp. 119–34. Heidelberg: Springer-Verlag.

Hook, E.B. (1983). Chromosome abnormalities and spontaneous fetal death following amniocentesis: further data and associations with maternal age. *Am. J. Hum. Genet.*, **35**, 110–16.

Jandial, V., Towler, C., Horne, C.H. & Abramovich, D.R. (1978). Plasma pregnancy-specific beta-glycoprotein in complications of early pregnancy. *Br. J. Obstet. Gynaecol.*, **85**, 832–6.

Joupilla, P., Seppala, M. & Chard, T. (1980). Pregnancy-specific beta-glycoprotein in complications of early pregnancy. *Lancet*, **1**, 667–8.

Knight, G.J., Palomaki, G.E., Haddow, J.E., Johnson, A.M., Osathanondh, R. & Canick, J.A. (1989). Maternal serum levels of the placental products hCG, hPL, SP1 and progesterone are all elevated in cases of fetal Down syndrome. *Am. J. Hum. Genet.*, **45**, A263.

Krazer, P.G., Golbus, M.S., Monroe, S.E., Finkelstein, D.E. & Taylor, R.N. (1991). First trimester aneuploidy screening using serum human chorionic gonadotropin (hCG), free αhCG, and progesterone. *Prenatal Diagn.*, **11**, 751–65.

Lenton, E.A., Grudzinskas, J.G., Gordon, Y.B., Chard, T. & Cooke, I.D. (1981). Pregnancy-specific beta 1-glycoprotein and chorionic gonadotrophin in early pregnancy. *Acta Obstet. Gynecol. Scand.*, **60**, 489–92.

Lin, T.M., Halbert, S.P., Kiefer, D., Spellacy, W.N. & Gall, S. (1974). Characterisation of four pregnancy-associated plasma proteins. *Am. J. Obstet. Gynecol.*, **118**, 223–36.

Macintosh, M.C.M. & Chard, T. (1992). First trimester biochemical screening for Down's syndrome. *Contemp. Rev. Obstet. Gynaecol.*, **4**, 185–90.

Macintosh, M.C.M. & Chard, T. (1993). Biochemical screening for Down's syndrome in the first trimester of pregnancy. *Fetal Mat. Med. Rev.*, **5**(4), 181–90.

Macintosh, M.C.M., Brambati, B., Chard, T. & Grudzinskas, J.G. (1993). First trimester maternal serum Schwangerschafts protein 1 (SP1) in pregnancies associated with chromosomal anomalies. *Prenatal Diagn.*, **13**(7), 563–8.

Merkatz, I., Nitowsky, H., Macri, J. & Johnson, W. (1984). An association between low maternal serum α-fetoprotein and fetal chromosomal abnormalities. *Am. J. Obstet. Gynecol.*, **148**, 886–94.

Nebiolo, L., Ozturk, M., Brambati, B., Miller, S., Wands, J. & Milunsky, A. (1990). First trimester maternal serum alpha-fetoprotein and human chorionic gonadotropin screening for chromosome defects. *Prenatal Diagn.*, **10**, 575–81.

Ozturk, M., Milunsky, A., Brambati, B., Sachs, E.S., Miller, S.L. & Wands, J.R. (1990). Abnormal maternal serum levels of human chorionic gonadotropin free subunits in trisomy 18. *Am. J. Med. Genet.*, **36**, 480–3.

Petrocik, E., Wassman, E.R., Lee, J.L. & Kelly, J.C. (1990). Second trimester maternal serum pregnancy specific beta-1 glycoprotein (SP1) levels in normal and Down syndrome pregnancies. *Am. J. Med. Genet.*, **37**, 114–18.

Schulz-Larsen, P. & Herz, J.B. (1978). Predictive value of pregnancy-specific beta1 glycoprotein in threatened abortion. *Eur. J. Obstet. Gynaecol. Reprod. Biol.*, **8**, 253–7.

Spencer, K. (1991). Pregnancy specific beta 1 glycoprotein in Down's syndrome screening: does it have any value? *Proc. ACB Meeting, 1991, Ann. Clin. Biochem.*, **C46**, 108.

Spencer, K., Macri, J.N., Aitken, D.A. & Connor, J.M. (1993). Free β-hCG as first-trimester marker for fetal trisomy. *Lancet*, **339**, 1480.

Sterzik, K., Wenske, C., Rossmanith, W. & Benz, R. (1986). Beta1-glycoprotein determination in normal and disturbed pregnancy. *Int. J. Gynaecol. Obstet.*, **24**, 65–8.

Tatarinov, Y.S. & Masyukevich, V.N. (1970). Immunochemical identification of new beta 1 globulin in the blood serum of pregnant women. *Bull. Exp. Biol. Med., USSR*, **69**, 66–9.

Teisner, B., Westergaard, J.G., Folkersen, J., Husby, S. & Svehag, S.E. (1978). Two pregnancy-associated serum proteins with pregnancy-specific β1-glycoprotein determinants. *Am. J. Obstet. Gynecol.*, **131**, 262–6.

van Lith, J.M.M. (1992). First-trimester maternal serum human chorionic gonadotrophin as a marker for fetal chromosomal disorders. *Prenatal Diagn.*, **12**, 495–504.

Wald, N.J., Cuckle, H.S., Densem, J. *et al.* (1988). Maternal serum screening for Down's syndrome in early pregnancy. *Br. Med. J.*, **297**, 883–7.

Wald, N.J., Cuckle, H.S. & Densem, J.W. (1989). Maternal serum specific β1-glycoprotein in pregnancies associated with Down's syndrome. *Lancet*, 450.

Westergaard, J.G., Teisner, B., Hau, J., Grudzinskas, J.G. & Chard, T. (1985). Placental function studies in low birth weight infants with and without dysmaturity. *Obstet. Gynaecol.*, **65**, 316–18.

Wurz, H., Geiger, W., Kunzig, H.J., Jabs-Lehmann, A., Bohn, H. & Luben, G. (1981). Radioimmunoassay of SP1 (pregnancy-specific beta1-glycoprotein) in maternal blood and in amniotic fluid in normal and pathological pregnancies. *J. Perinat. Med.*, **9**, 67–78.

12

Ultrasound and Down's syndrome

M. BRONSHTEIN AND Z. BLUMENFELD

Although more than 95% of the newborns with Down's syndrome are diagnosed by morphologic criteria, and despite intense efforts to develop non-invasive techniques for the prenatal diagnosis of Down's syndrome, less than 50 articles have been published on the ability of prenatal sonography to detect this condition.

All too commonly a 'precious' pregnancy achieved after treatment of long-standing infertility has a high risk on the basis of biochemical markers or maternal age. In such cases the information from ultrasonographic examination may be very important. Current information on the detection of Down's syndrome by prenatal sonography is summarized in Table 12.1. The reported sensitivity ranges from as low as 13–30% (Nyberg *et al.*, 1990a; Chitty *et al.*, 1991; Levi *et al.*, 1991) to over 70% (Benacerraf *et al.*, 1987, 1990a, 1992; Lockwood *et al.*, 1987; Ginsberg *et al.*, 1987; Nicolaides *et al.*, 1992). The main difference between the former articles which report a low sensitivity and the latter which report high sensitivity is the gestational week of ultrasound examination. Figure 12.1 summarizes the findings at different gestational ages. Sensitivity is highest in the early second trimester and lower after 18 weeks of gestation (Fig. 12.1) probably as a result of the disappearance of nuchal edema as pregnancy advances.

Sonographic markers of Down's syndrome other than nuchal edema

In addition to nuchal edema, several investigators have reported on short femur length or an abnormal ratio of biparietal diameter (BPD) to femur length (FL) associated with Down's syndrome (BPD/FL ratio) (Benacerraf *et al.*, 1987; Lockwood *et al.*, 1987). However, ten other publications could not reproduce these findings; for example:

181

Table 12.1. *The clinical data and sensitivity of Down's syndrome detection by prenatal sonography as reported in the literature: only those articles where the sensitivity was reported are included*

Author	Diagnosed	Out of	Sensitivity (%)	Weeks of gestation	Markers
Levi et al., 1991	5	25	20	>18	Gross
Ginsberg et al., 1990	9	12	75	14–20	BPD/FL, nuchal edema
Dicke et al., 1991	11	36	30	16–24	Gross
Nicolaides et al., 1992	10	13	76	10–14	Nuchal edema
Chitty et al., 1991	2	15	13	>18	Gross
Crane et al., 1991	12	16	75	14–21	Nuchal edema
Rodis et al., 1991	7	11	60	14–21	Short humerus
Nyberg et al., 1990a	31	94	33	>18	Gross
Benacerraf et al., 1992a	29	32	91	14–20	Nuchal edema and gross
Total	116	254	45		

BDP, biparietal diameter; FL, femur length.

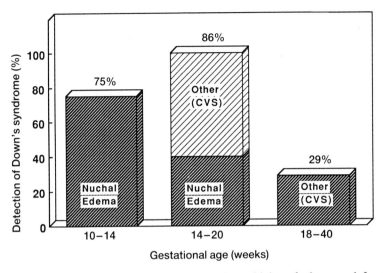

Fig. 12.1. Different sonographic markers and sensitivity of ultrasound for the detection of Down's syndrome at different gestational ages, as reported in the literature (see Table 12.1). CVS, cardiovascular system anomalies.

'We conclude that ultrasonographic screening of short femur is *less effective* for prenatal detection of Down's syndrome *than initially suggested.*' (Nyberg *et al.*, 1990b)

'We found a substantial difference in femur length of normal fetuses in our population compared to that reported by Benacerraf. Further, we were unable to demonstrate statistically discernible deviation of measured versus predicted femur lengths in Down syndrome cohort employing either formula recommended by Benacerraf or a formula calculated from our normal cohort.' (LaFollete *et al.*, 1989)

'The magnitude of femoral shortening in Down syndrome suggests that this measurement may be *only-marginally useful.*' (Lockwood *et al.*, 1991)

'The femur length in fetuses with Down syndrome *is slightly shorter* than normal and this difference may sometimes be difficult to demonstrate in all laboratories and all populations. It may be more difficult to use as a parameter when unaccompanied by any other finding.' (Benacerraf *et al.*, 1992).

Table 12.2 summarizes other possible sonographic markers of Down's syndrome, usually based on a small number of cases. The table also summarizes the probability of Down's syndrome associated with each

Table 12.2. *Sonographic markers for Down's syndrome detection, other than the nuchal signs: probability of Down's syndrome associated with each marker and the incidence of a specific marker in the population of fetuses with Down's syndrome*

	Down's syndrome	
	Probability (%)	Incidence in (%)
Cardiac	30–40 (CAVC)	10–30
Duodenal atresia	30–40	5–10
Hydronephrosis (>4 mm)	0.3–3.3	17–25
IUFGR	0.14	6
Hyperechogenic bowel:	2–41	5
Hydrocephalus	10	1–5
Short: frontal lobe dimensions, humerus, middle phalanx of the fifth digit ... and even short ear length.	?	?
Other: omphalocoele, NTD, CPC	?	?

IUFGR, intrauterine fetal growth retardation; NTD, neural tube defect; CPC, cyst of choroid plexus; CAVC, common atrio-ventricular canal. The association between 'short' organs and 'other' findings with Down's syndrome is questionable and, therefore, is not cited.

marker and the incidence of a specific marker in the population of fetuses with Down's syndrome. The association between 'short' organs (femur, frontal lobe, humerus, middle phalanx of the fifth digit, and ear) and Down's syndrome is questionable in light of the non-reproducibility of early reports on such possible associations.

Transvaginal sonography at 14–16 weeks of gestation

Scanning by transvaginal sonography (TVS) at 14–16 weeks of gestation provides high resolution and can identify nuchal edema and cystic hygromas before they disappear (usually by 18 weeks of gestation). The high resolution also allows detection of other malformations such as cardiac anomalies. We perform amniocentesis for karyotype assessment whenever *any* morphologic anomaly is detected, whether permanent or transient.

Between 1987 and 1993, 14 193 fetal examinations were performed by one examiner (M. Bronshtein) using TVS at 14–16 weeks of gestation in a selected population of private patients. Only 30% of this population was at high risk for fetal anomalies (maternal age >35 years, consanguinity, previous obstetric history, exposure to possible teratogens such as medications, X-rays, etc). The extensive sonographic examination included scanning of fetal face, eyes, fingers, and cardiac echo. The mean duration of the examination was 20–30 minutes.

More than 350 anomalous fetuses and over 560 anomalies were detected. Fifty six of these were cardiac anomalies, an incidence of 1:253. Forty two fetuses were dyskaryotic (1:330) and 20 of these were diagnosed as trisomy 21 (1:700). In addition there were 280 'transient' sonographic anomalies associated with a normal karyotype and a healthy neonate. These transient anomalies included cysts of the choroid plexus, cystic hygromas, fetal hydronephrosis, and abdominal cysts. Four cases of Down's syndrome were not identified by ultrasound; all of them were diagnosed by amniocentesis carried out because of advanced maternal age or biochemical markers (MSAFP, hCG, uE_3). Therefore, the sensitivity of TVS at 14–16 weeks of gestation for the detection of Down syndrome was 83% (20/24).

Table 12.3 summarizes the structural sonographic anomalies indicating

Table 12.3. *Sonographic markers of Down's syndrome*

	Number
Cervical region	
Septated hygroma	8
Non-septated cystic hygroma	4
Nuchal edema	4
Total	16
Non-cervical (other)	
Cardiac	
CAVA, VSD	3
Urinary	
Hydronephrosis, cyst	4
Cord	
Tumor of cord, omphalocoele	2
CNS	
Ventriculomegaly	1
Axilar cyst	1
Total	11
Normal sonographic appearance	4
Sensitivity = 20/24 = 83%	

CAVA, common atrio-ventricular canal; VSD, ventricular septal defect.

Table 12.4. *Comparison between septated and non-septated cystic hygroma*

	Septated	Non-septated
Incidence	34 (1/470)	270 (1/53)
Location	Posterior nuchal	Bilateral anterior cervical
Morphology	Reticular septae	Clear
Earliest week	9	13
Abnormal karyotype	78% (18/23)	4% (11/270)
Hydrops formation	64% (22/34)	0.7% (2/270)
Associated anomalies	67% (23/34)	6% (16/270)
'Take home baby' rate[a]	14% (5/34)	96% (259/270)

[a] Cases where no other associated anomalies were present in the non-septated group.

amniocentesis. The nuchal, cervical anomalies such as septated cystic hygroma (SCH), non-septated cystic hygroma (NSCH), and nuchal edema or thickening contributed 60% of the sonographic markers for Down's syndrome. Table 12.4 summarizes the difference between the SCH and NSCH, as previously described (Bronshtein *et al.*, 1993). The dyskaryosis is associated with 4% of cases of NSCH as opposed to 78% of cases with SCH. The association of webbed neck and dyskaryosis was 7%.

Figures 12.2 and 12.3 show the development of fetal cervical SCH at 10–18 weeks. In our experience, the origin of SCH is the nuchal edema appearing at 10–11 weeks. At 11–15 weeks, the cystic hygroma may develop along one of two pathways. (Fig. 12.2). The first, when associated with additional structural malformations (short bones, omphalocoele, cardiac and urinary tract anomalies), is usually associated with trisomies 13, 18 or 45XO. These may turn into fetal hydrops and the fetus dies around the 18th week of gestation. In the other pathway, in which no additional malformations can be detected, the cystic hygroma usually resolves (via a webbed neck) and later disappears. At 18–20 weeks these fetuses appear normal. These cases are often associated with trisomy 21 (80%). The sonographic appearance of the different morphologic dynamic figures is shown in Fig. 12.3.

The development of NSCH between 13 and 18 weeks is shown in Fig. 12.4. The NSCH usually appears after the 12th week. Due to its relatively high incidence (1 : 50) this may be a transient physiological phenomenon, but the absorbance is delayed in dyskaryotic fetuses. Most of the NSCH are detected at 13–16 weeks of gestation and usually resolve by 16–18

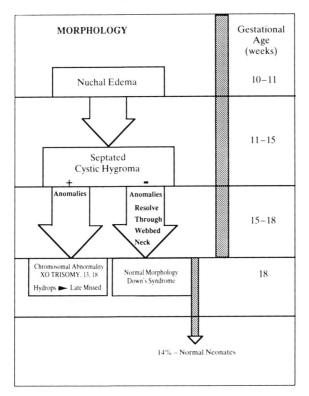

Fig. 12.2. Suggested flowchart of the morphological dynamics of SCH at 10–18 weeks of gestation.

weeks, through a transient stage of nuchal thickening. Most fetuses appear normal by 18 weeks, and 4% may have abnormal karyotype (Fig. 12.4).

Figure 12.5 describes the later development of webbed neck. Although most resolve by 18–19 weeks, in 7% it may be associated with trisomy 21.

Transient sonographic phenomena

One of the most important and clinically relevant findings in our series is the fact that 63% (17/27) of all the 'markers' of Down's syndrome were transient and disappeared at 17–20 weeks of gestation, at which time the result of karyotype assessment has been received. Eleven of the 20 diagnosed as Down's syndrome (55%) would not have been identified if the initial sonographic examination had been performed at, or later than, the 18th week. Figure 12.6 summarizes the sensitivity of the sonographic

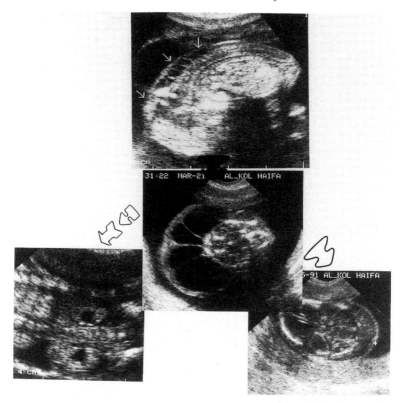

Fig. 12.3. Sonographic examples of the dynamic morphology of SCH: nuchal thickening at 10 weeks (upper panel); the classical septated CH (middle panel); hydrops fetalis and hydronephrosis (left lower panel); webbed neck without other anomalies, later completely resolved (right lower panel).

markers for the detection of Down's syndrome at different gestational ages. At 10–14 weeks of gestation the only sonographic marker for Down's syndrome is nuchal edema, with a sensitivity of about 75% (Fig. 12.6). At 14–16 weeks (the most appropriate gestational age for a systematic TVS examination) the appropriate markers are the nuchal findings (SCH, NSCH, nuchal thickening) on one hand, and all the other sonographic anomalies such as cardiac malformations, urinary tract anomalies, etc. At this gestational age, the sensitivity for detection of Down's syndrome is over 80%.

Sonographic screening at 18–22 weeks is inappropriate for detecting markers of Down's syndrome, since most of the early nuchal signs have disappeared and the later markers are not yet detectable. After the 24th

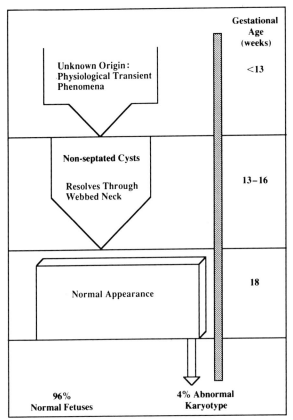

Fig. 12.4. Suggested flowchart of the morphological dynamics of NSCH at 13–18 weeks of gestation.

week, additional sonographic markers for Down's syndrome detection may be observed. These 'late' markers include duodenal atresia, late hydronephrosis, and hydrothorax. The overall sensitivity after 24 weeks is 50%.

Conclusions

The sonographic markers of fetal Down's syndrome vary with gestational age and are therefore only effective for detection of Down's syndrome at the appropriate age. The optimal gestational age for detection of Down's syndrome by sonographic markers is 14–16 weeks, and the recommended method is a detailed TVS examination. Until further experience is

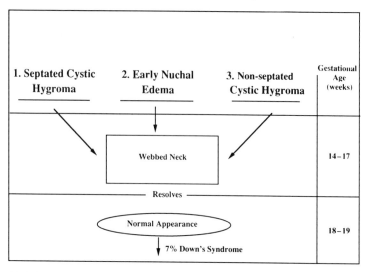

Fig. 12.5. Suggested flowchart of the morphological dynamics of webbed neck at 14–19 weeks of gestation.

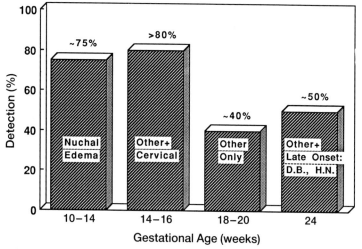

Fig. 12.6. The sensitivity and the relevant sonographic markers for the detection of Down's syndrome at different gestational ages according to the literature and our experience. D.B. double bubble; H.N. hydronephrosis.

acquired, karyotype assessment should be performed in every case of abnormal sonographic finding.

Ultrasound is an effective means for the detection of fetal Down's syndrome, with a sensitivity of over 80%, at least as good as maternal age and biochemical markers, and future integration and combination of maternal age, biochemical markers, and sonographic screening may yield the optimal non-invasive screening test for Down's syndrome.

References

Benacerraf, B.R., Gleman, R. & Frigoletto, F. (1987). Sonographic identification of second trimester fetuses with Down syndrome. *N. Engl. J. Med.*, **317**, 1371–6.

Benacerraf, B.R., Mandell, J., Estroff, J.A. & Harlow, B.C. (1990a). Fetal pyelectasis: a possible association with Down syndrome. *Obstet. Gynecol.*, **76**, 58–60.

Benacerraf, B.R., Harlow, B.L. & Frigoletto, F.D. (1990b). Hypoplasia of the middle phalanx of the fifth digit, a feature of the second trimester fetus with Down syndrome. *J. Ultrasound Med.*, **9**, 389–94.

Benacerraf, B.R., Nyberg, D., Bromley, B. & Frigolleto, F.D. (1992). Sonographic scoring index for prenatal detection of chromosomal abnormalities. *J. Ultrasound Med.*, **11**, 449–58.

Bronshtein, M., Bar-Hava, I., Blumenfeld, I., Bejar, J., Todler, V. & Blumenfeld, Z. (1993). The difference between septated and non-septated nuchal cystic hygroma in the early second trimester. *Obstet. Gynecol.*, **81**, 683–7.

Chitty, L.S., Hunt, G.H., Moore, J. & Lobb, M.D. (1991). Effectiveness of routine ultrasonography in detecting fetal structural abnormalities in a low risk population. *Br. Med. J.*, **303**, 1165–9.

Corteville, J.E., Dicke, J.M. & Crane, J.P. (1992). Fetal pelectasis and Down syndrome: is genetic amniocentesis warranted? *Obstet. Gynecol.*, **79**, 770–2.

Crane, J. & Gray, D.L. (1991). Sonographically measured nuchal skinfold thickness as screening tool for Down syndrome: result of prospective clinical trial. *Obstet. Gynecol.*, **77**, 533–9.

Dicke, J.M. & Crane, J.P. (1991). Sonographic recognition of major malformations and aberrant fetal growth in trisomic fetuses. *J. Ultrasound Med.*, **10**, 433–8.

Ginsberg, N., Cadkin, A., Pergament, E. & Verlinsky, Y. (1990). Ultrasonographic detection of second trimester fetus with trisomy 18 and 21. *Am. J. Obstet. Gynecol.*, **163**, 1186.

La Follette, L., Silly, R.A., Anderson, R. & Golbus, M.S. (1989). Fetal femur length to detect trisomy 21 – a reappraisal. *J. Ultrasound Med.*, **8**, 657–60.

Lettieri, L., Rodis, F., Vintzileos, A.M., Feeney, L., Ciarleglio, L. & Craffey, A. (1993). Ear length in second trimester aneuploid fetuses. *Obstet. Gynecol.*, **81**, 57–60.

Levi, S., Hyjazi, Y., Schaaps, P., Defoort, D., Coulon, R. & Buekens, P. (1991). Sensitivity and specificity of routine antenatal screening for congenital anomalies by ultrasound: the Belgian multicentric study. *Ultrasound Obstet. Gynecol.*, **1**, 102–10.

Lockwood, C., Benacerraf, B.R., Krinsky, A. *et al.* (1987). A sonographic screening method for Down syndrome. *Am. J. Obstet. Gynecol.*, **157**, 803–8.

Lockwood, C.J., Lynch, L. & Berkowitz, R.L. (1991). Ultrasonographic screening for the Down syndrome fetus (review). *Am. J. Obstet. Gynecol.*, **165**, 349–52.

Nicolaides, K.H., Azar, G., Byrne, D., Mansur, C. & Marks, K. (1992). Fetal nuchal translucency: ultrasound screening for chromosomal defects in first trimester of pregnancy. *Br. Med. J.*, **304**, 867–69.

Nyberg, D., Resta, R.G., Luthy, D.A., Hickok, D.H., Mahony, B.S. & Hirsh, J.H. (1990a). Prenatal sonographic findings of Down syndrome: review of 94 cases. *Obstet. Gynecol.*, **76**, 370–6.

Nyberg, D.A., Rosta, E.G., Hickok, D.E., Hollenbach, K.A., Luthy, D.A. & Malone, B.S. (1990b). Femur length shortening in the detection of Down syndrome: is prenatal screening feasible? *Am. J. Obstet. Gynecol.*, **162**, 1247–52.

Rodis, J.F., Vintzileos, A.M., Fleming, A.D., Ciarleglio, L. & Nardi, D.A. (1991). Comparison of humerus length with femur length in fetuses with Down syndrome. *Am. J. Obstet. Gynecol.*, **164**, 1051–6.

Scioscia, A.L., Pretorius, D.H., Buddrick, N.E., Cahill, T.C. & Axelrod, F.T. (1992). Second trimester ecogenic bowel and chromosomal abnormalities. *Am. J. Obstet. Gynecol.*, **167**, 889–94.

Prenatal diagnosis studies

In collaboration with Katherine Klinger at Integrated Genetics (Framingham, MA), a series of 69 maternal blood samples have been studied (Elias *et al.*, 1992b). In one group, a 20 ml blood sample was drawn *after* the diagnosis of fetal aneuploidy by first trimester CVS, second trimester CVS or second trimester amniocentesis (this group is of limited value because blood samples drawn after invasive procedures could contain fetal cells solely as a result of an iatrogenic feto-maternal bleed.) In a second group of patients, a 20 ml maternal blood sample was drawn immediately *prior* to the CVS or amniocentesis. All samples were flow sorted for NRBCs as described above. Coded slides were sent to Integrated Genetics in batches of two to six patient samples. Various combinations of chromosome-specific probes were used for FISH analysis: HL 10-10-8a, a repetitive sequence specific for the X centromere; pWe7.1 and pWe5.0, overlapping mid-long-arm regions specific for chromosome 18; 519, a 20 kb sequence on the distal long arm of chromosome 21; and pDP97, a repeat sequence that recognizes the centromere alphoid repeat DY23 of the Y chromosome (provided by David Page, Cambridge, MA). Because the number of nuclei in a 20 ml maternal blood sample that met the sorting criteria ranged widely from only about 300 to 50 000, and because during the process of slide preparation only 10 to 30% of these sorted nuclei were attached to each slide, it was generally not possible to perform FISH studies on a blood sample using all five chromosome-specific probes. Therefore, in those cases in which there was a high likelihood of finding fetal aneuploid cells (e.g. where the results of CVS or amniocentesis had already shown a fetal trisomy or there was ultrasonographic evidence of fetal anomalies), probes for 21 and 18 were used preferentially for that batch of samples. If the batch of samples did not include a high risk case (i.e. if the sample was drawn prior to CVS or amniocentesis solely on the basis of advanced maternal age), only X and Y chromosome-specific probes were used for the FISH analysis. If sufficient nuclei were available, additional chromosome-specific probes were used. In all cases the slides were scored by independent observers who were unaware of the fetal karyotype.

The cell shown in Fig. 13.3 was among those flow-sorted from a blood sample taken prior to CVS from a woman carrying a male fetus. The X-probe was labeled with biotin-II-dUTP and detected with avidin-Texas red; the Y-probe was labeled with digoxigenin-II-dUTP and detected with FITC-conjugated sheep-antidigoxigenin Fab fragments. A dual band pass

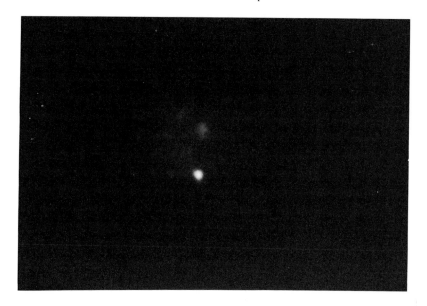

Fig. 13.3. Green hybridization signal with Y-probe (digoxigenin/antidigoxigenin-FITC) and red hybridization signal with X-probe (biotin/avidin-Texas red). Cell flow sorted from a blood sample taken prior to CVS from a women carrying a male fetus.

filter (Omega, Brattleboro, VT) was used to visualize FITC and Texas red simultaneously. Results were photographed directly from the microscope using a 35 mm camera and Kodak Gold 400 film. Although these methods allow detection of male cells in maternal blood, cells from a normal female fetus could not be distinguished from maternal cells because both display two X-probe signals.

Table 13.2 summarizes the FISH analyses of flow-sorted bloods from women carrying chromosomally abnormal fetuses among the 69 pregnancies studied (Elias *et al.*, 1992b). In this series, after each batch of samples was analyzed, the flow sorting as well as the FISH protocols were modified depending on the results of the previous runs. These changes were made to enhance the purity of sorted fetal NRBCs and to optimize conditions for FISH analysis. Because each batch of two to six samples was processed differently and because of the very small sample size, inferences concerning the sensitivity, specificity or predictive value of our methods cannot be drawn.

Two of our cases warrant highlighting. The first involves a 42-year-old woman referred for prenatal diagnosis at 10 weeks of gestation because

Table 13.2. *Summary of FISH analyses of flow-sorted maternal bloods from women carrying chromosomally abnormal fetuses, found among the 69 pregnancies studied*

Case	Procedure	Fetal karyotype	Trisomic cells detected	
			No.	(%)
1	Post CVS	47,XX, + 21	24/62	38.7
2	Post Amniocentesis	47,XX, + 21	21/113	18.6
3	Pre CVS	47,XX, + 18	25/295	8.5
4	Pre CVS	47,XX, + 21	3/104	2.8
5	Post Amniocentesis	47,XX, + 21	4/50	8.0
6	Pre CVS	47,XX, + 21	74/100	74.0
7	Post CVS	47,XXY	6/93	6.4
8	Pre CVS	47,XXY	0/93	0

of maternal age (case 3 in Table 13.2). Her two previous pregnancies resulted in the delivery of a normal female infant and the delivery of a set of normal twins, one male and one female. From a maternal blood sample obtained *prior* to CVS, flow-sorted fetal cells were analyzed by FISH with probes for chromosomes Y, X, 18, and 21 (Fig. 13.4). Again, slides were scored without knowledge of fetal karyotype. The results are shown in Table 13.3: Y-probe, 8.7% of the nuclei exhibited a single hybridization signal and 90.3% exhibited no signal; X-probe, 14.5% of the nuclei displayed a single hybridization signal and 86% of the nuclei displayed two hybridization signals; the 18-probe showed 86% to be disomic and 8.5% trisomic; and with the chromosome 21-probe, 95.2% of the nuclei showed two hybridization signals. These data indicate a male fetus with trisomy 18. The patient elected to terminate the pregnancy on the basis of cytogenetic results from CVS showing trisomy 18, and the diagnosis of 47,XY, + 18 was confirmed in the abortus. This was the first report of a fetal aneuploidy (47,XY, + 18) detected prospectively by isolating fetal cells from maternal blood (Price *et al.*, 1991).

The second case was that of a 42-year-old primigravida referred for prenatal diagnosis at 10 weeks of gestation because of maternal age (case 6 in Table 13.2). From a maternal blood sample obtained *prior* to CVS, flow-sorted fetal cells were analyzed simultaneously with probes for chromosomes 18 and 21 and scored for red or green signals using dual band pass filters. (Fig. 13.5). Again, slides were scored without knowledge

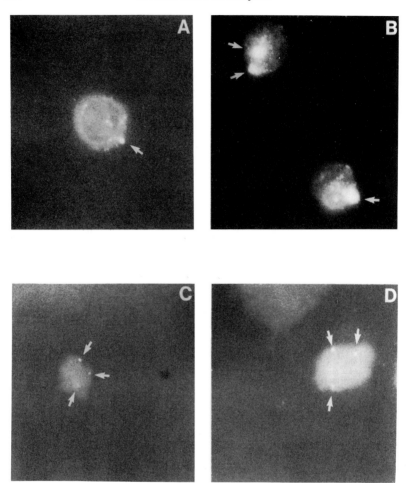

Fig. 13.4. Flow-sorted cells from case 3 hybridized to various chromosome-specific probes. Probes were labeled with biotin and visualized with fluorescein isothio-cyanate-streptavidin. All cells were isolated from a single maternal blood sample and analyzed in coded fashion. (**A**) Male cell of fetal origin. Fluorescent signal (arrow) in cell hybridized to pDP97-probe, which identifies the centromere alphoid repeat DYZ3 of the Y chromosome. (**B**) Female cell of maternal origin (upper left) showing two signals (two arrows) and male cell of presumed fetal origin (lower right) showing single signal (arrow). Cells hybridized to X-chromo-some-specific cosmid probe, which identifies a pericentromeric repeat sequence on the X chromosome. (**C** and **D**) Trisomy 18 fetal cells sorted from maternal blood. Fluorescent signals (three arrows) in cells hybridized to a chromosome 18-specific cosmid contig probe, which identifies a single-copy sequence on the distal long arm of chromosome 18. (Reproduced with permission from Price, J.O., Elias, S., Wachtel, S.S. *et al.* (1991). *Am. J. Obstet. Gynecol.*, **165**, 1731–37.)

Table 13.3. *Flow-sorted maternal blood specimen obtained before transabdominal CVS in a woman carrying a 47, X X, + 18 fetus: distribution of* in situ *hybridization signals for chromosome-specific probes*

Chromosome-specific probe	Hybridization signals per nucleus No. (%)				
	0	1	2	3	Total
Y[a]	93(90.3)	9 (8.7)	1 (1.0)	—	103
X[b]	—	17(14.5)	100(85.5)	—	117
18[c]	—	16 (5.4)	254(86.1)	25(8.5)	295
21[d]	—	3 (1.8)	158(95.2)	5(3.0)	166

Chromosome-specific probes used were:
[a] pDP97;
[b] HL10-10-8a;
[c] pWe 7.1 and pWe 5.0;
[d] 519.

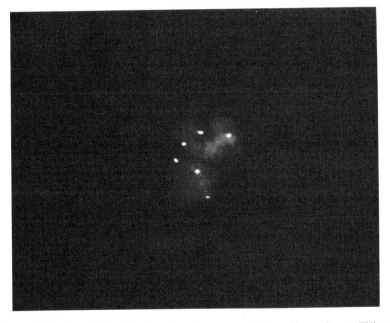

Fig. 13.5. Results of hybridization of a chromosome 21-specific probe set (Klinger *et al.*, 1992) to fetal NRBCs. Three hybridization signals can be visualized in each nucleus. Digital imaging microscopy was performed with a Zeiss epifluorescence microscope equipped with a cooled CCD camera (Photometrics PM512, Tucson, AZ), which was controlled by a PC. Gray scale images were captured with filter sets for DAPI and fluorescein (pseudocolored and merged for display).

Table 13.4. *Interphase FISH of NRBCs, flow sorted from maternal blood, indicating fetal 47,XX,+21*

Chromosome-specific probes	No. hybridization signals per nuclei				Total nuclei scored
	1	2	3	4	
18	1	98	2	0	101
21	0	25	74	1	100

of the fetal karyotype. The results are shown in Table 13.4: 18-probe, 98% of the nuclei exhibited two hybridization signals; 21-probe, 74% of the nuclei exhibited three hybridization signals. In aggregate, these data indicate a fetus with trisomy 21. Insufficient nuclei were available to prepare slides for X and Y FISH analyses; therefore, fetal sex determination was not attempted. The patient elected to terminate the pregnancy on the basis of the CVS results showing trisomy 21, and the diagnosis of 47,XX, +21 was confirmed in the abortus. This was the first report of a fetal trisomy 21 detected prospectively by isolating fetal cells from maternal blood (Elias *et al.*, 1992a).

In this case approximately three-quarters of the cells analyzed were determined to be fetal, the highest proportion we have thus far observed in any maternal blood sample. One possible explanation is that by chance the blood sample may have been drawn at a very early stage of spontaneous abortion and, hence, at a time when a feto-maternal bleed was occurring. This would be consistent with the known high frequency of autosomal trisomies, including trisomy 21, among first trimester spontaneous abortuses.

Conclusion

Ideally, the sensitivity, specificity and predictive value will ultimately prove sufficient to allow this non-invasive approach of isolating fetal cells from maternal blood to serve as the definitive diagnostic test for fetal aneuploidy. However, even if this stringent requirement is not met, we suggest that the method could play an important role in prenatal screening for fetal aneuploidy, either as an independent test or in combination with other tests. Our group (Phillips *et al.*, 1992) as well as others (Cuckle and Wald, 1992; Haddow *et al.*, 1992; Wald *et al.*, 1992a) have shown that for women less than 35 years of age the combination of maternal serum α-fetoprotein (MSAFP), human chorionic gonadotropin (hCG) and unconjugated estriol (uE_3) in the second trimester is an effective screening test for fetal Down's syndrome and other aneuploidies, with a sensitivity (detection rate) of about 60%. The test selects about 5% of women requiring amniocentesis for definitive diagnoses. It now appears that in the first trimester MSAFP, uE_3, pregnancy-associated plasma protein A(PAPP-A) and pregnancy-specific β-glycoprotein (SP1) levels are reduced and hCG levels raised in pregnancies associated with fetal Down's syndrome (Cuckle *et al.*, 1988, 1992; Bogart *et al.*, 1989; Brock *et al.*, 1990; Nebiolo *et al.*, 1990; Ozturk *et al.*, 1990; Wenger *et al.*, 1990; Brambati *et al.*, 1991; Crandall *et al.*, 1991; Johnson *et al.*, 1991; Wald *et al.*, 1992b). Accordingly, the role of flow sorting and FISH analysis of NRBCs may prove to be that of a *screening* test, either alone or in combination with other markers, to identify patients at increased risk for fetal chromosomal abnormalities who would then proceed to either CVS or amniocentesis for definitive prenatal diagnosis.

Acknowledgements

The authors wish to acknowledge their collaborators at the University of Tennessee, Memphis (J.O. Price, S.S. Wachtel, M. Dockter, A. Tharapel, L.P. Shulman, O.P. Phillips, C.M. Meyers, C. Grevengood, J. Dungan) and at Integrated Genetics, Framingham, MA (K. Klinger, D. Shook). Supported in part by National Institutes of Health contracts HD8-2903 and HD8-2904 (S.E.) and a University of Tennessee Chair of Excellence (J.L.S.).

References

Benacerraf, B.R., Gelman, R. & Frigoletto, F.D. (1987). Sonographic identification of second-trimester fetuses with Down's syndrome. *N. Engl. J. Med.*, **317**, 1371–6.

Bianchi, D.W., Flint, A.F., Pizzimenti, M.F. *et al.* (1990). Isolation of fetal DNA from nucleated erythrocytes in maternal blood. *Proc. Natl. Acad. Sci. USA*, **87**, 3279–83.

Bianchi, D.W., Mahr, A., Zickwolf, G.L. *et al.* (1992a). Detection of fetal cells with 47,XY, +21 karyotype in maternal peripheral blood. *Hum. Genet.*, **90**, 368–70.

Bianchi, D.W., Zickwolf, G.K., Geifman, O.H. *et al.* (1992b). Erythroid-specific antibodies enhance separation of fetal nucleated erythrocytes from maternal blood. *Prenatal Diagn.,* **12**, S2.

Bogart, M.H., Golbus, M.M., Sorg, N.D. *et al.* (1989). Human chorionic gonadotropin levels in pregnancies with aneuploid fetuses. *Prenatal Diagn.,* **9**, 379–84.

Brambati, B., Lanzani, A. & Tului, L. (1991). Ultrasound and biochemical assessment of first trimester pregnancy. In *The embryo: Normal and Abnormal Development and Growth.* ed. M. Chapman, J.G. Grudzinskas & T. Chard, p. 181. London: Springer-Verlag.

Brock, D.J.H., Barron, L., Holloway, S. *et al.* (1990). First trimester maternal serum biochemical indicators in Down syndrome. *Prenatal Diagn.,* **10**, 245–251.

Bruch, J.F., Metezeau, D., Garcia-Fonknechten, N. *et al.* (1991). Trophoblast-like cells sorted from peripheral maternal blood using flow cytometry: a multiparametric study involving transmission electron microscopy and fetal amplification. *Prenatal Diagn.,* **10**, 787–98.

Cacheux, V., Milesi-Fluet, C., Tachdjian, G. *et al.* (1992). Detection of 47,XYY trophoblast fetal cells in maternal blood by fluorescence *in situ* hybridization after using immunomagnetic lymphocyte depletion and flow cytometry sorting. *Fetal Diagn. Ther.,* **7**, 190–4.

Camaschella, C., Alfarno, A., Gattardi, E. *et al.* (1990). Prenatal diagnosis of fetal haemoglobin Lepore–Boston disease on maternal peripheral blood. *Blood,* **75**, 2101–6.

Covone, A.E., Johnson, P.M., Mutton, D. *et al.* (1984). Trophoblast cells in peripheral blood from pregnant women. *Lancet,* **i**, 841–3.

Covone, A.E., Kozma, R., Johnson, P.M. *et al.* (1988). Analysis of peripheral maternal blood samples for the presence of placental-derived cells using Y-specific probes and McAb H315. *Prenatal Diagn.,* **8**, 591–607.

Crandall, B.F., Golbus, M.S., Goldberg, J.D. *et al.* (1991). First-trimester maternal serum unconjugated oestriol and alpha-fetoprotein in fetal Down's syndrome. *Prenatal Diagn.,* **11**, 377–80.

Cuckle, H.S. & Wald, N.J. (1992). HCG, estriol and other maternal blood markers of fetal aneuploidy. In *Maternal Serum Screening for Fetal Genetic Disorders*, ed. S. Elias & S. Simpson, pp. 87–107. New York: Churchill Livingstone.

Cuckle, H.S., Wald, N.J., Barkai, G. *et al.* (1988). First trimester biochemical screening for Down's syndrome. *Lancet,* **2**, 851–2.

de Grouchy, J. & Trubuchet, C. (1971). Transfusion foeto-maternelle de lymphocytes sanguins et detection du sexe du foetus. *Ann. Genet.,* **14**, 133–7.

Elias, S. & Simpson, J.L. (1992). Amniocentesis and induced abortion for genetic indications. In *Genetic Disorders and the Fetus.* ed. A. Milunsky, p. 33. Baltimore: Johns Hopkins University Press.

Elias, S., Price, J., Dockter, M., Wachtel, S., Tharapel, A. & Simpson, J.L. (1992a). First trimester prenatal diagnosis of trisomy 21 in fetal cells from maternal blood. *Lancet,* **340**, 1033.

Elias, S., Price, J., Klinger, K. *et al.* (1992b). Prenatal diagnosis of aneuploidy using fetal cells isolated from maternal blood. *Am. J. Hum. Genet.,* **51**, A4.

Gänshirt-Ahlert, D., Börjesson-Stoll, M., Burschyk, M. *et al.* (1992). Noninvasive prenatal diagnosis: triple density gradient, magnetic activated cell sorting and FISH prove to be an efficient and reproducible method for detection of fetal aneuploidies from maternal blood. *Am. J. Hum. Genet.,* **51**, A48.

Grossett, L. Barrelet, V. & Odartchenko, N. (1974). Antenatal fetal sex determination from maternal blood during early pregnancy. *Am. J. Obstet. Gynecol.,* **120**, 60–63.

Haddow, J.E., Palomaki, G.E., Knight, G.J. *et al.* (1992). Prenatal screening for Down's syndrome with use of maternal serum markers. *N. Engl. J. Med.,* **327**, 588–593.

Herzenberg, L.A., Bianchi, D.W., Schroder, J. *et al.* (1979). Fetal cells in the blood of pregnant women: detection and enrichment by fluorescence-activated cell sorting. *Proc. Natl. Acad. Sci. USA,* **76**, 1453–5.

Holzgreve, W., Gänshirt-Ahlert, D., Dohr, A. *et al.* (1992). Magnetically activated cell sorting for the isolation of fetal cells from maternal circulation. *Prenatal Diagn.,* **12**, S17.

Iverson, G.M., Bianchi, D.W., Cann, H.M. *et al.* (1981). Detection and isolation of fetal cells from maternal blood using the fluorescence-activated cell sorter (FACS). *Prenatal Diagn.,* **1**, 61–73.

Johnson, A., Cowchock, F.S., Darby, M. *et al.* (1991). First trimester maternal serum alpha-fetoprotein and chorionic gonadotropin in aneuploid pregnancies. *Prenatal Diagn.,* **11**, 443–50.

Klinger, K., Landes, G., Shook, D. *et al.* (1992). Rapid detection of chromosome aneuploidies in uncultured amniocytes by using fluorescence *in situ* hybridization (FISH). *Am. J. Hum. Genet.,* **51**, 55–65.

Lo, Y-M.D., Wainscot, J.S., Gilmer, M.D.G. *et al.* (1989). Prenatal sex determination by DNA amplification from maternal peripheral blood. *Lancet,* **ii**, 1363–1365.

Lo, Y-M.D., Patel, P., Sampietro, M. *et al.* (1990). Detection of single-copy fetal DNA sequence from maternal blood. *Lancet,* **335**, 1463–4.

Mueller, U.W., Hawes, C.S. & Wright, A.E. (1990a). Isolation of fetal trophoblast cells from peripheral blood of pregnant women. *Lancet,* **336**, 197–200.

Nebiolo, L., Ozturk, M., Brambati, B. *et al.* (1990). First-trimester maternal serum alpha-fetoprotein and human chorionic gonadotropin screening for chromosome defects. *Prenatal Diagn.,* **10**, 575–81.

Ozturk, M., Milunsky, A., Brambati, B. *et al.* (1990). Abnormal maternal serum levels of human chorionic gonadotropin free subunits in trisomy 18. *Am. J. Med. Genet.,* **36**, 480–3.

Phillips, O.P., Elias, S., Shulman, L.P. *et al.* (1992). Maternal serum screening for fetal Down syndrome in women less than 35 years of age using alpha-fetoprotein, human chorionic gonadotropin and unconjugated estriol: a prospective two-year study. *Obstet. Gynecol.,* **80**, 353–8.

Price, J., Elias, S., Wachtel, S.S. *et al.* (1991). Prenatal diagnosis using fetal cells isolated from maternal blood by multiparameter flow cytometry. *Am. J. Obstet. Gynecol.,* **165**, 1731–7.

Schroder, J. & de la Chapelle, A. (1972). Fetal lymphocytes in maternal blood. *J. Hematol.,* **39**, 153–62.

Schroder, J., Tiilikainen, A. & de la Chapelle, A. (1974). Fetal leukocytes in the maternal circulation after delivery. *Transplantation,* **17**, 346–60.

Siebers, J.W., Knauf, I. & Hillemans, H.G. (1975). Antenatal sex determination in blood from pregnant women. *Humangenetik,* **28**, 273–80.

Simpson, J.L. & Elias, S. (1992). Isolating fetal erythroblasts from maternal blood with identification of fetal trisomy by fluorescent *in situ* hybridization. *Prenatal Diagn.,* **12**, S34.

Tharapel, A.T., Jaswaney, V., Dockter, M. *et al.* (1989). Can fetal cells in maternal blood be selected through cytogenetic means? *Am. J. Hum. Genet.*, **45**(S), 271.

Tharapel, A.T., Anderson, K.P., Simpson, J.L. *et al.* (1993). Are all terminal ZQ deletions interstitial? Reevaluation of a deleted X-chromosome in a proband and her mother by southern blotting and by multiple FISH analyses. *Fetal Diagn. Ther.*, in press.

Tipton, R.E., Tharapel, A.T., Change, H.T., Simpson, J.L. & Elias, S. (1990). Rapid chromosome analysis using spontaneously dividing cells derived from umbilical cord blood (fetal and neonatal). *Am. J. Obstet. Gynecol.*, **161**, 1546–8.

Wachtel, S.S., Elias, S., Price, J. *et al.* (1991). Fetal cells in the maternal circulation: isolation by multiparameter flow cytometry and confirmation by PCR. *Hum. Reprod.*, **6**, 1466–9.

Wald, N.J., Cuckle, H.S., Densem, J.W. *et al.* (1988). Maternal serum screening for Down's syndrome in early pregnancy. *Br. Med. J.*, **297**, 883.

Wald, N.J., Kennard, A., Densem, J.W. *et al.* (1992a). Antenatal maternal serum screening for Down's syndrome: results of a demonstration project. *Br. Med. J.*, **305**, 391–4.

Wald, N.J., Stone, R., Cuckle, H.S. *et al.* (1992b). First trimester concentrations of pregnancy associated plasma protein A and placenta protein 14 in Down's syndrome. *Br. Med. J.*, **305**, 28.

Walknowska, J., Conte, F.A. & Grumback, M.M. (1969). Practical and theoretical implications of fetal/maternal lymphocyte transfer. *Lancet*, **i**, 1119–22.

Wenger, D., Ming, P., Holzgreve, W. *et al.* (1990). First trimester maternal serum alpha-fetoprotein screening for Down syndrome and other aneuploidies. *Am. J. Med. Genet.*, Suppl. **7**, 89–90.

Wessman, M., Ylinen, K. & Knuutila, S. (1992). Fetal granulocytes in maternal venous blood detected in *in situ* hybridization. *Prenatal Diagn.*, **12**, 993–1000.

Wilson, R.D. & Langlois, S. (1992). Non-invasive prenatal sex determination for X-linked genetic disease by DNA amplification from maternal blood. *Prenatal Diagn.*, **12**, S177.

Yeoh, S.C., Sargent, I.L., Redman, C.W.G. *et al.* (1991). Detection of fetal cells in maternal blood. *Prenatal Diagn.*, **11**, 117–23.

Zilliacus, R., de la Chappelle, A., Schroder, J. *et al.* (1975). Transplacental passage of foetal blood cells. *Scand. J. Haematol.*, **15**, 333–8.

14

Rapid detection of chromosome aneuploidies in uncultured fetal cells using fluorescence *in situ* hybridization

T. BRYNDORF, B. CHRISTENSEN, Y. XIANG
AND J. PHILIP

Introduction

Prenatal detection of Down's syndrome has been a goal for decades. The discovery by Lejeune *et al.* (1959), of an extra chromosome 21 in the cells of individuals with Down's syndrome and the subsequent demonstration that chromosome analysis could be performed on amniotic fluid cells (Steele and Breg, 1966) spurred the development of today's routine cytogenetic screening of fetal tissue samples for numerical and structural chromosome aberrations. However, cytogenetic analysis is expensive, takes 7–14 days to obtain, and the pregnancy is subjected to risk when sampling the necessary fetal tissue. That is why only pregnancies at increased risk for fetuses with chromosome abnormalities are offered prenatal diagnosis.

Identification of risk pregnancies has evolved considerably. Initially, advanced maternal age was used as the primary risk parameter. Identification of pregnancies at risk for carrying fetuses with Down's syndrome by maternal screening protocols using biochemical markers (Merkatz *et al.*, 1984) is now gaining wide acceptance. Furthermore risk pregnancies can be identified by sonographic screening. No matter how a pregnancy at increased risk is identified, a fetal genetic diagnosis subsequently has to be established. Currently diagnosis is obtained only by cytogenetic analysis of fetal tissue.

Lately a new method for prenatal detection of numerical aberrations has evolved: fluorescence *in situ* hybridization (FISH) with chromosome-specific probes using uncultured fetal cells. Because the cell culture necessary for conventional chromosome analysis is avoided, FISH assays are less expensive and faster than conventional cytogenetics. FISH will allow early exclusion or diagnosis of Down's syndrome, and consequently an earlier answer in affected pregnancies. However, fetal tissue sampling has to be performed whether FISH analysis or conventional chromosome analysis is performed; and FISH analysis has some diagnostic limitations in comparison with cytogenetics.

We carried out a study with the aim of assessing the detection power of a FISH assay – not only for Down's syndrome but also for numeric aberrations of chromosomes 13, 18, X and Y. We used the five probes described by Klinger *et al.* (1992) for a prospective clinical trial comparing FISH analysis of uncultured amniotic fluid cell and mesenchymal chorionic villus cell samples with conventional chromosome analysis.

Materials and methods

Cells

Uncultured amniotic fluid cells Cells were processed by a modification of the method described by Klinger *et al.* (1992). The amniotic fluid cells were washed and resuspended in phosphate-buffered saline. A 25 µl sample of this suspension was placed on a slide heated to 37 °C. The cells on each slide were then processed *in situ* by the addition of 25 µl 100 mM KCl and incubated at 37 °C for 15 minutes. The hypotonic solution was replaced by 100 µl of 30% 3:1 fixative (methanol:acetic acid), 70% 75 mM KCl for 5 minutes at room temperature. The solution was decanted and 3:1 fixative (methanol:acetic acid) was added. The slides were dried at 60 °C for 5 minutes. The attached cells were washed in phosphate-buffered saline and dehydrated in ethanol.

Uncultured chorionic villus cells Single-cell suspensions from mesenchymal chorionic tissue were established by a two-step enzyme treatment as previously described (Smidt-Jensen *et al.*, 1989; Bryndorf *et al.*, 1993). Following enzyme treatment the cell suspensions were washed twice in Hank's balanced salt solution and then processed in the same way as the amniotic fluid cell suspensions.

Probes, hybridization and detection

The chromosome 13-, 18-, and 21-specific probes were developed from unique sequence regions (Klinger *et al.*, 1992). The three probes were all three-cosmid contigs containing 80 000–109 000 base pairs of non-overlapping DNA. The X chromosome set was composed of a single cosmid which hybridizes to the paracentromeric region on the X chromosome (Ward *et al.*, 1993). The Y-probe was derived from the repetitive clone pDP97 (provided by D. Page, Whitehead Institute for Biomedical Research, Cambridge, MA, USA), a subclone of the alpha-satellite repeat present in the cosmid Y97 (Wolfe *et al.*, 1985). The probes were labelled by nick-translation with biotin-11-dUTP (except the chromosome X-probe). Hybridization under suppression conditions and detection were performed as described by Klinger *et al.* (1992). All experiments were carried out with simultaneous detection of the X-probe (directly labelled with resorufin) and the Y-probe (biotin/avidin-FITC).

Quantitative analysis

Two technicians evaluated 30 and 20 different hybridized nuclei per probe for each sample, respectively. The number of nuclei displaying one, two, three or four hybridization signals was recorded. Overlapping nuclei were not scored. Patchy and diffuse signals were included in the evaluation only if they were well separated. Split-spots (i.e. signals in a paired arrangement) were scored as one signal if the distance between the signals was less than the width of one of these signals or as two signals if the distance was larger.

Blind study design

Consecutive samples from consenting pregnant women referred to our laboratory for prenatal diagnosis were evaluated in parallel by cytogenetic analysis and FISH analysis. Cytogenetic analysis was carried out using 13 ml amniotic fluid and 15 mg chorionic villus tissue; the remaining fluid and tissue was used for FISH analysis. Three chorionic villus samples from women having their pregnancies terminated because of previously diagnosed fetal trisomy 21 were added to the trial in a blind fashion. The FISH analyses were carried out blindly. Both amniotic fluid and chorionic villus samples were coded and stored without the knowledge of the indication for the prenatal testing and the karyotype of the sample. Blood-contaminated amniotic fluid samples were not analyzed. Amniotic fluid samples ≥ 5 ml were hybridized with all five probes, samples between 3–5 ml were hybridized with the chromosome 21-, 18-, and 13-probes, and samples < 3 ml were hybridized with the 21- and 18-probes. The X- and Y-probes were only used after amniotic fluid sample number 44 and chorionic villus sample number 61 were received.

Results

Blinded study on uncultured amniocytes

The amniotic fluid study involved 257 pregnant women. Four women had only 13 ml or less fluid withdrawn, consequently no FISH analysis was performed. Of the remaining 253 samples, an average of 4.7 ml (1–8 ml) amniotic fluid was used for FISH analysis. A final diagnosis was not obtained for 47 samples: 30 (12%) samples were not hybridized because of visible blood or other contaminants in the amniotic fluid; two samples (1%) were abandoned because the chromosome 13 hybridization and the chromosome 13, X and Y hybridizations for unexplained reasons did not show any signals; and 15 samples (6%) were abandoned because there were less than 50 scorable nuclei at one or more of the hybridizations. The results of the FISH analysis of the remaining 206 samples are summarized in Table 14.1. Eleven samples were not hybridized with the chromosome 13-probe because the amniotic fluid volumes were below 3 ml. Hybridization was successfully carried out for 97 samples with the X- and Y-probes. In samples disomic with respect to the probed autosomal chromosomes, an average of about 90% (range 68–100%) of the scored nuclei demonstrated two signals, while approximately 2% (0–20%) had three hybridization signals. By contrast, in the samples trisomic for chromosomes 18 and 21, 68% and 72% of the nuclei exhibited three

Table 14.1. *Current prenatal FISH studies in Copenhagen*

		% nuclei (range)		
Probe	Karyotyping	With two signals	With three signals	No. individuals
Uncultured amnion				
13	Disomy 13	90 (68–100)	2 (0–16)	195
18	Disomy 18	91 (72–100)	2 (0–16)	205
18	Trisomy 18	28	68	1
21	Disomy 21	90 (62–100)	1 (0–20)	205
21	Trisomy 21	24	72	1
Uncultured chorion				
13	Disomy 13	94 (70–100)	1 (0–8)	262
18	Disomy 18	95 (78–100)	1 (0–8)	262
21	Disomy 21	95 (82–100)	1 (0–6)	257
21	Trisomy 21	19 (12–28)	80 (68–88)	4

[a] 50 nuclei were stored for each hybridization.

signals, respectively, while 28% and 24% had two signals, respectively. In the karyotypically male samples 97% (80–100%) of the nuclei had one X- and one Y-signal each; 95% (90–100%) of the nuclei in the karyo-typically female samples had two X-signals each.

One of the samples gave potentially discrepant results by karyotyping and FISH. However, the sample was abandoned because the total number of hybridizable nuclei was only 18. The sample's karyotype was 47, XX, +21. The scoring result for this sample's chromosome 21 hybridization was 14 nuclei with two signals each and 4 nuclei with three signals each.

Blinded study on uncultured chorionic villus cells

The chorionic villus study involved 272 pregnant women. Ten women had only 15 mg or less tissue sampled, consequently no FISH analysis was performed. Of the remaining 262 samples, an average of 11.9 mg (2–15 mg) tissue was used for FISH analysis. All hybridizations were successful. Hybridization with the X- and Y-probes was carried out for 202 samples. The results are summarized in Table 14.1. In samples disomic with respect to the probed chromosomes, an average of about 95% (range 70–100%) of the scored nuclei demonstrated two signals, while approxi-mately 1% (0–8%) had three hybridization signals. By contrast, in the samples trisomic for chromosome 21, 80% (68–88%) of the nuclei exhibited three signals, while 19% (12–28%) had two signals each. In the karyotypically male samples, 98% (86–100%) had one X- and one Y-signal each; 97% (90–100%) of the nuclei in the karyotypically female samples had two X-signals each.

Discussion

The purpose of this study was to assess the detection power of a FISH assay for numeric aberrations of chromosomes 13, 18, 21, X and Y. We detected 1 case of trisomy 21 and 1 case of trisomy 18 in the amniotic fluid trial and 4 cases of trisomy 21 in the chorionic villus study (3 of the latter cases were added to the trial from women having their pregnancies terminated because of previously diagnosed fetal trisomy 21). However, a much larger database is necessary to allow proper statistical analysis. In order to prove with 95% probability that the sensitivity or specificity of a FISH assay is greater than 95%, the assay has to correspond with conventional karyotyping in 99 out of 100 samples with trisomy 21 (Conover, 1980). In order to prove that the assay sensitivity or specificity is above 99%, a FISH assay has to correspond with conventional

Table 14.2. *Prenatal FISH studies in the literature*

Prenatal FISH assays	Tissue	Pro- or retrospective	Chromosome(s)	Probe types	No. samples	Aneuploidies by FISH/conventional karyotyping
Guyot et al., 1988	Amnion	Retro-	Y	Repetitive	54	1/1
Zheng et al., 1992	Amnion	Retro-	21	Locus-specific cosmid contig	49	4/4
Evans et al., 1992	Chorion	Pro-	13, 18, 21	Locus-specific cosmid contigs	47	1/1
Lebo et al., 1992	Amnion	?	X and Y 13/21, 18, X and Y	Repetitive Repetitive	25 (13/21-probe) 100 (18-, X-, Y-probes)	2/2
Lebo et al., 1992	Chorion	?	13/21, 18, X and Y	Repetitive	10	1/1

karyotyping in 499 out of 500 samples with trisomy 21. It is evident that a multi-centre trial is necessary to assess the detection power of a FISH assay. However, the literature and our own experiences do give some indications about the performance of prenatal FISH analysis.

Klinger *et al.* (1992) reported the first major prospective study comparing a five-probe FISH assay on uncultured amniocytes with conventional chromosome analysis. The five probes used were specific for chromosomes 13, 18, 21, X and Y. The first clinical application of this technology was reported by Ward *et al.* (1993). The sensitivity of the assay was 93.9%, the specificity was greater than 99.9%, the false-negative rate was 6.1% and the false-positive rate was 0.03%. These are impressive numbers, but it has to be noted that the Ward group received 4500 samples but only reported results on 3901 of these. Samples were not processed because of (i) visible blood or other contaminant in the amniotic fluid (104); and (ii) insufficient volume (69). Of the 4327 hybridized samples, 426 (9.8%) were uninformative because of (i) suspected maternal cell contamination; (ii) lack of sufficient numbers of hybridizable nuclei; (iii) technical problems in sample processing; and (iv) hybridization patterns that did not meet the reporting criteria for normals and abnormals.

There have been several reports of smaller trials comparing prenatal FISH assays on uncultured cells with conventional chromosome analysis on cultured cells. These studies are summarized in Table 14.2. Guyot *et al.* (1988) reported a retrospective study of FISH detection of numerical aberrations of chromosome Y on 54 uncultured amniotic fluid samples. One sample with XYY syndrome was detected. Zheng *et al.* (1992) also reported a retrospective study comparing a FISH assay on chromosome 21 only in uncultured amnion with conventional chromosome analysis. They analyzed 49 cases and 4 out of 4 trisomy 21 cases were correctly detected by the FISH assay. Evans *et al.* (1992) reported a prospective study using a FISH assay with the five probes described by Klinger *et al.* (1992) on 47 uncultured chorionic villus cell samples. One out of one trisomy 21 case was correctly identified by the FISH assay. Lebo *et al.* (1992) reported a pro- or retrospective study using repetitive probes specific for chromosomes 13 + 21, 18, X and Y on uncultured amniotic fluid cells and uncultured chorionic villus cells. Out of the 25 uncultured amniotic fluid samples hybridized with the 13 + 21-probe and the 100 samples hybridized with the 18-, X- and Y-probes, 1 case of XXY syndrome and 1 case of trisomy 21 were correctly identified. Out of the 10 uncultured chorionic villus samples hybridized with all four probes, 1 case of trisomy 18 was correctly identified.

Table 14.3. *Previous prenatal FISH studies in Copenhagen*

Copenhagen experiences	Tissue	Pro- or retrospective	Chromosome(s)	Probe types	No. samples	Aneuploidies by FISH/conventional karyotyping
Christensen *et al.*, 1992	Amnion	Retro-	18 and 1	Repetitive	33	3/3
Bryndorf *et al.*, 1992	Amnion	Retro-	21	Locus-specific yeast artificial chromosome	20	8/8
Copenhagen group, unpublished	Amnion	Pro-	21	Locus-specific cosmid contig	210	3/3
Bryndorf *et al.*, 1993	Chorion	Retro-	18	Repetitive	50	3/3
			13 and 21	Locus-specific yeast artificial chromosomes		
Bryndorf *et al.*, 1994	Chorion	Pro-	21	Locus-specific cosmid contig	60	2/2

Repetitive probes generally yield well-defined and intense FISH signals. In our own first study on uncultured amniocytes, therefore, we used repetitive probes specific for chromosomes 18 and 1 (Christensen *et al.*, 1992; Table 14.3). In a retrospective study of 33 samples, we identified two samples with trisomies 18 and one with trisomy 18 and 1 (i.e. the sample was triploid). No repetitive probe is specific only for chromosome 21. Therefore, we used locus-specific probes for FISH screening for Down's syndrome on uncultured amniotic fluid samples. Initially we used a large (500 000 base pair) chromosome 21-specific yeast artificial chromosome (Bryndorf *et al.*, 1992; Potier *et al.*, 1992). Retrospectively we were able to identify correctly samples from eight Down's syndrome fetuses. However, the FISH signals were not optimal being too large and diffuse to discern effectively. In collaboration with Becton Dickinson Immunocytometry Systems we subcloned another large chromosome 21-specific yeast artificial chromosome into smaller cosmids (Bryndorf *et al.*, 1994). Empirically we decided which combination of cosmids produced the most intense and well-defined signals. At the same time we employed the cell-preparation technique described by Klinger *et al.* (1992). This combination of improved probe and sample preparation enabled us to screen prospectively 210 uncultured amnion samples. Three trisomy 21 cases were easily identified.

Our first studies on uncultured chorionic villus samples used a combination of yeast artificial chromosomes specific for chromosomes 13 and 21 and a repetitive chromosome 18-specific probe. In a prospective series of 50 samples, we identified two samples with trisomy 21 and one triploid sample. However, as with the uncultured amnion samples, the signals generated by the yeast artificial chromosome probes were rather large and diffuse making signal scoring complicated. Therefore, we tried the chromosome 21-specific cosmid contig probe already mentioned (Bryndorf *et al.*, 1994). We readily identified two samples with trisomy 21 in a prospective series of 60 samples.

The above data indicate that prenatal FISH assays have the potential for clinical implementation. In small trials, all numerical abnormalities have been detected by FISH and in the large amnion trial described by Ward *et al.* (1993) the specificity was very high (99.9%), while the sensitivity was lower (93.9%). However, the problem of the many 'non-reported samples' for the amnion assay has to be solved or circumvented before this assay is used clinically. In the trial described by Ward *et al.* (1993), 12% of the samples received with adequate volume for FISH were not reported on and in our trial so far 19% of samples have been 'non-reportable'. The main reason for the samples being 'non-reportable' was suspected maternal-cell contamination. In our trial, 12% of specimens could not be analyzed at all because of visible blood or other contaminants in the amniotic fluid. Maternal leukocytes in amniotic fluid samples are not a major problem for conventional chromosome analysis since leukocytes do not 'plate' during *in vitro* cell culture. However, *all* cells including leukocytes are analyzed when performing FISH on uncultured cells. Christensen *et al.* (1993) showed that FISH should not be used for chromosome enumeration of uncultured amniotic fluid samples that are macroscopically blood-stained. Numerical aberrations might be overlooked. Moskowitz *et al.* (1993) showed that the maternal cell contamination problem can be reduced by using a very strict amniocentesis protocol, among other things taking care to avoid damage to the placenta. But the problem of maternal cell contamination still exists. One solution could be to differentially stain leukocytes and amniocytes or to remove the leucocytes artificially.

If the problem of maternal-cell contamination is solved for the amnion-FISH assay and multi-centre trials show that FISH performs satisfactorily on uncultured amniotic fluid samples and/or on uncultured chorionic villus samples, it still remains to be decided how to use FISH prenatally: whether to use FISH as a diagnostic tool and/or as a screening tool. The answer to this question will depend on ethical considerations taking into account (i) the risk of inducing a miscarriage by amniocentesis and chorionic villus sampling; (ii) the diagnosis achieved; and (iii) economics.

Risk The risk of inducing a miscarriage by amniocentesis and chorionic villus sampling will apply whatever analyses are performed on the sampled tissue. However, if the FISH assay is used as a screening tool, it may only be necessary to sample a fraction of the fetal tissue that is sampled today. To our knowledge, nobody knows the fetal risk of sampling, for example, 5 ml of amniotic fluid. In the future, the risk of sampling fetal tissue for FISH analysis may even be eliminated totally by isolating fetal cells from maternal blood (Bianchi *et al.*, 1990).

Diagnosis If conventional chromosome analysis is substituted by FISH assays using probes specific for chromosomes 13, 18, 21, X and Y, then certain rare, serious disorders involving regions outside those hybridized to, for example, Cri-du-Chat syndrome, will not be diagnosed. Whiteman and Klinger (1991) calculated that using a FISH assay with probes specific for chromosomes 13, 18, 21, X and Y only 66% of all prenatal abnormalities including balanced translocations and variants detected by conventional

The Sheffield laboratory

The Sheffield laboratory services six Health Districts and part of a seventh in the north of the Region and, additionally, provides services for two Districts in the adjacent Yorkshire Region. The combined catchment area yields some 29 000 pregnancies per annum. Down's syndrome screening has been introduced progressively throughout the catchment area only after extensive consultation with the clinical services. This has, inevitably, resulted in a gradual uptake of screening with the Districts coming on-stream at different times and with slightly differing policies. The eventual aim, however, is for a uniform policy throughout the catchment area.

Policy

Discussions between the screening laboratory, cytogenetics service, obstetricians and midwives have resulted in a common preferred policy of serum screening for all mothers, regardless of age, at 14–16 weeks of gestation. The routine offer of amniocentesis to mothers over the age of 35 years has been discontinued although the option has been retained for mothers over the age of 40 years. This policy was, in part, dictated by the funding provided by the Authority whereby monies were made available for the biochemical element of the screening programme but no additional monies were made available for the resultant cytogenetic examinations which were deemed to be included within existing numbers.

The point at which amniocentesis would be offered was set at a mid-trimester risk of 1:200, which should yield an intervention rate of about 4.5%, equivalent to the proportion of all pregnancies occurring in women between the ages of 35 and 40 years, and equating with the age-related full-term risk at 36 years.

It was agreed that the report from the screening laboratory would quote the actual risk level, but that risks greater than 1:200 would be flagged as of 'high risk', and risks less than 1:200 as 'low risk'. The terms 'screen positive' and 'screen negative' are avoided as these could be misleading and open to misinterpretation.

Information

The screening programme represents a change in the policy for prenatal diagnosis which had been in existence for a number of years. For this reason, it was felt necessary to embark on a programme of education for all health-care professionals. The programme included explanation of the scientific basis of the screening programme and its expected yield, and a detailed discussion of counselling. It was accepted that, with the increasing trend for first hospital attendances to be delayed until 18 weeks of gestation, the burden of education and the initial counselling would fall on the community professionals.

In support of the education programme of seminars and discussion groups, two leaflets were produced: one for health-care professionals and one for patients. The latter was widely disseminated in hospital clinics and health centres. Use has also been made of a patient information video for use in hospital antenatal clinics and health centres. The programme has also received mention on local radio and television.

As the screening programme has progressed, up-date leaflets have been prepared for circulation to all clinics detailing the results obtained, together with relevant information from other centres, both within the Region and on a national basis. Where appropriate, additional information has also been included from the European Down's Syndrome Screening Group.

Sample collection

With the existing serum screening programme for neural tube defect (NTD) in operation throughout the catchment area of the laboratory, sample collection for Down's syndrome screening presented no problems. The only significant change was that of blood sample collection at 14–16 weeks of gestation rather than the 16–18 weeks of gestation preferred for NTD screening.

It was decided to assess the risk in relation to the best estimate of gestation available at the time of blood collection. This was either based on last menstrual period or from ultrasonographic examination. Few of the antenatal clinics performed routine early 'dating' scans, but where these were available they would form the definitive assessment of gestational age. When an early scan had not been performed, and a later scan caused a revision of the gestational age by more than 10 days, the risk factor is recalculated.

The influence of gestational-age assessment on the risk factor calculation is best illustrated by reference to three districts within the catchment area. Review of the 'high-risk' flags over a 2-month period showed significant differences which can be related to local obstetric practice. In one District where practice dictated an early dating scan, the 'high risk' rate was 3.8%; in a second, where 30% of samples were submitted from the community and dating scans were performed on about half of the hospital attendees, the 'high risk' rate was 4.8%; whilst in the third, where 80% of samples were submitted from the community and only 5% of patients had early scans, the rate was 7.0%.

Assay

Following early reports of various biochemical screening protocols, initial trials were conducted in 1990 utilising AFP and free β-subunit of hCG. The trials, with sera stored from the existing prenatal screening programme, gave results which were in agreement with other centres (Macri *et al.*, 1990; Spencer, 1991). Further work established median values for free β-hCG at the relevant weeks of gestation and, in collaboration with other laboratories, established the parameters needed for calculation of risk (Spencer *et al.*, 1992).

With these trials completed and a programme for the risk calculation added into the laboratory information system, prospective screening was commenced in one District in October 1990. This was extended to a second District in 1991, and a third in 1992. In addition to the full District screening, facilities were also made available for patients to be screened in the other Districts served by the laboratory on an individual request basis. Two further Districts have commenced full screening programmes during 1993 and the remaining Districts in the catchment area will commence in the next few months when the full counselling and information systems are available.

The gradual introduction of biochemical screening throughout the catchment area of the laboratory has allowed the protocols and the information systems to be modified in the light of experience. The need for adequate counselling has been emphasised, as has the need for improvements in the assessment of gestational age.

Results observed

In the two years since the screening programme has been operational, 10 415 screened pregnancies have delivered. Eighteen trisomies have been ascertained: 13 trisomy 21 and 5 trisomy 18 cases, an incidence of 1:800 and 1:2080, respectively. The incidence rates agree with the expected incidence of these chromosome anomalies in the general population, suggesting that the assessment procedures are effective and give a complete picture of the local birth incidence.

A classification of 'high risk' was made for 459 pregnancies (4.4%), with risk estimates in excess of 1:200 at mid-trimester. This percentage is in keeping with the calculated intervention level which was designed to give an amniocentesis rate no higher than that associated with maternal age-directed amniocentesis.

Included within the high-risk pregnancies were 16 of the trisomies: 11 trisomy 21 and all 5 cases of trisomy 18, a detection rate of 85% for trisomy 21 and 100% for trisomy 18, and an overall trisomy detection rate of 89%. This represents a significant advance on the trisomy detection rate of 20% achieved by the age-alone protocol. The incidence of fetal trisomy detected by biochemical screen-directed amniocentesis of 1:29 is also considerably higher than the 1:85 rate obtained by maternal age-directed amniocentesis.

Audit

Any screening programme must have a comprehensive system of audit. The screening laboratory, and the obstetric services, should have a complete picture of the effects of the screening programme, with an assessment of its successes and its failures.

Identification of all trisomic pregnancies can only be obtained by gathering information from a number of sources. These include the birth anomalies register maintained by each District Director of Public Health, the relevant cytogenetic laboratory, and the hospital delivery suites. This information can be supplemented by an estimate of the expected number of trisomies obtained by application of the age-related incidence (Cuckle *et al.*, 1987) to the age profile of pregnancies screened. Table 15.1 shows the combined age profile of pregnancies in two Districts served by the Sheffield laboratory for 1 year. The expected number of Down's syndrome pregnancies obtained from the age profile confirms that the number ascertained is likely to be complete, with five expected in the observed age mix of pregnancies, and five ascertained from the combination of information sources.

Audit will allow modifications to the risk calculation and the operational policy, as well as yielding information for health-care professionals involved with counselling.

In addition to audit within the catchment area, audit of the programme throughout the Region will allow comparison to be made between assay

Table 15.1. *Age profile of pregnancies and Down's syndrome ascertained in two Districts for* 1991

| | Pregnancies | Down's syndrome | |
		Rate (1 in)	Expected No.
Age profile			
48	1	11	0.0909
47	0	15	0
46	0	21	0
45	0	28	0
44	3	37	0.0811
43	2	49	0.0408
42	7	65	0.1077
41	8	85	0.0941
40	18	112	0.1606
39	18	146	0.1233
38	41	189	0.2169
37	37	242	0.1529
36	47	307	0.1531
35	80	384	0.2083
34	106	474	0.2264
33	89	574	0.1551
32	154	683	0.2255
31	203	796	0.2550
30	236	909	0.2596
29	309	1018	0.3035
28	291	1119	0.2601
27	298	1208	0.2467
26	343	1286	0.2667
25	375	1351	0.2776
24	299	1404	0.2130
23	310	1447	0.2142
22	261	1481	0.1762
21	200	1507	0.1327
20	200	1528	0.1309
19	139	1544	0.0900
18	140	1556	0.0900
17	74	1565	0.0473
16	27	1572	0.0172
15	12	1578	0.0076
Total	4327		5.02
Corrected to mid-trimester			6.18

Ascertained Down's syndrome
Mid-trimester	2
Postnatal	3
Expected number	5

protocols. This might suggest changes to established practice and the development of a more unified approach to the screening programme.

References

Cuckle, H.S., Wald, N.J. & Thompson, S.G. (1987). Estimating a woman's risk of having a pregnancy associated with Down's syndrome using her age and serum alpha-fetoprotein level. *Br. J. Obstet. Gynaecol.*, **94**, 387–402.

Macri, J.N., Kasturi, R.V., Krantz, D.A. *et al.* (1990). Maternal serum Down's syndrome screening: free beta protein is a more effective marker than human chorionic gonadotropin. *Am. J. Obstet. Gynaecol.*, **163**, 1248–53.

Spencer, K. (1991). Evaluation of an assay for the free beta subunit of choriogonadotropin and its potential value in screening for Down's syndrome. *Clin. Chem.*, **37**, 809–14.

Spencer, K., Coombes, E.J., Mallard, A.S. & Milford Ward, A. (1992). Free beta human choriogonadotropin in Down's syndrome screening: a multicentre study of its role compared with other biochemical markers. *Ann. Clin. Biochem.*, **29**, 506–18.

Wald, N.J. & Cuckle, H.S. (1987). Recent advances in screening for neural tube defects and Down's syndrome. In *Baillière's Clinical Obstetrics and Gynaecology*, vol. I, ed. C. Rodeck, pp. 649–76. London: Baillière and Tindall.

Wald, N.J., Cuckle, H.S., Densem, J.W. *et al.* (1988). Maternal serum screening for Down's syndrome in early pregnancy. *Br. Med. J.*, **297**, 883–7.

Wald, N.J., Kennard, A., Densem, J.W. *et al.* (1992). Antenatal maternal screening for Down's syndrome: result of a demonstration project. *Br. Med. J.*, **305**, 391–4.

Wilson, J.M.G. & Jungner, G. (1968). Principles and practice of screening for disease. *Public Health Papers* 34. Geneva: WHO.

16

Organization of screening programs: the Californian experience

M.S. GOLBUS, L. LUSTIG AND G.C. CUNNINGHAM

Introduction

Since prenatal diagnosis of genetic disorders was introduced into clinical practice in the late 1960s, there has been a need for suitable screening of the pregnant population to identify those pregnancies at highest risk of having an aneuploid fetus. Because of the known association of maternal age and the risk of fetal trisomy, the classic screening test has been the mother's age. It is currently accepted medical practice to advise pregnant women above a cut-off age (35 years in the United States) about their increased risk of a trisomic fetus and to offer prenatal diagnosis by one of the currently available invasive diagnostic tests (amniocentesis or chorionic villus sampling, CVS). Another screening test became available with the demonstration of an association between low levels of maternal serum α-fetoprotein (MSAFP) and fetal Down's syndrome (Merkatz et al., 1984). MSAFP screening was shown to be effective (New England study, 1989) and to detect approximately 20% of Down's syndrome fetuses (Lustig et al., 1988). MSAFP screening has been widely added to maternal age screening to identify those pregnancies at highest risk for a chromosomally abnormal fetus.

The Genetic Disease Branch of the Department of Public Health of the State of California instituted an MSAFP screening program with a goal of providing voluntary screening to all pregnant women in California between 15 and 20 menstrual weeks. The program objectives were defined as providing (i) information to the patients about the availability of testing, and the benefits, risks and limitations of the testing; (ii) assistance to clinicians in utilizing the program and in interpreting the results; (iii) a network of laboratories and prenatal diagnosis programs through which program participants could obtain all necessary tests and procedures;

(iv) centralized organization and computerization; and (v) a fiscal basis for the program. The Genetic Disease Branch was greatly assisted in developing a program to meet these objectives by technical committees consisting of clinical geneticists and laboratory supervisors, physician representatives of the California Medical Association and the American College of Obstetricians and Gynecologists, and representatives of the Spina Bifida Association and the Down's Syndrome Parents Association. Broad-based participation in designing the MSAFP program helped establish wide and rapid acceptance when the program was implemented.

Activities prior to testing

The California MSAFP screening program was grafted onto an already existing statewide prenatal diagnosis program. This latter program, under the auspices of the Genetic Disease Branch, consisted of 20 prenatal diagnosis centers, predominantly at University medical centers, each serving a catchment area of the state's 500 000 annual deliveries in 1986 (600 000 deliveries by 1990). Those prenatal diagnosis centers which were capable of meeting the Genetic Disease Branch standards (see below) were invited to become regional MSAFP Screening Program co-ordinating centers and 14 such centers were established. Each regional MSAFP center hired a co-ordinator (mostly genetic counselors but some registered nurses) who was charged with providing an education program for hospital staffs, community clinics and physician office staffs in a specific catchment area. Committees were organized which included Genetic Disease Branch staff, clinical geneticists, laboratory supervisors and community representatives and were charged with developing educational material for both patients and physicians, informed consent forms and standards for the laboratories, the co-ordinating centers and the staff of the co-ordinating centers. The Genetic Disease Branch also developed specimen collection kits and directions and contracted with a small number of laboratories to provide statewide testing. It was felt that by having a small number of laboratories it would be easier to maintain quality control.

Two aspects of establishing the program warrant further comment. The first was a decision by the Genetic Disease Branch to computerize the entire program and to mandate statewide reporting of fetuses and neonates with chromosome abnormalities and neural tube defects. This has made possible evaluation of the program and the grafting onto the program of various research projects to answer significant clinical questions (Lustig *et al.*, 1988; Waller *et al.*, 1990; Haddow *et al.*, 1993). The second aspect was a decision by the Genetic Disease Branch to set standards not only for the assay laboratories but also for the regional co-ordinating centers and their staff. The centers were required to have a board-certified clinical geneticist as director, genetic counselors who were board eligible or certified, and to provide services, including amniocentesis, level II consultative sonography, pregnancy termination (or referral) and cytogenetics, and to collect pregnancy outcome data on at least 90% of the patients counseled.

Standards were also developed for the physicians in the centers. Currently, these include the following requirements. Amniocentesis was to be provided by an obstetrician gynecologist or an individual from another specialty supervised by an obstetrician gynecologist. The operator had to have performed 100 supervised ultrasound-guided second trimester amniocenteses, to be performing at least 50 amniocenteses annually, to be trained to provide level I sonography and to have reported an individual adverse outcome rate for a 6-month period to the Genetic Disease Branch. Consultative ultrasonography was to be provided by a board-certified radiologist or an obstetrician gynecologist who had completed a maternal fetal medicine or ultrasonography fellowship or who had 6-month's sonography training in a unit doing at least 2000 second trimester examinations annually. The provider had to have done 500 detailed sonograms on patients referred for the detection of fetal anomalies and to perform 200 such examinations annually. Transcervical CVS was to be performed by a board-certified obstetrician gynecologist with specific training in prenatal diagnosis who/had performed 50 supervised transcervical CVSs and who continued to do 50 CVSs annually. Transabdominal CVSs was to be performed by a board-certified obstetrician gynecologist with specific training in prenatal diagnosis who had performed 50 supervised transabdominal CVSs or was approved for amniocentesis and had performed 10 supervised transabdominal CVSs or was approved for percutaneous umbilical blood sampling (PUBS) and had performed five supervised transabdominal CVSs, and who continued to do 50 CVSs annually. PUBS was to be performed by a board-certified obstetrician gynecologist who had approval for amniocentesis and who had performed 15 supervised PUBSs and who continued to perform 10 PUBSs annually. The establishment of such statewide standards had contributed to minimizing the procedure complication rates.

Program results

The California MSAFP screening program started in 1986 and has progressed from screening 22% of all eligible births in 1986 to screening 69% of all eligible births in 1992. Cut-off levels were established such that 4–4.5% of patients screened are referred for follow-up of an abnormal AFP serum level. Table 16.1 presents the number of patients screened,

Table 16.1. *AFP-related services provided at regional co-ordinating centers*

	1987	1992	Total
Total AFP	7552	12 281	62 574
Genetic counseling/ultrasound	6435	12 111	60 777
Amniocentesis	3663	6334	32 445
Abnormalities detected	286	433	2241

receiving genetic counseling and sonography examinations, receiving amniocentesis, and being diagnosed as carrying an abnormal fetus in 1987, 1992 and for the length of the program.

A reasonable estimate of the financial costs and benefits of the California MSAFP screening program can be made. The Center for Disease Control estimated the lifetime costs for spina bifida as $250 000 in 1985 dollars, discounted by 5% (MMWR 21 April, 1989), and a review of 20 studies on the lifetime costs of care for a Down's syndrome individual suggests $403 962 as a conservative cost estimate in California. In fiscal year 1989–90, the California MSAFP program was responsible for the prevention of 62 cases of open spina bifida and 29 cases of Down's syndrome with a cost avoidance of $30 573 004. Discounting at 3% per annum for 40 years results in a net present value of costs avoided of $14 057 877. The total savings are actually greater because the MSAFP program is also responsible for the prenatal detection of many other fetal birth defects. A more elaborate cost–benefit analysis considering replacement costs, lost productivity, etc. reported for similar programs would increase this figure. The total state expenditure in fiscal year 1989–90 for this program was $13 142 862, not including abortion costs which are not covered under the program.

The future

In the late 1980s, two further analytes, human chorionic gonadotropin (Bogart *et al.*, 1987) and unconjugated estriol (Canick *et al.*, 1988), were identified as potentially increasing the sensitivity of the screening provided by MSAFP in detecting the fetus with Down's syndrome. Triple marker screening utilizing these three markers and correcting for their inter-correlations have indicated a marked improvement in the efficiency of the screening process (Haddow *et al.*, 1992; Phillips *et al.*, 1992; Cheng *et al.*, 1993; Wald *et al.*, 1993). The Genetic Disease Branch is in the process of converting the California program to a multiple analyte screen with the education process to start in July 1994 and multiple analyte testing to start in September 1994.

Another consideration raised by multiple analyte testing is whether it should be applied to all pregnancies and not just those of women less than 35 years of age. An in-press manuscript resulting from a collaborative study by the Genetics Disease Branch and the Foundation for Blood Research (Scarborough, Maine) suggests that this might be the most appropriate public health policy. The California MSAFP screening program is now considering the ramifications of such a change. The future course is not yet charted but appears challenging and exciting to all involved in the prenatal detection of genetic disorders.

References

Bogart, M.J., Pandian, M.R. & Jones, O.W. (1987). Abnormal maternal serum chorionic gonadotropin levels in pregnancies with fetal chromosome abnormalities. *Prenatal Diagn.*, 7, 623–30.

Canick, J.A., Knight, G.J., Palomaki, G.E. *et al.* (1988). Low second trimester maternal serum unconjugated oestriol in pregnancies with Down's syndrome. *Br. J. Obstet. Gynaecol.*, 95, 330–3.

Cheng, E.Y., Luthy, D.A., Zebelman, A.M. *et al.* (1993). A prospective evaluation of a second trimester screening test for fetal Down syndrome using maternal serum alpha-fetoprotein, hCG, and unconjugated estriol. *Obstet. Gynecol.*, 81, 72–7.

Haddow, J.E., Palomaki, G.E., Knight, G.J. *et al.* (1992). Prenatal screening for Down's syndrome with use of maternal serum markers, *N. Engl. J. Med.*, 327, 588–93.

Haddow, J.E., Palomaki, G.E., Knight, G.J. *et al.* (1993). Prenatal screening to reduce amniocentesis in pregnant women age 35 and older: a multicenter prospective non-intervention trial, submitted for publication.

Lustig, L., Clarke, S., Cunningham, G. *et al.* (1988). California's experience with low MSAFP results. *Am. J. Med. Genet.*, 31, 211–22.

Merkatz, I.R., Nitowsky, H.M., Macri, J.N. *et al.* (1984). An association between low maternal serum alpha-fetoprotein and fetal chromosomal abnormalities. *Am. J. Obstet. Gynecol.,* **148**, 886–94.

New England Regional Genetics Group Prenatal Collaborative Study of Down Syndrome Screening (1989). Combined maternal serum alpha-fetoprotein measurements and age to screen for Down syndrome in pregnant women under age 35. *Am. J. Obstet. Gynecol.,* **160**, 578–81.

Phillips, O.P., Elias, S., Shulman, L.P. *et al.* (1992). Maternal serum screening for fetal Down syndrome in women less than 35 years of age using alpha-fetoprotein, hCG, and unconjugated estriol: a prospective 2-year study. *Obstet. Gynecol.,* **80**, 353–8.

Wald, N.J., Kennard, A., Densem, J.W. *et al.* (1993). Antenatal maternal serum screening for Down's syndrome: results of a demonstration project. *Br. Med. J.,* **305**, 391–4.

Waller, K., Lustig, L. & Hook, E. (1990). Gestational age at maternal serum alpha-fetoprotein screening and the detection of Down syndrome. *Am. J. Hum. Genet.,* **47**, 581–2.

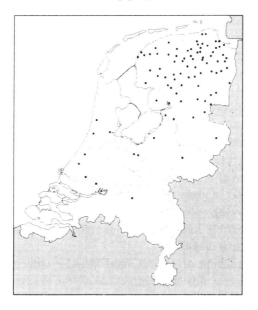

Fig. 17.3. The Netherlands. Serum samples were sent to the University Hospital, Groningen from the places marked with a dot.

attendant contacted the woman on the same day or on the next day in person or by telephone. We informed the women who were screen-positive for Down's syndrome of the age-related and the calculated risk. If the result was screen-negative, we provided information about the risk levels only if the women were over 36 years of age, to enable them to make a well-founded decision about their 'right' to undergo amniocentesis.

The results of karyotyping were known within 2 weeks of amniocentesis, the amniotic fluid AFP results within 2 days and the results of the third-level ultrasound were available immediately. The screen-positive rate for Down's syndrome was 6.7%. We found nine fetuses with trisomy 21, two with trisomy 18, one with Turner's syndrome, one with trisomy 13, one triploidy, as well as two fetuses with NTD and two with an omphalocoele. We missed at least three infants with trisomy 21 and one with NTD.

With a risk cut-off for Down's syndrome of 1 in 250 at term, the expected proportion of screen-positives is usually around 5%, and 55% of the fetuses with Down's syndrome would be detected (Wald *et al.*, 1988). These percentages would increase if more older women were to be included, because maternal age plays an important role in determining

Table 17.1. *Age-specific characteristics of serum screening: the cutoff for Down's syndrome risk $\geq 1:250$*

Age (years)	Screen-positive (%)[a]	Detection of Down's syndrome (%)[b]
20	3.4	47.1
24	3.8	48.5
28	5.0	52.9
32	9.0	62.3
36	21.1	77.3
40	49.8	92.0
44	86.5	99.0

[a] Percentage of the screened population.
[b] Calculated according to Crossley *et al.* (1991), with the medians and standard deviation of maternal serum AFP and hCG from the University Hospital, Groningen.

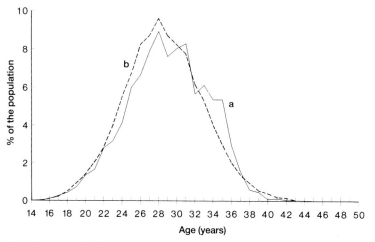

Fig. 17.4. The age distribution of (*a*) the screened population at term and (*b*) other pregnant women in the north-eastern part of the Netherlands (data from the Central Office for Statistics, The Hague).

the risk of fetal Down's syndrome (Table 17.1). As we had a 6.7% screen-positive result, we examined the age distribution in our population. The 33- to 36-year-old age group appeared to be over-represented compared to the rest of the pregnant population in our area (Fig. 17.4). These women form the borderline group for prenatal diagnosis as indicated by advanced maternal age, the cut-off point being 36 years of age in the Netherlands (Kloosterman, 1987).

Another cause for the high number of screen-positives might have been the fact that 27% of the women had no ultrasound dating. The screen-positive rate in this group was 8.6%, compared to 6.1% in the women with ultrasound dating.

It is essential to keep the time interval between serum screening and amniocentesis to a minimum because serum screening usually causes some distress if the result is positive (Abuelo *et al.*, 1991; Katz-Rothman, 1991; Roelofsen *et al.*, 1993).

A major concern in a situation with so many different referring sources and, therefore, often a small number of samples per source is how to provide adequate information for the women. We make this as uniform as possible by sending each 'new' source the written information we offer to pregnant women at our hospital. A 24-hour telephone service was available at the Department of Obstetrics and Gynaecology of the University Hospital Groningen for those who had questions about serum screening in general or about their own screening results. However, because population-wide screening is discouraged by the Dutch Government, information about such a screening programme only reaches those who ask for serum screening.

Maternal serum screening is cost-effective (Sheldon and Simpson, 1991; Wald *et al.*, 1992). The cost attributable to serum screening in the decentralized system is negligible. It is cheaper to send a sample than for the woman to visit the hospital herself. The extra cost of developing an automated system for follow-up and for providing adequate information was less than US $2500.

We conclude that reliable maternal serum screening for Down's syndrome and NTD is feasible in a strongly decentralized obstetric system such as that in the Netherlands. A programme based on individual requests is also effective. In such circumstances, it is important to keep screening centralized. This ensures the availability of adequate prescreening information for the participants, high-quality biochemical tests and complete follow-up of the pregnancy outcome.

References

Abuelo, D.N., Hopmann, M.R., Barsel-Bowers, G. & Goldstein, A. (1991). Anxiety in women with low maternal serum alpha-fetoprotein screening results. *Prenatal Diagn.*, **11**, 381–5.

Annual Report Committee of the Working Party on Prenatal Diagnosis (1992). *Annual Report*, 1989. Utrecht: Working Party on Prenatal Diagnosis of the Dutch Society of Obstetrics and Gynaecology and the Dutch Society of Clinical Genetics.

Beekhuis, J.R. (1993). Maternal serum screening for fetal Down's syndrome and neural tube defects. A prospective study, performed in the north of the Netherlands. Thesis. Groningen: Dijkhuizen Van Zanten bv.

Beekhuis, J.R. & Mantingh, A. (1990). Maternale serum alfa-foetoproteine screening. *Ned. Tijdschr. Obstet. Gynaecol.*, **103**, 232–4.

Beekhuis, J.R., van Lith, J.M.M., van Loon, A.J. & Mantingh, A. (1991). Foetale echografie en neurale-buisdefecten: morfologische diagnose zonder klinische zekerheid (Letter). *Ned. Tijdschr. Geneeskd*, **135**, 340.

Beekhuis, J.R., Mantingh, A., de Wolf, B.T.H.M., van Lith, J.M.M. & Breed, A.S.P.M. (1993). Maternal serum screening for fetal neural tube defects and Down's syndrome; first Dutch experience. *Ned. Tijdschr. Geneeskd.*, **137**, 1303–7.

Crossley, J.A., Aitken, D.A. & Connor, J.M. (1991). Prenatal screening for chromosome abnormalities using maternal serum chorionic gonadotropin, alpha-fetoprotein, and age. *Prenatal Diagn.*, **11**, 83–101.

Gezondheidsraad (1988). *Neuraalbuisdefecten.* 's Gravenhage: Gezondheidsraad, p. 116.

Katz-Rothman, B. (1991). The tentative pregnancy: prenatal diagnosis and the future of motherhood. In *Screening in Prenatal Diagnosis*, ed. A. Mantingh, A.S.P.M. Breed, J.R. Beekhuis & J.M.M. van Lith, pp. 53–61.

Kloosterman, M.D. (1987). *Prenatale diagnostiek in de eerste helft van de zwangerschap.* Apeldoorn: Medicom.

Korff de Gidts, S. & Doppenberg, H. (1993). De organisatie van de abortushulpverlening in Nederland anno 1993. *Med. Contact*, **48**, 110–12.

Los, F.J. (1980). Serum-AFP-screening op foetale neuraalbuisdefecten. Thesis. Meppel: Krips Repro.

Macri, J.N. (1991). Is screening a wolf in sheep's clothing? How experience in a large scale program has revealed pitfalls and perils but led to benefits. In *Screening in Prenatal Diagnosis*, ed. A. Mantingh, A.S.P.M. Breed, J.R. Beekhuis & J.M.M. van Lith, pp. 11–24. Groningen: Academic Press.

Ministerie van Welzijn, Volksgezondheid en Cultuur (1989). *Beleidsstandpunt bevolkingsonderzoek neurale buisdefecten.* WVC kenmerk DGV gz/E en I/23513. Rijswijk: WVC.

Ris, M. (1986). Obstetrical care in the Netherlands. The place of midwives and specific aspects of their rôle. In *Perinatal Care Delivery Systems*, ed. M. Kaminsky, G. Bréart, P. Buekens, H.J. Huisjes, G. McIlwaine & H.K. Selbmann, pp. 167–77. Oxford: Oxford University Press.

Roelofsen, E.E.C., Kamerbeek, L.I., Tijmstra, Tj., Beekhuis, J.R. & Mantingh, A. (1993). Women's opinions on the offer and use of maternal serum screening. *Prenatal Diagn.*, **13**, 741–7.

Sheldon, T.A. & Simpson, J. (1991). Appraisal of a new scheme for prenatal screening for Down's syndrome. *Br. Med. J.*, **302**, 1133–6.

Wald, N.J., Cuckle, H.S., Densem, J.W. et al. (1988). Maternal serum screening for Down's syndrome in early pregnancy. *Br. Med. J.*, **297**, 883–7.

Wald, N.J., Cuckle, H.S., Densem, J.W., Kennard, A. & Smith, D. (1992). Maternal serum screening for Down's syndrome: the effect of routine ultrasound scan determination of gestational age and adjustment for maternal weight. *Br. J. Obstet. Gynaecol.*, **99**, 144–9.

18

Organisation of screening programmes: the French experience

F. MULLER AND A. BOUÉ

Pregnancy care in France is based on clinical follow-up, maternal serum screening and ultrasound examination. At the first clinical examination the parameters investigated include blood group and serum antibodies for toxoplasmosis, rubella, syphilis, hepatitis B and HIV. Maternal serum α-fetoprotein (MSAFP) screening is not used because of the low incidence (1/2000) of neural tube defects (NTD) in France. Ultrasound examinations are performed at 10, 22 and 32 weeks. Amniocentesis for fetal karyotyping is offered to women aged 38 years or more and is actually performed in 60% of these cases.

There are 60 cytogenetic laboratories (public and private) in France. The population is 56 million and in a typical year there are around 750 000 live births; around 1100 occurrences of trisomy 21 at birth; 200 000 terminations of pregnancy for social reasons (before the 12th week); 30 000 prenatal diagnoses (cytogenetics, monogenic diseases); 1000 terminations of pregnancy for anomalies detected by laboratory analysis; and an unknown number of terminations of pregnancy for anomalies detected by ultrasound.

Development of prenatal diagnosis in France

Amniocentesis and prenatal diagnosis were introduced in France in 1972. As of 1980, amniocentesis for fetal karyotyping was made available free of charge to patients aged 38 years and over, patients with a previous child affected by a chromosomal anomaly, and parents carrying a balanced structural anomaly. Between 1980 and 1990, 113 000 karyotypes were performed for reasons of maternal age (in 1991, 60% of mothers > 38 years underwent amniocentesis), leading to the diagnosis of 2800 chromosomal anomalies including 2100 cases of trisomy 21.

Universal application of screening based on maternal age (patients > 38 years) would lead to diagnosis of only 25% of trisomy 21 cases. In women under 38, trisomy 21 screening is now often based on ultrasound findings, the detection efficiency of which is difficult to evaluate.

In France, ultrasound examination is highly developed and is paid for by the social security system. A 1987 study of the Provence–Alpes–Côte d'Azur region showed that only 1% of pregnant women did not undergo ultrasound scanning and that 70% had at least three scans. The sensitivity of ultrasound in screening for malformations depends on the timing of the scan, the malformation sought, the equipment and the competence of the operator. In 1985, karyotyping after abnormal ultrasound findings was organized. Between 1985 and 1990, 12 000 karyotypes were determined, leading to the diagnosis of 1300 (11%) chromosomal anomalies, including 350 cases of trisomy 21. Large variations in incidence were related to the type of ultrasound finding.

The efficiency of ultrasound findings in the detection of chromosomal anomalies was studied in 1989 and 1990 (Table 18.1). Of 45 750 cytogenetic analyses, 6850 were indicated by ultrasound anomalies. This led to the diagnosis of 720 chromosomal anomalies (10.5%). Analyses were performed in 35 000 patients aged over 38 years, leading to the diagnosis of 842 (2.4%) chromosomal anomalies. Ultrasound signs are therefore four times more efficient than maternal age as an indicator for chromosomal anomaly screening. However, trisomy 21 cases represent only 28% of chromosomal anomalies identified by ultrasound. Moreover, 25% of trisomy 21 cases diagnosed at 16 weeks do not reach term (Hook et al.,

Table 18.1. *Cytogenetic prenatal diagnosis in France; cumulative results from 1989–90*

Indications	No. diagnoses (%)	No. chromosome anomalies (%)
Maternal age > 38 years	35 000 (76.5)	842 (50.9)
Unexpected finding at ultrasound	6 850 (15)	720 (43.5)
Previous pregnancy with chromosome anomaly	2 760 (6)	29 (1)
Chromosome anomaly in parent	1 140 (2.5)	62 (3.7)
Total	45 750 (100)	1 653 (100)

Association Française pour le Dépistage et la Prévention des Handicaps de l'Enfant.

1989) and it is likely that most trisomy 21 fetuses detected by ultrasound will die *in utero* or in the perinatal period.

How many cases of trisomy 21 are potentially detectable by ultrasound examination? What is the real efficiency of screening for minor ultrasound signs associated with trisomy 21 in a general population? At present it is impossible to answer these questions in a general public health programme. It was in this general context (karyotyping for patients over 38 and widespread use of ultrasound) that maternal serum markers were incorporated in the programme of screening for trisomy 21.

Frequency of trisomy 21

Trisomy 21 is a topical subject in Paris since its prevalence has increased in recent years, as revealed by the register of congenital malformations started in 1987 and transmitted to the European EUROCAT register (J. Goujard, personal communication). Between 1981 and 1990, De Vigan observed that 738 cases of trisomy 21 (births and terminations of pregnancy) were notified out of 361 204 births and 1365 terminations of pregnancy carried out because of detected malformations (De Vigan *et al.*, 1992). This is an overall prevalence of 1/490. Over the same period, 415 trisomic live infants were reported (prevalence 1/870). However, a progressive increase in the number of cases of trisomy 21 was observed in the Paris area: from 50 in 1981 to 109 in 1990. Hence, the yearly number of live trisomic births has remained relatively constant (39 in 1981, 34 in 1990), despite the undeniable advance of prenatal screening (Fig. 18.1).

Analysis of demographic data reveals an increase in maternal age over the last decade in the Paris area. In 1981, 62.2% of pregnant women were less than 30 years of age, whereas this proportion had dropped to 50.2% in 1989. The corresponding figures for women of 35 to 38 years were 7.3% in 1981 and 10.6% in 1989. In 1981, 3.7% of pregnant women were aged 38 years or more, compared with 8.4% in 1989. In Paris, 83% of pregnant women of 38 or over underwent amniocentesis in 1990. The maternal age-related increase in the number of cases of trisomy 21 in the Paris area is worrrying, particularly as it has not been halted by prenatal screening over the last decade.

Maternal serum screening for trisomy 21

Maternal AFP screening has not been implemented in France because of the low frequency of neural tube defects (1/2000). hCG screening was

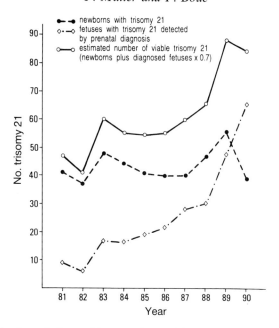

Fig. 18.1. Number of trisomy 21 cases observed in Paris (and suburbs) from 1981 to 1990.

implemented following the observations of Bogart *et al.* (1987). Studies were performed prospectively in some maternity units (1988–90) and were expanded in 1991 to include 14 towns (obstetrics, laboratories, cyto-genetics). The organisation, funding and expansion of this programme are currently under discussion. The following screening-related difficulties have been observed.

Technical problems of hCG measurement Most assay kits were designed for early diagnosis of pregnancy and, therefore, measure low hCG values. They may be unsuitable for second trimester screening (60 000 IU/l). A study by the French Society of Clinical Biology showed that eight laboratories reported widely differing hCG values for the same serum sample (Table 18.2). Correlation between two assays may be good ($r^2 = 0.95$), even though one may be unsuitable for elevated hCG values. Figure 18.2 shows the correlation curve for assays A and B. Residuals analysis (Fig. 18.3) shows that assay B exhibits 45% scatter around the correlation curve above an hCG value of 30 000 IU/l, whereas below this level the error is only 20%. Screening for trisomy 21 during the second

Table 18.2. *The result of analysis of the*
same serum sample for hCG
measurement in eight different
laboratories: a study by the French
Society of Clinical Biology

Technique	Serum hCG (IU/l)
1	26 800
2	19 000
3	35 200
4	31 300
5	45 400
6	30 565
7	31 137
8	29 100

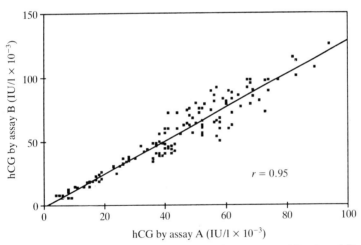

Fig. 18.2. Correlation for hCG measurement between two kits, A and B.

trimester depends on accurate determination of hCG values in the range
30 000–60 000 IU/l. Therefore, in trisomy 21 screening, quality control
must be stringent.

Gestational age-related variations During the second trimester, hCG
values decrease with gestational age. In our prospective study, gestational
age was verified in most (>90%) patients during the first trimester by
ultrasound examination.

F. Muller and F. Boué

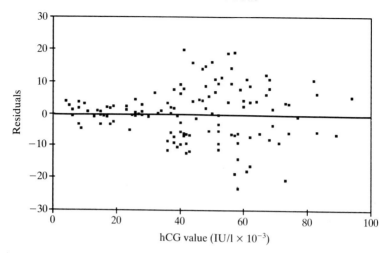

Fig. 18.3. Comparison between kit A and kit B for hCG measurement. Results are expressed as residuals.

The difference between screening and diagnosis This difference is still incompletely understood in France, in contrast to countries that have practised AFP screening since 1976. Maternal anxiety related to this misunderstanding (by the patient or clinician) is a major problem.

Results of prospective hCG screening

Between 1988 and 1990, the protocol of our study was based on maternal blood sampling at 15–17 weeks and hCG measurement by a kit designed for high hCG levels (Clonatec-Paris). Normal values were established with 12 500 samples. Amniocentesis was offered when hCG levels were over the 95th percentile for patients <35 years, over the 80th percentile for patients of 35–36 years, and over the 70th percentile for patients of 37 years. Patients aged over 38 years were not included in this study. During this period, 23 459 patients were tested (singleton pregnancies). The outcome is known in 95% of cases. Three groups of patients can be distinguished: those under 35 years of age, those aged from 35 to 37, and those over 38. The results are shown in Table 18.3: in the group of 16 873 patients aged less than 35 years, 61% of trisomy 21 cases were detected with a 5% amniocentesis rate; in the 4152 patients aged 35 and 36 years, 20% of karyotypes led to the detection of 74% cases of trisomy 21. Patients over 38 years represent a special group because karyotyping is offered in

Table 18.3. *Results of trisomy* 21 *screening with maternal hCG in*
1989–90

Maternal age (years)	No. women tested	No. women selected	Trisomy 21 with hCG > cut-off level	Total trisomy 21
<35	16 873	766 (4.5%)	19 (61%)	31
35–37	4 152	838 (20%)	17 (74%)	23
≥38	2 434	1217 (50%)	34 (94%)	36

all cases but is sometimes refused because of the risk of amniocentesis. If an hCG cut-off at the 50th percentile were to be chosen, amniocentesis would be performed in only 50% of these cases and the trisomy detection rate would be 94%. In this age group, hCG assay can be used as an aid to making decisions.

Since 1992, hCG assay has been combined with maternal age to give a risk factor (Muller *et al.*, 1993). We have determined the risk of trisomy 21 related to maternal age in a prospective study based on 20 000 cases of known outcome. When this risk is > 1/100, amniocentesis is offered.

Improvement of trisomy 21 screening

Two options for improvement of trisomy 21 screening are a combination of hCG and other markers (AFP and/or oestriol) or hCG assay used in conjunction with ultrasound.

Evaluation of AFP measurement

NTD detection Eleven cases (4 anencephaly, 7 spina bifida) of NTD were observed in 24 500 pregnancies. Eight were detected by ultrasound examination performed at 22–24 weeks and 3 cases of spina bifida were observed at birth. AFP screening would at best benefit these 3 cases.

Trisomy 21 screening Retrospective measurement shows that in 57 cases, 22 (38%) had AFP values above the median. The combination of AFP and hCG therefore would not significantly increase the effectiveness of

F. Muller and F. Boué

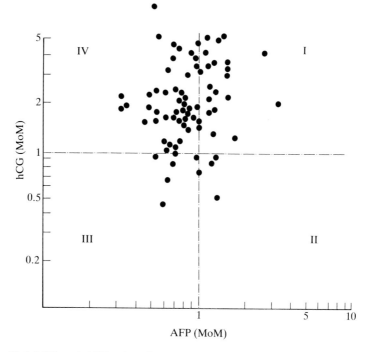

Fig. 18.4. hCG and AFP values for maternal serum in each case of fetal trisomy 21. Results are expressed as MoM.

trisomy 21 screening as compared with hCG assay alone. In Fig. 18.4, a plot of the multiple of the median (MoM) for hCG versus AFP levels in 57 cases of trisomy 21 has been divided into four areas. Area IV corresponds to the classical situation in trisomy 21: high hCG values associated with low AFP values. Area I corresponds to trisomy 21 cases with high hCG values associated with high AFP values. In these cases, AFP would not improve screening efficiency. Area II corresponds to trisomy 21 cases with low hCG values and high AFP values; these cases would never be detected by maternal screening. Area III corresponds to cases with low hCG values and low AFP values; these cases would be detected only by AFP screening.

As most cases of trisomy 21 have high hCG values and low AFP values, they are detected by this combination. But in cases with AFP > 1 MoM (38% of cases), the combination of hCG and AFP does not increase trisomy 21 detection rate and may even decrease it.

Benefits of ultrasound examination

Ultrasound examination is useful in several ways:

(1) accurate determination of gestational age, thereby eliminating mis-classification
(2) screening for signs associated with trisomy 21 in patients with borderline hCG values; this resulted in detection of 10 cases of trisomy 21 in addition to 37/57 cases detected by hCG examination of patients with low hCG values (< 5th percentile); this can detect trisomy 18 or fetal death.

In our study population, fetal or neonatal death (with normal karyotype) was observed in 1.3% of cases. When hCG was < 5th percentile, fetal or neonatal death was observed in 2.2% of cases, and when hCG was < 1st percentile, the frequency of fetal or neonatal death was 6.4%. In our study population, the frequency of trisomy 18 was 0.06%. When hCG was < 5th percentile, the frequency was 0.3%, and when it was < 1st percentile, the frequency was 1.6%. The risk of trisomy 18 is multiplied by 50 when hCG < 1st percentile.

Conclusion

Rather than multiply laboratory tests, we prefer to use ultrasound examination to minimise the inevitable limitation of a test based on cut-off values. The aim of French Public Health policy is effective co-ordination of obstetrics, laboratory tests and cytogenetics, allowing detection of around 80% of cases of trisomy 21 and identification of other fetal anomalies.

References

Bogart, M.H., Pandian, M.R. & Jones, O.W. (1987). Abnormal maternal serum chorionic gonadotropin levels in pregnancies with fetal chromosomal abnormalities. *Prenatal Diagn.*, **7**, 623–30.

De Vigan, C., Vodovar, V., Dufouil, C. & Goujard, J. (1992). La trisomie 21 dans la population Parisienne: evolution 1981–1990. *Bull. Epidémiol.*, **38**, 182–3.

Hook, E.B., Topol, B.B. & Cross, P.K. (1989). The natural history of cytogenetically abnormal fetuses detected at midtrimester amniocentesis which are not terminated electively: new data and estimates of the excess and relative risk of late fetal death associated with 47, +21 and some other abnormal karyotypes. *Am. J. Hum. Genet.*, **45**, 855–61.

Muller, F., Aegerter, P. & Boué, A. (1993). Prospective maternal serum human chorionic gonadotrophin screening for the risk of fetal chromosome anomalies and of subsequent fetal and neonatal death. *Prenatal. Diagn.*, **13**, 29–43.

19

The United Kingdom National External Quality Assessment Scheme for screening for Down's syndrome

J. SETH AND A.R. ELLIS

Introduction

The assessment of the quality of laboratory performance has long been a feature of clinical biochemistry and National External Quality Assurance Schemes (UK NEQAS) covering all major laboratory disciplines are provided from several different centres in the United Kingdom. The Edinburgh NEQAS centre provides schemes for several peptide hormones, tumour markers and maternal serum screening for neural tube defects. Participation is by subscription and is available to all laboratories. The majority of participants are from within the National Health Service, but there are also a significant number of participants from commercial laboratories, overseas laboratories and manufacturers.

The UK NEQAS for screening for Down's syndrome

The need for an external quality assessment scheme for laboratories interested in screening for Down's syndrome became apparent in the late 1980s. In response to requests from laboratories already performing such screening, a preliminary study was undertaken for 6 months, commencing in the autumn of 1990, in 35 laboratories. Although the study was of limited scope and duration, it did provide an objective view of laboratory practice and performance in the UK and was sufficiently well received by participants to encourage us to move towards establishing a full UK NEQAS for screening for Down's syndrome (the Down's NEQAS). The data obtained from the NEQAS cannot be used to make firm recommendations as to the best strategy for screening for Down's syndrome – only prospective clinical trials are able to do this – but they do raise several points of concern regarding laboratory practice.

Materials and methods

Pool type

All pools are of human serum or plasma. The donations used to prepare a pool are tested and shown to be negative for hepatitis B surface antigen, anti-hepatitis C virus and anti-human immunodeficiency virus. The pools are filtered to sterility (0.2 μm) and sodium azide (0.05% w/v) is added as a bacteriostat. Pools are prepared so as to contain α-fetoprotein (AFP), intact human chorionic gonadotrophin (hCG), the free β-subunit of hCG (free β-hCG) and unconjugated oestriol (uE$_3$) at concentrations expected in mid-term affected and unaffected pregnancies. The concentration ranges covered are 7.5–45 kU/l BS 72/227 (AFP); 21–84 kU/l IRP 75/537 (intact hCG); 12–75 U/l IRP 75/551 (free β-hCG); and 0.4–7.6 nmol/l (uE$_3$). Two types of pool are used to achieve these concentrations.

Pregnancy serum The majority of pools used are prepared from donations of human, mid-trimester pregnancy serum or plasma. The advantage of the use of such pools is that they are very similar to, if not identical with, patient specimens. The use of such pools should therefore ensure that the performance of a laboratory with the quality control material is a true reflection of its performance with patient specimens. The principal disadvantage is that it is difficult to obtain material that is at increased risk of Down's syndrome. Indeed, if a large number of donations are included in a pool then the concentrations of each analyte tend towards the median. A limited number of pools at apparently high risk of Down's syndrome can be prepared by selecting patient specimens that have been shown themselves to represent an increased risk. An alternative approach that we have recently tried is to prepare pools from first trimester pregnancy serum, but to designate these pools as being of mid-trimester. Such pools can have very low concentrations of AFP and uE$_3$ and very high concentrations of intact hCG and free β-hCG. Donations of serum from a mother bearing a fetus proved to be affected by Down's syndrome are likely to be available only very occasionally, although we have been fortunate to have obtained one such donation.

Spiked male serum Male serum has virtually undetectable concentrations of the four analytes and so may be a suitable base material for the preparation of pools containing known additions of analyte. The base material used for the other NEQASs operated from Edinburgh is pooled

Table 19.1. *Relative concentration of free β-hCG in samples of purified hCG*

Source of hCG	Free β-hCG content[a]
R. Iles, St Bartholomew's Hospital, London	84
Scripps Laboratories, San Diego, USA	40
Scipac Ltd, Sittingbourne, Kent	41

[a] Units IRP 75/551 per 20 000 units IRP 75/537.

serum obtained at therapeutic venesection (TV serum) of subjects suffering from either polycythaemia or haemochromatosis. Such material has been shown to behave in a similar fashion to normal serum in immunoassays. Limited use has been made of such material in the Down's NEQAS. Suitable AFP concentrations can be achieved by adding known amounts of the British Standard 72/227 (a gift from the National Institute of Biological Standards and Control), and solutions of pure oestriol (Sigma Chemical Co. Ltd) can be used to obtain the desired uE$_3$ concentrations. However, obtaining suitable preparations of hCG has not been possible so far. The principal difficulty lies in the exceedingly low concentration of free β-hCG in maternal serum relative to the concentration of intact hCG. Typically, a maternal serum with a concentration of intact hCG of 20 000 IU/l (IRP 73/537) would have a free β-hCG concentration of approximately 12 U/l (IRP 75/551). We have been fortunate to obtain gifts of three preparations of hCG, all purified from human pregnancy urine. The materials we have tried, and an estimate of their free β-hCG content, are shown in Table 19.1, which shows that all three materials contain a relative excess of free β-hCG. Our experience, albeit with only a limited number of preparations, suggests that it may not be possible to prepare hCG to the required standard. We have decided to make no further use of such material.

Pools are prepared in sufficient volume to permit distribution on several occasions. Each pool is divided into 500 μl volumes and stored at −30 °C until despatch. Specimens of three different pools are posted at ambient temperature to participating laboratories every 4 weeks. Participants then have 3 weeks in which to analyse the specimens according to their normal protocol and return their results. Each specimen is supplied with relevant clinical details so that participants can report the results of their analyses in concentration units and after conversion to multiples of their median for the gestational age stated. Participants also calculate a risk of Down's syndrome and report this together with an indication as to whether or not any further action would be taken.

Details of participation

There are currently 73 participating laboratories, but it is not possible to determine what proportion of all laboratories performing Down's screening are participating in the NEQAS. Most participants are National Health Service laboratories, as shown in Table 19.2. The numbers of participants using various combinations of analytes (test panel) are shown in Table 19.3. Although the most popular analyte combination is AFP plus intact hCG, the fastest growing combination is AFP plus free β-hCG.

Table 19.4 shows that there are several different methods in use for the measurement of AFP and hCG. Pharmacia DELFIA is the most popular method for determining AFP whilst over one third of participants use the Kodak AMERLEX-M Second Trimester kit for the measurement of hCG. Assays for hCG can be classified as those measuring the free β-subunit

Table 19.2. *Location and type of participating laboratories*

Laboratory type	No.
Service, United Kingdom	62
Service, overseas	6
Manufacturer, United Kingdom	3
Manufacturer, overseas	2
Total	73

Table 19.3. *Combinations of analyte used in deriving risk estimates*

Test panel	No. participants
AFP alone	6
Intact hCG alone	1
AFP and intact hCG	35
AFP and free β-hCG	17
AFP, intact hCG and uE_3	13
AFP, free β-hCG and uE_3	1

Table 19.4. *Methods used for the determination of AFP and intact hCG*

Method	No. Laboratories	
	AFP	hCG
Abbott IMX	4	5
Boehringer ENZYMUN	6	3
Clonatec E.I.A.		1
D.P.C. RIA	1	
Hybritech TANDEM-E	1	
Hybritech TANDEM-R	1	1
I.D.S. OMNIA	8	1
In-House IRMA	8	2
In-House RIA, Double Antibody	5	3
In-House RIA, Single Antibody	3	
Kodak AMERLEX-M, Second Trimester	9	18
Kodak AMERLITE	5	2
North East Thames Regional Health Authority RIA	4	
Pharmacia DELFIA	17	8
Roche COBAS CORE	2	
Serono MAIAclone		4
Undefined method		1

(free β-hCG) or predominantly the intact heterodimer hormone (intact hCG) or both species together (total hCG) (Sturgeon *et al.*, 1992). As the concentration of β-subunit relative to intact hCG is negligible in second trimester pregnancy serum, this study does not distinguish between intact and total assays, and we will refer to these as intact assays, this being the major hCG species measured.

All 17 participants that measure free β-hCG do so by means of the C.I.S. β-IRMA and all 13 laboratories measuring uE$_3$ use the Kodak AMERLEX-M Second Trimester kit.

Survey by questionnaire

All participants in February, 1992 were surveyed by questionnaire and all new participants are requested to complete the questionnaire. The questionnaire was designed to study methods of data reduction, and topics covered include:

(1) methods of correcting assayed concentrations for maternal weight etc.
(2) medians

(3) age-related risk of Down's syndrome
(4) algorithm used to calculate risk of Down's syndrome
(5) population parameters used in the calculation
(6) risks calculated from dummy data supplied as multiples of the median (MoM).

Results

Analyses of serum pools

Participants return the results of their determinations on serum pools in concentration units and after conversion to MoMs. These data are then analysed by methods common to all the schemes operated from Edinburgh (Hanning *et al.*, 1991). The spread of results is indicated by the geometric coefficient of variation (GCV). Table 19.5 shows the mean, overall GCVs for all four analytes. There is excellent overall, between-laboratory agreement for results in concentration units, as evidenced by the low GCVs. Agreement alters little upon conversion of intact hCG results to MoMs, but does worsen somewhat for the other analytes, especially for free β-hCG and uE_3. Note that for these two analytes the GCVs are *within-method* GCVs as only one method is used in each case.

Table 19.6 shows the method-related, between-laboratory GCVs for AFP and intact hCG for methods that have five or more users (major methods). All major methods provide good between-laboratory agreement, with the Pharmacia DELFIA method proving to be very good in that respect.

Table 19.5. *Mean, overall GCVs for results in concentration units and after conversion to MoMs*

Analyte	Mean GCV (%) for results in	
	Units[a]	MoMs
AFP	10.5	12.7
Intact hCG	13.4	13.8
Free β-hCG	6.3	9.1
uE_3	13.1	19.8

GCV: geometric coefficient of variation.
[a] Units used are: AFP, kU/l BS 72/227; intact hCG, U/l IRP 75/537; β-hCG, U/l IRP 75/551; uE_3, nmol/l.

Table 19.6. *Overall, within-method, between-laboratory GCVs for AFP and intact hCG methods*

Method	Mean GCV (%) for	
	AFP[a]	Intact hCG[a]
I.D.S. OMNIA	7.3	
In-House IRMA	10.5	
Kodak AMERLEX-M 2T	10.6	8.5
Kodak AMERLITE	7.1	
Pharmacia DELFIA	5.4	5.8

[a] Results expressed in concentration units as in Table 19.5.

Table 19.7. *AFP: method-related BIAS (median and interquartile range) for results in kU/l and in MoMs*

Method	BIAS (%) results in	
	kU/l	MoM
I.D.S. OMNIA	+0.6 (−1.5, +7.2)	−2.9 (−7.8, +1.3)
In-House IRMA	−3.4 (−11.0, −0.4)	−0.4 (−8.2, +4.4)
Kodak AMERLEX-M 2T	−0.1 (−3.2, +5.6)	+0.3 (−0.8, +2.0)
Pharmacia DELFIA	+2.6 (−0.5, +5.7)	−1.1 (−4.1, +0.8)

BIAS: between method differences in cumulative mean deviation from the expected value.

Between-method differences in cumulative mean deviation from the expected value (the BIAS) are indicators of the relative accuracy of methods. Tables 19.7 and 19.8 show such BIAS data for the major methods for AFP and intact hCG. Equivalent data are not available for free β-hCG or uE$_3$: each has only one method and therefore sets its own expected value. The between-method differences in median BIAS are small for AFP, for results both in kU/l and in MoMs. The two major methods for intact hCG do show a significant difference in BIAS for results in U/l, but this difference appears to be removed upon conversion of results to MoMs.

Table 19.8. *Intact hCG: method-related BIAS (median and interquartile range) for results in U/l and in MoMs*

	BIAS (%) for results in	
Method	U/l	MoM
Kodak AMERLEX-M 2T	+2.8 (−7.2, +5.9)	−1.3 (−9.0, +2.5)
Pharmacia DELFIA	−12.5 (−13.4, −9.7)	0 (−7.1, +0.8)

BIAS: between method differences in cumulative mean deviation from the expected value.

Estimates of the risk of Down's syndrome from serum pools

Each specimen has clinical details associated with it; therefore, participants are able to use the results of their analyses and the clinical details to calculate a risk of Down's syndrome for each specimen and to indicate whether or not further action would be taken.

The risk estimates can be regarded as test results and subjected to statistical analysis. Table 19.9 shows the mean, trimmed arithmetic coefficients of variation (CVs) of the risk estimates, divided according to test panel. The spread of risk estimates is reasonable for those laboratories measuring AFP alone but increases as hCG and then uE_3 are included. This is partly a result of the accumulation of analytical errors. The actual risk estimates vary according to the test panel used, so it may not be strictly correct to compare the mean CVs. Furthermore, it has been suggested that if the discriminatory power of a test panel improves as analytes are added, then a concomitant increase in the spread of risk estimates is acceptable. However, the spread of risks is of great significance

Table 19.9. *Within-test panel, between-laboratory agreement in risk estimates*

Test panel	Mean CV[a] (%)
AFP only	18.5
AFP and intact hCG	31.1
AFP and free β-hCG	27.0
AFP, intact hCG and uE_3	46.3

[a] Mean trimmed arithmetic coefficient of variation.

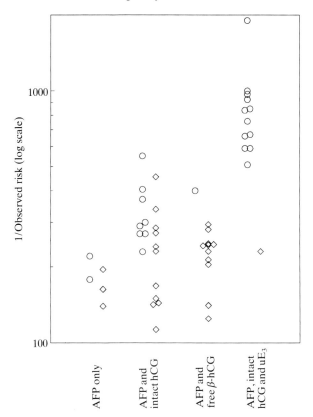

Fig. 19.1. Spread of risk estimates and recommendations for further action on a specimen of pooled serum (DO46, distribution 16). ○, No further action recommended; ◇, further action recommended.

when the mean risk is close to laboratories' cut-off points. Figure 19.1 shows that the overall spread of risks can be wide (for example, the range for the AFP + intact hCG group is from 1 in 115 to 1 in 550) and that this variability can lead to disagreement in recommendation for further action. As expected, higher risks generally lead to further action whilst lower risks do not, although there is a 'grey area' caused by the variation in the individual laboratory's chosen cut-off (see below). Table 19.10 summarises the recommendations for action on three specimens of similar mean risk. Clearly, there can be a marked lack of between-laboratory, within-test panel consensus in the interpretation.

The effect of the spread of risk estimates upon interpretation can also be clearly seen in Fig. 19.2. This shows the risk estimates reported on a

Table 19.10. *Mean and coefficient of variation (CV) of risk estimates and recommendations for further action on three specimens of pooled serum*

Test panel	Specimen D046			Specimen D047			Specimen D048		
	Mean (CV, %)	FA	NFA	Mean (CV, %)	FA	NFA	Mean (CV, %)	FA	NFA
AFP only	175 (17.4)	3	3	166 (11.4)	3	3	163 (10.9)	3	3
AFP and intact hCG	242 (37.1)	11	8	394 (34.0)	4	15	557 (26.9)	2	17
AFP and free β-hCG	251 (17.3)	11	1	338 (11.6)	9	2	372 (12.0)	2	10
AFP, intact hCG and uE$_3$	765 (29.9)	1	12	1244 (35.9)	1	12	1283 (30.0)	1	12

CV, coefficient of variation; FA, number of laboratories recommending further action; NFA, number of laboratories not recommending further action.

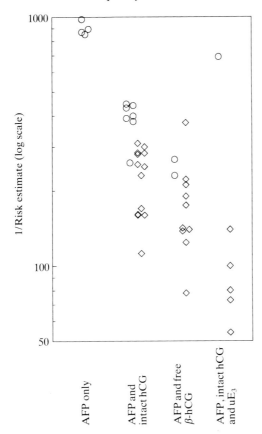

Fig. 19.2. Spread of risk estimates and recommendations for further action on a specimen of serum from a known case of Down's syndrome. ○, No further action recommended; ◇, further action recommended.

specimen of serum obtained from a mother carrying a fetus with chromosomally proved Down's syndrome. In this particular case, none of the participants measuring AFP alone identified this specimen as being at high risk, whereas five out of six measuring AFP, intact hCG and uE_3 (the triple test) and 10 out of 12 measuring AFP and free β-hCG did so. However, only 13 out of 20 participants measuring AFP and intact hCG recommended further action on this specimen.

Data obtained from the questionnaire

The questionnaire concerning methods of data reduction has been issued to 74 laboratories, and to date 55 have replied. The data obtained from the questionnaires give cause for concern regarding many stages of the process of calculation of the risk.

Medians in use

As noted above, conversion of the NEQAS results from concentration units to MoMs invariably results in some worsening of between-laboratory agreement. This is perhaps a rather unexpected observation as one of the original reasons for the conversion of AFP results to MoMs was to reduce between-laboratory scatter. However, the reliability of immunoassays has improved dramatically over recent years and good International Standards for AFP and hCG are now available.

There will inevitably be some imprecision in the median itself so if the between-laboratory differences are small then dividing a result in concentration units by a median will result in an MoM with somewhat larger imprecision than either of its component parts. However, the NEQAS results can show considerable increases in GCVs, particularly for free β-hCG and uE_3, raising the possibility of the use of inappropriate medians by some laboratories.

Figure 19.3 shows the medians currently in use in individual laboratories. Where between-method differences exist for results in concentration units, one would expect similar method-related differences in medians. There will also be some population-related differences in medians and, as noted

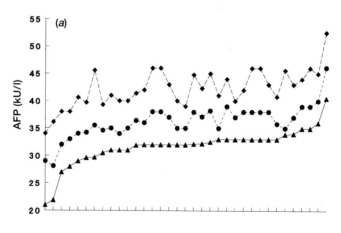

Laboratories ranked by 16-week median

Fig. 19.3. Medians in use for (*a*) AFP, (*b*) intact hCG, (*c*) free β-hCG and (*d*) uE_3. Individual laboratories ranked in order of 16-week median (▲). Medians for 17 weeks (●) and 18 weeks (◆) are also shown.

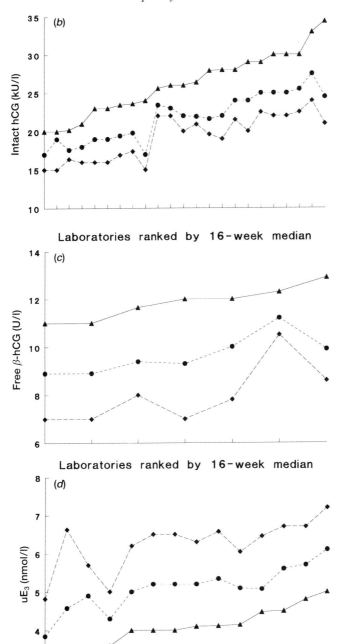

Laboratories ranked by 16-week median

Laboratories ranked by 16-week median

Laboratories ranked by 16-week median

above, the derivation of medians is also subject to some error. In the case of AFP, the between-method differences are small and there is relatively good between-laboratory agreement in medians (Fig. 19.3a). Excluding three obvious outliers, the 16-week medians are in the range 27–36 kU/l.

The range of medians for intact hCG is somewhat greater (20–34 kU/l), but as noted above, there can be significant differences between results obtained by the various methods. Users of Pharmacia DELFIA (a method giving relatively low results) appear to be using low, and probably appropriate, medians. However, the medians reported by users of the Kodak AMERLEX-M Second Trimester kit (a method giving relatively high results) range from 20–33 kU/l. Conversion of intact hCG results to MoMs has very little effect upon between-laboratory agreement, so it would seem that most participants are using appropriate medians.

The situation is different again for free β-hCG and for uE_3. Here only one method is used for each analyte, so there can be no between-method differences and yet there is invariably a marked worsening of between-laboratory agreement upon conversion of results to MoMs. Figure 19.3c, d show the medians for free β-hCG and uE_3. There are marked between-laboratory differences in median, particularly for uE_3 (overall range 3.08–5.0 nmol/l at 16 weeks). It seems, therefore, that some laboratories may be using inappropriate medians for free β-hCG and uE_3.

Most participants have established their own medians and some are using data obtained from colleagues. However a number are using data obtained from kit inserts, apparently without local validation. The number of results used to establish in-house medians is of concern in some cases. It has been suggested (Special Report, 1985) that at least 100 results should be used to establish a median, yet Table 19.11 shows that a significant number of laboratories have used fewer results. In addition, not all

Table 19.11. *Number of results used to establish 16-week medians in participating laboratories*

No. of results	No. of participants			
	AFP	Intact hCG	Free β-hCG	uE_3
< 100	5	3	2	4
100–300	4	3	4	1
300–500	4	2		1
500–1000	7	5	1	2
> 1000	13	5		2

Table 19.12. *Numbers of participants applying corrections for maternal weight*

Analyte	Mandatory correction	Corrected for if weight is known	Never corrected for
AFP	2	24	15
Intact hCG	1	3	10
Free β-hCG	0	7	3
uE$_3$	0	3	12

participants keep a regular check on their medians. For example, 28% of respondents check their AFP medians no more than yearly.

Correcting for maternal weight

It has been reported (Wald *et al.*, 1981) that MSAFP is significantly negatively correlated with maternal weight, and that the false-positive rate in screening for neural tube defects (NTD) could be improved if borderline positive results were corrected for weight. This procedure has been extended into screening for Down's syndrome. Table 19.12 shows that most participants correct their AFP results for maternal weight when it is known, but use uncorrected values if the weight is unavailable. A smaller number of laboratories correct hCG and uE$_3$ results for maternal weight. Three formulae are used to apply the weight correction:

$$[\text{Param}]_{\text{Corr}} = \frac{[\text{Param}]_{\text{Meas}}}{(C_1 - (C_2 \times W))} \tag{19.1}$$

$$[\text{Param}]_{\text{Corr}} = \frac{[\text{Param}]_{\text{Meas}}}{(10^{(C_3 - (C_4 \times W))})} \tag{19.2}$$

$$[\text{Param}]_{\text{Corr}} = \frac{[\text{Param}]_{\text{Meas}}}{(C_5 \times C_6^W)} \tag{19.3}$$

where Param = analyte concentration, or result, after conversion to MoMs; Meas = Param as measured; Corr = Param after correction; W = maternal weight; C_1 to C_6 are constants.

Equation 19.2 is used by the majority of participants, but there is a lack of consensus in the constants to be used. Calculations with dummy data have shown that it is possible to vary the risk calculated on the basis

Table 19.13. *Additional risk modifiers and the number of participants applying corrections*

Risk modifier	Mandatory correction	Corrected for if known	Not corrected for
Diabetes	3	11	41
Racial origin	2	5	48
Multiple pregnancy	11	11	33
Family history of Down's or NTD	1	6	48
Threatened abortion	0	1	54
Smoking habit	0	2	53

of AFP alone by up to 25%, simply by choosing the highest and lowest constants.

Correcting for other risk modifiers

Some participants correct their calculations for a number of other risk modifiers. The numbers of participants applying corrections for the various modifiers are shown in Table 19.13. As with weight correction, there is a lack of consensus and it may be of particular concern to note the number of laboratories that apply corrections on an inconsistent basis, that is only if the status of the risk modifier is known.

Calculation of the risk of Down's syndrome

Forty-three participants gave details of how they calculated the risk of Down's syndrome. Three laboratories (all of whom consider AFP only) simply look up the risk from the appropriate tables (Cuckle *et al.*, 1987) and two calculate a discrimination index. The remaining 38 all calculate likelihood ratios, by means of a variety of software (Table 19.14). The users of in-house software derived their programs from information available in the literature (Cuckle *et al.*, 1987; Wald *et al.*, 1988; Reynolds and Penney, 1990; Crossley *et al.*, 1991).

Whatever the source of the software, few participants have derived their own population parameters (mean and standard deviation of [log] MoM for normal and affected populations, plus all the possible correlations). Most rely on data either supplied with their software or available in the literature. Only 13% of respondents said that they established their

Table 19.14. *Source of software used to calculate risk*

Source	No. laboratories
In-house	18
Alpha, Shire Management Services, Highlands Road, Shirley, Solihull, West Midlands, UK	10
T. Reynolds, Department of Medical Biochemistry, Cardiff Royal Infirmary, Newport Road, Cardiff CF4 1SZ, UK	7
Purchased, non-commercial	1
CIS Risk Calculator	1
Wallac Multicalc	1

own AFP parameters for affected pregnancies, while only 15% have done so for intact hCG and none at all for free β-hCG or uE_3. This may seem rather surprising as it has been long recognised in clinical biochemistry that laboratories should always establish their own reference ranges. However, with the low incidence of Down's syndrome, it could take laboratories a very considerable time to derive their own parameters. Therefore, the best practical solution is to use the published data. Of course, the reliance upon published work raises the possibility of existing data becoming enshrined, despite changes in practice.

Similarly, most participants rely on the data presented by Cuckle *et al.* (1987) for the age-related (*a priori*) risk of Down's syndrome, sometimes with minor adjustments to allow for variations in their local population. Thus of the 30 participants who indicated their *a priori* risk at term, 27 fall in the range of 1 in 1300 to 1 in 1400 at age 25; 1 in 900 to 1 in 970 at age 30; and 1 in 380 to 1 in 440 at age 35. The three remaining laboratories indicated wildly out of consensus figures, suggesting that they may have misinterpreted the question.

These differences combine to account for some of the spread of calculated risks. This was demonstrated by asking participants to derive risks from data supplied to them as MoMs, that is with all sources of error other than the algorithm and associated constants removed. Figure 19.4 shows the spread of risks calculated by laboratories performing the triple test. Clearly, the between-laboratory agreement is very much better than when laboratories actually perform the analyses (compare with Figs. 19.1, 2), but it might be possible to improve between-laboratory agreement by reaching a consensus as to the most appropriate algorithm and population parameters.

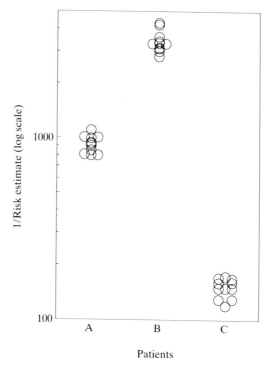

Fig. 19.4. Risks calculated by laboratories performing the 'triple test' from data supplied as MoMs.

Interpretation of risks

Most laboratories (75%) offer an interpretation of the calculated risk to their clinicians. The questionnaire asked participants what risk they considered to represent a cut-off point for determining whether or not to take further action. Figure 19.5 shows that there is some spread of these cut-offs. This reflects local policy decisions regarding the desired detection rates, and, of course, this will contribute to the apparent lack of consensus of interpretation shown by the NEQAS (Fig. 19.1).

Conclusions

The UK NEQAS provides an audit of laboratory practice and performance in screening for Down's syndrome in the United Kingdom. Early data have revealed some marked between-laboratory, within-test panel differences in calculated risks. They serve as a reminder that good laboratory

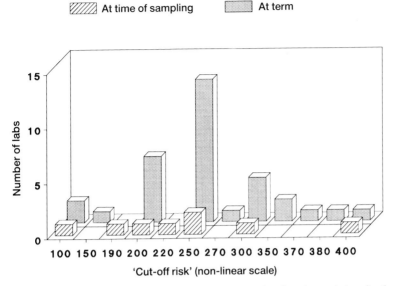

Fig. 19.5. Risk estimates taken to be the cut-off point for determining further action.

practice depends not only on analytical accuracy and precision but also on the use of reliable reference and population data. It seems likely that the variability in risk estimates would be reduced in particular if laboratories took greater care in establishing correct medians and then continuously monitored their medians. Furthermore, some consensus needs to be reached as to the necessity for, and methods of, correcting the observed analyte concentrations for maternal weight and other factors.

References

Crossley, J.A., Aitken, D.A. & Connor, J.M. (1991). Prenatal screening for chromosome abnormalities using maternal serum chorionic gonadotrophin, alpha-fetoprotein and age. *Prenatal Diagn.*, **11**(2), 83–101.

Cuckle, H.S., Wald, N.J. & Thompson, S.G. (1987). Estimation of a woman's risk of having a pregnancy associated with Down's syndrome using her age and serum alpha-fetoprotein level. *Br. J. Obstet. Gynaecol.*, **94**, 387–402.

Hanning, I., Seth, J., Bacon, R.R.A., Hunter, W.M. & Al-Sadie, R. (1991). Progress in immunoassays for serum prolactin: evidence from the UK External Quality Assessment Scheme (EQAS) 1980–1989. *Ann. Clin. Biochem.*, **28**, 91–7.

Reynolds, T.M. & Penney, M.D. (1990). The mathematical basis of multivariate risk screening: with special reference to screening for Down's syndrome. *Ann. Clin. Biochem.*, **27**, 452–8.

Special Report (1985). Maternal serum alpha-fetoprotein screening for neural tube defects: results of a consensus meeting. *Prenatal Diagn.*, **5**, 77–81.

Sturgeon, C.M., Seth, J. & Al-Sadie, R. (1992). EQA for tumour marker assays: strategy in the United Kingdom. *J. Tumor Marker Oncol.*, **7**, 91–102.

Wald, N.J., Cuckle, H.S., Boreham, J. & Terzian, E. (1981). The effect of maternal weight on maternal serum alpha-fetoprotein levels. *Br. J. Obstet. Gynaecol.*, **88**, 1094–6.

Wald, N.J., Cuckle, H.S., Densem, J. *et al.* (1988). Maternal serum screening for Down's syndrome in early pregnancy. *Br. Med. J.*, **297**, 883–8.

Note added in proof

The data presented in this chapter were gathered over the 2-year period up to May 1993. Screening practice in the United Kingdom is, however, a continually evolving process and recent NEQAS data reflect some significant changes. These include a marked increase in the number of laboratories participating, particularly those measuring AFP and free β-hCG (from 17 in 1993 to 27 in 1994). In addition, there is some evidence that laboratories are checking and adjusting their medians. Conversion of intact hCG results from U/l to MoMs now causes a significant decrease in overall GCVs whilst converting uE_3 results has little effect upon the GCVs. This represents an improvement since 1993 (see Table 19.5) and is almost certainly caused by the laboratories checking their medians for these analytes carefully and adjusting them when necessary. It was encouraging to note the results of a survey carried out in June 1993 which revealed that a number of laboratories had checked and adjusted their medians in response to the data produced by the UK NEQAS.

20

Training obstetricians and midwives to offer serum screening for Down's syndrome

T.M. MARTEAU

The objectives of prenatal screening and diagnosis include allowing the widest possible range of informed choice to women and couples at risk of having a child with an abnormality and providing reassurance and reducing the anxiety associated with reproduction (Royal College of Physicians, 1989). Unfortunately, most research has focussed upon developing the technology, to the neglect of the effects of the technology on women. There have been few studies on how obstetricians and midwives are dealing with these tests.

To achieve the objectives of prenatal screening, it is essential to address the training needs of staff. In this chapter I shall explore how obstetricians and midwives are meeting the challenges posed by prenatal screening for Down's syndrome, in particular, and for other fetal abnormalities. Some of the problems that health professionals face in achieving the objectives of screening will be described, together with some possible solutions.

Obstetricians and midwives have two key roles in providing prenatal screening for fetal abnormalities including Down's syndrome: first, to facilitate informed decision-making at all stages of the process; and second, to provide emotional support. Observational studies of obstetricians and descriptive studies of women's experiences of screening show that these roles are not always performed well.

Facilitating informed decision-making

Two of the decisions which may confront pregnant women are whether to undergo testing and, for those receiving a positive diagnosis, whether to continue with the pregnancy.

Presenting tests

The decision about whether to undergo prenatal screening for a fetal abnormality should be made by the pregnant woman on the basis of good information (Black Report, 1979; Royal College of Physicians, 1989). Yet women's knowledge of screening tests in pregnancy is often inadequate. For example, 2 days postpartum, 39% of women could not correctly state whether they had undergone AFP screening for spina bifida (Marteau *et al.*, 1988b). Women undergoing routine antenatal care frequently report their wish for more information about tests than is generally given (Reid, 1988). Women's knowledge may be poor for one of several reasons: they are not given information; information is given but misunderstood or forgotten; or information that is given may be misleading or incorrect.

Observational studies of obstetricians and midwives presenting prenatal screening and diagnostic tests show that often very little, and sometimes misleading, information is given. In one study, routine consultations between 102 pregnant women and their obstetricians or midwives were tape-recorded to determine how maternal serum α-fetoprotein (MSAFP) screening tests for neural tube defects and Down's syndrome were presented (Marteau *et al.*, 1992a). Overall, little information was provided about the test, the conditions being screened for and the meaning of either a positive or a negative test result.

In contrast with the routine presentations of MSAFP screening, obstetricians gave much more information when describing amniocentesis to women at increased risk of chromosome abnormalities because of their age (Marteau *et al.*, 1993). Presentations focussed upon the risks of fetal abnormality and the risks of pregnancy loss following amniocentesis. These risks were frequently contrasted. Equivalent probabilities tended to be described as low in relation to fetal loss and high in relation to Down's syndrome. Implicit in obstetricians' presentations was an assumption that all women would or should undergo the procedure. Information concerning the range of conditions detected with routine amniocentesis was infrequently given; the conditions themselves were never described. In summary, information pertinent to decisions of whether to undergo amniocentesis was most often presented in a way to encourage uptake of the test, as opposed to fostering informed decision-making. Possible explanations for not providing more information include: lack of knowledge about the tests on the part of the staff; reluctance to give information for fear of making women anxious; and lack of skills at providing information.

While these problems are increasingly recognised, little is known about how to improve practice. The task that confronts health professionals who implement screening programmes is how best to inform people about serious events of low probability without causing undue alarm or false reassurance.

We have recently developed a brief training package intended to improve obstetricians' and midwives' presentations of prenatal screening. Training involved a 1-hour session, centred around video-taped scenes of midwives and obstetricians presenting different aspects of prenatal testing. The training session also provided written information about giving information and about routine prenatal screening and diagnostic tests. In addition, half the study participants were given individual feedback on their performances. Preliminary results of this multi-centre trial show that the training was effective: those trained had better communication skills and presented more information than the untrained control group. This was particularly so for those receiving individual feedback on their consultations. These results suggest that presentations can be improved with minimal training. The effects are likely to be enhanced if training was incorporated into continuing education for staff.

Written information

Information is more likely to be understood and remembered if presented orally *and* in writing rather than orally alone (for review, see Ley, 1988). Many clinics prepare leaflets to describe the tests they offer. This information may influence, sometimes unintentionally, the decisions women make about testing. In an analogue study, non-pregnant women were less likely to intend to undergo prenatal testing when they were provided with detailed information about Down's syndrome than when they were given the standard leaflet with no information about Down's syndrome (Price, 1993). This raises questions about what information should be provided, and in what form. Any research on this question needs first to define the objectives of presenting information. These may include increasing knowledge and producing good quality decision-making concerning the use of tests. The effects of information can then be evaluated against these pre-set criteria.

Decisions about whether to continue with a pregnancy

A few women who undergo prenatal testing will receive a positive diagnosis of a fetal abnormality. Such women and their partners are then confronted with a decision about whether to continue with the pregnancy. One factor likely to influence their decisions will be perception of the severity of the condition. Discussion about these issues is sometimes initiated by obstetric staff. In some centres, such parents will be referred to a geneticist or a paediatrician.

The counselling approach taken by obstetricians and geneticists differs. Obstetricians are more likely to counsel directly, particularly in the direction of terminating the pregnancy (Marteau *et al.*, 1994). With Down's syndrome, for example, a marked discrepancy was evident between the approaches taken by obstetricians, geneticists and genetic counsellors: 32% of obstetricians, 57% of geneticists and 94% of genetic counsellors reported counselling non-directively, defined in this study as presenting positive and negative aspects of the condition equally. These results suggest that counselling will vary according to the health professional concerned. Such counselling is likely to vary both in the information given about conditions and in the extent to which the counselling is directed. We do not know how these differences in counselling are reflected in clinical practice. Nor do we know the extent to which counselling influences couples' decisions. Evidence of influence comes from a descriptive study of couples' decisions about termination following diagnosis of a sex chromosome anomaly (Holmes-Siedle *et al.*, 1987). Of 18 couples counselled by obstetricians, 14 terminated their pregnancies in contrast with 11 of the 22 seen by geneticists. These numbers are small, and the study was uncontrolled. More research is needed to determine how counselling may affect decisions about whether to continue or interrupt a pregnancy, and the short- and long-term consequences for the family.

Emotional support

Distress is evident in some women at all stages of screening, from making a decision about initial testing to dealing with the consequences of a late termination for fetal abnormality. The issues confronting parents in these circumstances are considered below.

Deciding whether to undergo tests

Many factors influence the use of tests. These include attitudes towards termination, knowledge about the tests, perceptions of risk and the perceived burden of the condition for which screening is being offered (for review, see Marteau and Slack, 1992). Presentation of this information may also be important. When counselling was offered on the same day as amniocentesis, significantly more women underwent the procedure than if counselling took place a day or more before (Lorenz *et al.*, 1985). However, little is known about the quality of these decisions, or whether parents regretted or were satisfied with their decisions.

Awaiting test results

Awaiting the results of amniocentesis or chorionic villus sampling is an anxious period (Green, 1990). Various suggestions have been made as to how to reduce anxiety. Some clinics invite all women to attend at a pre-set date to receive their results. Others ask women to telephone at a pre-arranged time, to avoid them fearing the conveyance of bad news every time the telephone rings.

Receipt of positive results on screening

Being recalled following a routine prenatal screening test is frequently the cause of high levels of anxiety (for review, see Marteau and Slack, 1992). This is particularly marked in those who have not previously considered themselves at increased risk, such as younger women (Marteau *et al.*, 1988a). Women may remain anxious even where no abnormality is evident following further tests, and this sometimes continues until after the baby is born (Marteau *et al.*, 1992b).

Receipt of positive results on diagnostic tests

A small proportion of those undergoing prenatal diagnostic testing will receive a positive result. This news is invariably received with shock and distress, as illustrated in vivid personal accounts of the event (Statham, 1987; Brown, 1989). Those receiving positive results have great need of information and support in deciding whether to continue or to interrupt the pregnancy. The majority of women in this situation choose to terminate the pregnancy.

Termination of affected pregnancies

Terminating a pregnancy for a fetal abnormality causes acute grief as well as some relief. The psychological effects are often more serious than terminations for social reasons (Lloyd and Laurence, 1985).

In a prospective study of women undergoing terminations of pregnancy because of a fetal abnormality, Iles (1989) found that women often experienced guilt at destroying a life and at opting out of rearing a disabled child. Therefore, women undergoing terminations for spina bifida, whose babies might have survived, had poorer psychological outcomes than women whose babies were anencephalic and hence unable to survive beyond birth.

Iles also found that adjustment was more difficult the later in pregnancy that the termination occurred. Black (1989) followed up women whose pregnancies ended after prenatal diagnosis, either following a decision to terminate the pregnancy, or following a procedure-induced miscarriage. The main finding was a large individual variation in adjustment. As was found by Iles (1989), women who lost a pregnancy later in gestation showed the greatest mood disturbances, as did women with less social support from their partners and friends.

In a study of 48 women who underwent terminations of pregnancies for neural tube defects and chromosome abnormalities, 77% experienced an acute grief reaction akin to that after stillbirth or neonatal death (Lloyd and Laurence, 1985). Six months after the pregnancy had ended, 46% remained depressed and some required psychiatric support. In a 2-year follow-up of couples who had undergone termination for fetal abnormalities, 20% of the 84 women interviewed were still affected and experienced regular bouts of crying, sadness and irritability (White-van Mourik *et al.*, 1992).

None of these studies provided data on comparative groups, such as women undergoing terminations for non-medical reasons, women continuing with pregnancies, or women having healthy babies. For example, severe psychological reactions are more common following the birth of a healthy child than following terminations for non-medical reasons (Brewer, 1977). Until direct comparisons are made, conclusions regarding the extent of distress that can be directly attributed to terminations for fetal abnormalities must be tentative.

The special needs of women receiving positive test results are slowly being recognised by the formation of support groups at both local (Blumenthal, 1990) and national levels. One such group is SATFA (Support Around Termination for Abnormality). This was formed by women who had undergone terminations for fetal abnormalities but who felt that their needs were not met by the routine care offered to them.

Birth of a child with an abnormality

Even with full coverage by screening programmes, some parents will give birth to an affected child. There are two reasons for this: first, some parents decide to continue with the pregnancy; second, not all fetal abnormalities will be detected. The consequences of each may differ.

Birth of child with an expected abnormality Some parents decide to continue with a pregnancy following prenatal diagnosis of an abnormality. Both Whelton (1990) and Farrant (1985) describe vividly the problems for parents who decide not to terminate a pregnancy where the fetus has a diagnosed abnormality. These problems include not only the distress of coping with a disabled child but also having to defend their decision to disapproving health professionals. The experiences of one such family has been described by their general practitioner (Watkins, 1989); the family decided to continue a pregnancy with an anencephalic fetus. This account suggests that continuing with a pregnancy, especially if the baby will not survive, is a preferable option for some couples, with fewer psychological effects than termination.

Birth of a child with an abnormality that was unexpected In those who undergo serum screening for Down's syndrome, around 40% of affected fetuses will be those of women who have received a low-risk or negative result on testing. There have been no formal studies of the effects of false-negative results for parents participating in any prenatal screening programmes, including serum screening for Down's syndrome, AFP screening for open neural tube defects and fetal anomaly scanning.

It is not known whether adjustment to the birth of an affected child is any different for parents who underwent screening as compared with those who did not. There are reports of parents of children with Down's syndrome not detected by screening who are angry, some of whom are planning to take legal action (The Independent, 1992; Parsons *et al.*, 1992). These parents may be more angry than others at the birth of their children with Down's syndrome. Alternatively, the natural anger of these parents (Gath, 1985) may become focussed on the screening programme.

Training staff so that they can provide fuller information about tests may ameliorate some of the difficulties described above. More support might be provided if the medical and nursing staff received help with their own emotional difficulties following diagnosis and termination of pregnancies with fetal problems (Statham, 1992). Health professionals dealing with prenatal screening programmes may find particular difficulty in dealing with patients whose values are at odds with their own. Whelton (1990) describes the need for staff to respect parents' choices, including the choice not to abort a fetus with an abnormality incompatible with life.

Some training in providing support for women is carried out by the voluntary sector. This usually involves seminars led by women with experience of terminations for fetal abnormality. These provide a focus for discussion and an opportunity for staff to examine their own feelings towards caring for women following diagnosis of a fetal abnormality. While it appears to be helpful, such training should be made more systematic prior to evaluation and possible implementation.

Conclusions

Technical competence at prenatal screening for Down's syndrome has outstripped our knowledge of how best to provide such services. To meet the objectives of prenatal testing services, all obstetric and midwifery staff should be given some training in how to present tests, and how best to support women at all stages of the process. The most effective and efficient ways of providing this have yet to be established. Meanwhile, clinics can address the educational and emotional needs of obstetric and midwifery staff of all grades, perhaps in group settings. Meeting the training needs of obstetric and midwifery staff is a prerequisite to meeting the needs of pregnant women confronting the fast-evolving field of prenatal testing for Down's syndrome.

Few of the problems now confronting health professionals and pregnant women were anticipated by those developing the tests. For example, we still do not know the best way to inform women that they have a low risk for Down's syndrome. Should they be told that their result is negative, or that it indicates a low risk for Down's syndrome, or should they be given the actual risk figures? Which would best reduce anxiety while avoiding false reassurance?

Introducing these tests into routine practice brings in their wake many dilemmas and problems. It is no longer tenable to delay research on the effects of a screening programme until after it has been introduced into clinical practice. Those evaluating new tests need to ensure that research on how best to deliver a screening service to women is conducted in parallel with research on the safety and efficacy of such tests.

No matter how good a test, screening of uninformed patients by unprepared staff is a recipe for confusion or sometimes disaster. This is potentially avoidable.

Acknowledgements

This chapter was written while the author was supported by a programme grant from the Wellcome Trust entitled 'Psychological and social aspects of the new genetics'.

References

Black, R.B. (1989). A 1 and 6 month follow-up of prenatal diagnosis patients who lost pregnancies. *Prenatal Diagn.*, 9, 795–804.

Black Report, DHSS (1979). *Report of the Working Group on the Screening for Neural Tube Defects*. London: Her Majesty's Stationery Office.

Blumenthal, D. (1990). Prenatal choice. *J. Am. Med. Assoc.*, 263, 1916–17.

Brewer, C. (1977). Incidence of post-abortion psychosis: a prospective study. *Br. Med. J.*, 274, 476–77.

Brown, J. (1989). The choice: a piece of my mind. *J. Am. Med. Assoc.*, 262, 2735.

Farrant, W. (1985). Who's for amniocentesis? The politics of prenatal screening. In *Sexual Politics of Reproduction*, ed. H. Homans, pp. 96–137. London: Gower.

Gath, A. (1985). Parental reactions to loss and disappointment: the diagnosis of Down's syndrome. *Devel. Med. Child Neurol.*, 27, 392–400.

Green, J. (1990). Calming or harming? A critical review of psychological effects of fetal diagnosis on pregnant women. *The Galton Institute Occasional papers*, 2nd series, No. 2. London: The Galton Institute.

Holmes-Siedle, M., Rynanen, M. & Lindenbaum, R. (1987). Parental decisions regarding termination of pregnancy following prenatal detection of sex chromosome abnormality. *Prenatal Diagn.*, 7, 239–44.

Iles, S. (1989). The loss of early pregnancy. In *Psychological Aspects of Obstetrics and Gynaecology*, ed. M. Oates, *Ballière's Clinical Obstetrics and Gynaecology*, 3, 769–90.

The Independent (1992). *The Right to a Perfect Baby*. Editorial, 22 August.

Ley, P. (1988). *Communicating with Patients: Improving Communication, Satisfaction and Compliance*. London: Croom Helm.

Lloyd, J. & Laurence, K.M. (1985). Sequelae and support after termination of pregnancy for fetal malformation. *Br. Med. J.*, 290, 907–9.

Lorenz, R.P., Botti, J.J., Schmitt, C.M. & Ladda, R.L. (1985). Encouraging patients to undergo prenatal genetic counselling before the day of amniocentesis. *J. Reprod. Med.*, 30, 933–5.

Marteau, T.M. & Slack, J. (1992). Psychological implications of prenatal diagnosis for patients and health professionals. In *Prenatal Diagnosis and Screening*, Ch. 39. ed. D.J.H. Brock, C.H. Rodeck & M.A. Ferguson-Smith. London: Churchill Livingstone.

Marteau, T.M., Kidd, J., Cook, R. *et al.* (1988a). Screening for Down's syndrome. *Br. Med. J.*, 297, 1469.

Marteau, T.M., Johnston, M., Plenicar, M., Shaw, R.W. & Slack, J. (1988b). Development of a self-administered questionnaire to measure women's knowledge of prenatal screening and diagnostic tests. *J. Psychosom. Res.,* **32**, 403–8.

Marteau, T.M., Kidd, J., Cook, R. *et al.* (1988c). Screening for Down's syndrome (letter). *Br. Med. J.,* **297**, 1469.

Marteau, T.M., Slack, J., Kidd, J. & Shaw, R.W. (1992a). Presenting a routine screening test in antenatal care: practice observed. *Public Health,* **106**, 131–41.

Marteau, T.M., Cook, R., Kidd, J. *et al.* (1992b). The psychological effects of false-positive results in prenatal screening for fetal abnormality: a prospective study. *Prenatal Diagn.,* **12**, 205–14.

Marteau, T.M., Plenicar, M. & Kidd, J. (1993). Obstetricians presenting amniocentesis to pregnant women: practice observed. *J. Reprod. Infant Psychol.,* **11**, 3–10.

Marteau, T.M., Drake, H. & Bobrow, M. (1994). Counselling following diagnosis of fetal abnormality: the differing perspectives of obstetricians, clinical geneticists and genetic nurses. *J. Med. Genet.,* in press.

Parsons, L., Richards, J. & Garlick, R. (1992). Screening for Down's syndrome. *Br. Med. J.,* **305**, 1228.

Price, H. (1993). A Comparison of the Effects of Written and Pictorial Information about Down Syndrome upon Attitudes towards Down Syndrome, Antenatal Screening and Termination. Thesis completed as part of an intercollated intercollegiate BSc in Psychology. University of London.

Reid, M. (1988). Consumer-oriented studies in relation to prenatal screening tests. *Eur. J. Obstet. Gynecol. Reprod. Biol.,* **28**, 79–92.

Royal College of Physicians (1989). *Prenatal Diagnosis and Genetic Screening. Community and Service Implications.* London: Royal College of Physicians.

Statham, H. (1987). *Cold Comfort.* The Guardian, 24 March.

Statham, H. (1992). Professional understanding and parents' experience of termination. In *Prenatal Diagnosis and Screening,* ed. D.J.H. Brock, C.H. Rodeck & M.A. Ferguson-Smith, pp. 697–702. London: Churchill Livingstone.

Watkins, D. (1989). An alternative to termination of pregnancy. *Practitioner,* **203**, 990–1.

Whelton, J.M. (1990). Sharing the dilemmas: midwives' role in prenatal diagnosis and fetal medicine. *Professional Nurse,* **July**, 514–18.

White-van Mourik, M.C.A., Connor, J.M. & Ferguson-Smith, M.A. (1992). The psychosocial sequelae of a second-trimester termination of pregnancy for fetal abnormality. *Prenatal Diagn.,* **12**, 189–204.

Table 21.3. *Maternal serum free β-hCG values in
fetal aneuploidy cases compared with 83 matched
contemporaneous controls, expressed in MoM*

Case	Free β-hCG ng/ml	MoM	Chromosomal abnormality
1	242.5	3.34	+21
2	158.7	2.18	+21
3	87.0	0.93	+21
4	191.2	2.63	+21
5	71.8	1.12	+21[a]
6	238.4	2.55	+21
7	217.0	3.41	+21
8	81.0	1.12	+21
9	91.8	1.14	+21
10	63.6	1.13	+21
11	142.7	1.97	+21
12	35.0	0.62	+21
13	66.0	0.80	t(q21;q21)
14	9.8	0.14	+18
15	8.8	0.09	+18
16	12.2	0.12	+13

[a] The fetus was also affected by Krabbe disease.

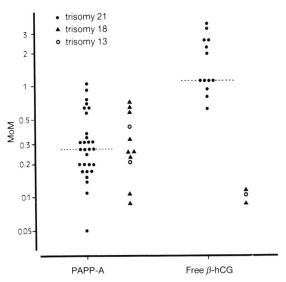

Fig. 21.2. First trimester maternal serum PAPP-A and free β-hCG values (MoM) in pregnancies with fetal aneuploidy (trisomy 21, 18, 13). The median values (dotted lines) are shown.

highest detection rate (78.9%) is achieved when the three parameters are combined (95% CI: 64.9–92.8).

Discussion

Prenatal screening for Down's syndrome, based on measurement of placental and fetal compounds in maternal serum, is in widespread use. Various combinations of maternal age and measurements of AFP, unconjugated oestriol (uE$_3$), and total or free β-subunit hCG are very effective. Detection rates range from 48% to more than 70% with false-positive rates of about 5% (Wald *et al.*, 1988; Macri *et al.*, 1990; Nørgaard-Pedersen *et al.*, 1990; Haddow *et al.*, 1992; Phillips *et al.*, 1992; Wald *et al.*, 1992a). However, late termination of an affected fetus is the major drawback of screening at this stage of pregnancy. The feasibility of first-trimester screening has been evaluated in several studies (Cuckle *et al.*, 1988; Milunsky *et al.*, 1988; Johnson *et al.*, 1991; Kratzer *et al.*, 1991; van Lith *et al.*, 1991; Brambati *et al.*, 1992; Spencer *et al.*, 1992; Wald *et al.*, 1992b; Aitken *et al.*, 1993; Fuhrmann *et al.*, 1993; Pescia *et al.*, 1993) (Fig. 21.3). Brambati *et al.* (1986) were the first to report an association of low MSAFP levels with fetal aneuploidy at 8–11 weeks: in

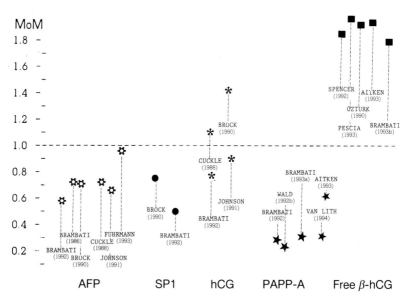

Fig. 21.3. Down's syndrome: first trimester serum median AFP, SP1, hCG, PAPP-A, and free β-hCG levels in 14 studies.

all 8 cases of trisomy 21 and in 7 of the 9 other aneuploidies the AFP values were below the normal median. These results were confirmed by an international collaborative study based on 22 Down's syndrome cases. This also showed that serum AFP and uE_3, but not total hCG, are potential markers in first-trimester screening (Cuckle *et al.*, 1988). The trends to lower levels of AFP and uE_3 in Down's syndrome cases were also reported by Brock *et al.* (1990) in cases at 7–14 weeks of gestation. However, no significant differences between the medians for affected and unaffected pregnancies were observed.

Another possible marker of fetal aneuploidy is Schwangerschafts protein 1 (SP1). SP1 concentrations are higher in the second trimester and lower in the first trimester when the fetus has Down's syndrome (Brock *et al.*, 1990; Brambati *et al.*, 1991). The median SP1 of the abnormal group (0.5 MoM) was found to be significantly lower than that of the normal group (1.0 MoM) in 30 pregnancies at 6 to 12 weeks with abnormal fetal karyotype (Macintosh *et al.*, 1993b). This relationship was maintained for the Down's syndrome cases (0.43 MoM) and for anomalies other than trisomy 18 (0.43 MoM) but not for trisomy 18 (1.1 MoM).

The most probable candidates for first-trimester fetal aneuploidy screening are PAPP-A and free β-hCG. In a study on 20 fetal aneuploidies at 6–9 weeks we have shown PAPP-A levels lower than the median of the normal population in all cases, and in 7 of the 13 Down's syndrome cases (55%) the values were less than or equal to the 5th centile (Brambati *et al.*, 1991). To explore whether PAPP-A might be useful in screening for Down's syndrome pregnancies, Wald *et al.* (1992b) measured concentrations in the same sera used in a previous study to evaluate AFP, total hCG, and uE_3. Concentrations of PAPP-A were significantly lower in Down's syndrome cases (0.23 MoM) than in controls, and in 12 of 19 women with an affected fetus (63%) PAPP-A levels were below the 10th centile value for the controls. Our two series (Brambati *et al.*, 1993a,b) have further confirmed the association between depressed early pregnancy serum PAPP-A levels and fetal aneuploidies. A detection rate up to 71% for the combination of age and PAPP-A is similar to the figures reported in second trimester studies (Brambati *et al.*, 1993b). Moreover, an investigation of cases, most of which were 14 weeks, found a comparable level of PAPP-A in Down's syndrome cases (0.40 MoM) and suggests that this marker might still be appropriate in the first week of the second trimester (Muller *et al.*, 1993).

A major reservation about the efficacy of PAPP-A in first trimester screening is the possibility that some of the abnormal pregnancies detected

Table 21.4. *Maternal age-specific risks for Down's syndrome at CVS and amniocentesis*[a]

Maternal age	Incidence at CVS (%)	Incidence at amniocentesis (%)	Difference (%)
44	5.6	3.6	40
40	1.8	1.3	27
38	1.0	0.8	17
36	0.6	0.5	13
35	0.4	0.4	0

[a] Modified from Ferguson-Smith and Yates (1984) and Hook *et al.* (1988).

would have proceeded to miscarriage. However, the results of the Muller study (1993) make this unlikely: PAPP-A levels were depressed in affected fetuses in whom Down's syndrome was ascertained after amniocentesis or at term (Muller *et al.*, 1993). Moreover, the difference is lower in younger mothers, and no losses of Down's syndrome fetuses would be expected between the time of CVS and amniocentesis at and below age 35 (Table 21.4).

Screening for chromosomal abnormalities in the first trimester is enhanced by the measurement of free β-hCG. This analyte is also the best single marker for Down's syndrome in the second trimester. In a population of consecutive women in early pregnancy (7–13 weeks), free β-hCG levels were significantly increased (1.88 MoM) in 13 cases of trisomy 21 and significantly reduced in 5 cases of trisomy 18 (Spencer *et al.*, 1992). These observations were confirmed by pooling with 25 additional cases (2.2 MoM) (Macri *et al.*, 1993). The combination of free β-hCG and PAPP-A further increases the detection rate to 80% for a 5% false-positive rate (Brambati *et al.*, 1993b).

Conclusion

More first trimester studies are required to fully define the sensitivity and specificity of PAPP-A and free β-hCG in the detection of fetal aneuploidies. Recent results suggest that PAPP-A alone or in combination with free β-hCG might provide an efficient tool to extend screening policies for fetal aneuploidies into the first trimester.

References

Aitken, D.A., McCaw, G., Crossley, J.A. *et al.* (1993). First trimester biochemical screening for fetal chromosome abnormalities and neural tube defects. *Prenatal Diagn.*, **13**, 681–9.

Barkai, G., Shaki, R., Pariente, C. & Goldman, B. (1987). First trimester alpha-fetoprotein levels in normal and chromosomally abnormal pregnancies. *Lancet*, **ii**, 389.

Brambati, B., Simoni, G., Bonacchi, I. & Piceni, L. (1986). Fetal chromosomal aneuploidies and maternal serum alpha-fetoprotein levels in first trimester. *Lancet*, **ii**, 165–6.

Brambati, B., Lanzani, A. & Tului, L. (1991). Ultrasound and biochemical assessment of first trimester pregnancy. In *The Embryo*, ed. M. Chapman, J.G. Grudzinskas & T. Chard, pp. 181–94. London: Springer-Verlag.

Brambati, B., Chard, T., Grudzinskas, J.G., Macintosh, M.C.M., Lanzani, A. & Bonacchi, I. (1992). Potential first trimester biochemical screening tests for chromosome anomalies. *Prenatal Diagn.*, **12**(Suppl): S4.

Brambati, B., Macintosh, M.C.M., Teisner, B. *et al.* (1993a). Low maternal serum levels of pregnancy associated plasma protein A (PAPP-A) in the first trimester in association with abnormal fetal karyotype. *Br. J. Obstet. Gynaecol.*, **100**, 324–6.

Brambati, B., Tului, L., Bonacchi, I., Shrimanker, K., Suzuki, Y. & Grudzinskas, J.G. (1993b). Serum PAPP-A and free beta hCG are first trimester screening markers for Down's syndrome (Abstract). *Hum. Reprod.*, **8**(Suppl. 1): 183.

Brock, D.J.H., Barron, L., Holloway, S., Liston, W.A., Hillier, S.G. & Seppala, M. (1990). First-trimester maternal serum biochemical indicators in Down syndrome. *Prenatal Diagn.*, **10**, 245–51.

Cuckle, H.S., Wald, N.J., Barkai, G. *et al.* (1988). First-trimester biochemical screening for Down syndrome. *Lancet*, **ii**, 851–2.

Ferguson-Smith, M. & Yates, J.R.W. (1984). Maternal age specific rates for chromosome aberrations and factors influencing them: report of a collaborative European study on 52 965 amniocenteses. *Prenatal Diagn.*, **4**, 5–44.

Fuhrmann, W., Altland, K., Jovanovic, V. *et al.* (1993). First-trimester alpha-fetoprotein screening for Down syndrome. *Prenatal Diagn.*, **13**, 215–18.

Haddow, J.E., Palomaki, G.E., Knight, G.J. *et al.* (1992). Prenatal screening for Down's syndrome with use of maternal serum markers. *N. Engl. J. Med.*, **327**, 588–93.

Hook, E.B., Cross, P.K., Jackson, L.G., Pergament, E. & Brambati, B. (1988). Maternal age-specific rates of 47, +21 and other cytogenetic abnormalities diagnosed in the first trimester of pregnancy in chorionic villus biopsy specimens: comparison with rates expected from observations at amniocentesis. *Am. J. Hum. Genet.*, **42**, 797–807.

Johnson, A., Cowchock, F.S., Darby, M., Wapner, R. & Jackson, L.G. (1991). First trimester maternal serum alpha-fetoprotein and chorionic gonadotropin in aneuploid pregnancies. *Prenatal Diagn.*, **11**, 443–50.

Kratzer, P.G., Golbus, M.S., Monroe, S.E., Finkelstein, D.E. & Taylor, R.N. (1991). First-trimester aneuploidy screening using serum human chorionic gonadotropin (hCG), free alpha hCG, and progesterone. *Prenatal Diagn.*, **11**, 751–65.

Macintosh, M.C.M., Brambati, B., Chard, T. & Grudzinskas, J.G. (1993a). Predicting fetal chromosome anomalies in the first trimester using pregnancy associated plasma protein-A: a comparison of statistical methods. *Meth. Inform. Med.*, **32**, 175–9.

Macintosh, M.C.M., Brambati, B., Chard, T. & Grudzinskas, J.G. (1993b). First-trimester maternal serum Schwangerschafts protein 1 (SP1) in pregnancies associated with chromosomal anomalies. *Prenatal Diagn.*, **13**, 563–8.

Macri, J.N., Kasturi, R.V., Krantz, D.A. et al. (1990). Maternal serum Down syndrome screening: free beta protein is a more effective marker than human chorionic gonadotrophin. *Am. J. Obstet. Gynecol.*, **163**, 1248–53.

Macri, J.N., Spencer, K., Aitken, D. et al. (1993). First-trimester free beta (hCG) screening for Down syndrome. *Prenatal Diagn.*, **13**, 557–62.

Milunsky, A., Wands, J., Brambati, B., Bonacchi, I. & Currie, K. (1988). First trimester maternal serum alpha-fetoprotein screening for chromosome defects. *Am. J. Obstet. Gynecol.*, **159**, 1209–13.

Muller, F., Cuckle, H., Teisner, B. & Grudzinskas, J.G. (1993). Serum PAPP-A levels are depressed in women with fetal Down syndrome in early pregnancy. *Prenatal Diagn.*, **13**, 633–6.

Nørgaard-Pedersen, B., Olesen Larsen, S., Arends, J., Svenstrup, B. & Tabor, A. (1990). Maternal serum markers in the screening for Down's syndrome. *Clin. Genet.*, **37**, 35–43.

Ozturk, M., Milunsky, A., Brambati, B., Sachs, E.S., Miller, S.L. & Wands, J.R. (1990). Abnormal maternal serum levels of human chorionic gonadotropin free subunits in trisomy 18. *Am. J. Med. Genet.*, **37**, 114–18.

Pescia, G., Marguerat, Ph., Weihs, D. et al. (1993). First trimester free beta human chorion gonadotropin (Fβ-hCG) and SP1 as markers for fetal chromosomal disorders: a prospective study of 250 women undergoing CVS. *Conference on Screening for Down's syndrome.* 24–26 May, London, Abstract Book, p. 45.

Phillips, O.P., Elias, S., Shulman, L.P., Andersen, R.N., Morgan, C.D. & Simpson, J.L. (1992). Maternal serum screening for fetal Down syndrome in women less than 35 years of age using alpha-fetoprotein, hCG and unconjugated estriol: a prospective 2-year study. *Obstet. Gynecol.*, **80**, 353–8.

Sinosich, M.J., Teisner, B., Folkersen, J., Saunders, D.M. & Grudzinskas, J.G. (1982). Radioimmunoassay for pregnancy-associated plasma protein A. *Clin. Chem.*, **5**, 777–86.

Spencer, K., Macri, J.N., Aitken, D.A. & Connor, J.M. (1992). Free β-hCG as first-trimester marker for fetal trisomy. *Lancet*, **339**, 1480.

van Lith, J.M.M., Mantingh, J.R., Beekhuis, J.R. & de Bruijn, H.W.A. (1991). First trimester CA 125 and Down's syndrome. *Br. J. Obstet. Gynaecol.*, **98**, 493–4.

van Lith, J., Grudzinskas, J.G., Mantingh, A. et al. (1994). Maternal serum PAPP-A levels in pregnancies with chromosomally normal and abnormal fetuses. *Br. J. Obstet. Gynaecol.*, in press.

Wald, N.J., Cuckle, H.S., Densem, J.W. et al. (1988). Maternal serum screening for Down syndrome in early pregnancy. *Br. Med. J.*, **297**, 883–7.

Wald, N.J., Kennard, A., Densem, J.W., Cuckle, H.S., Chard, T. & Butler, L. (1992a). Antenatal maternal serum screening for Down's syndrome: results of a demonstration project. *Br. Med. J.*, **305**, 391–4.

Wald, N.J., Stone, R., Cuckle, H.S. et al. (1992b). First trimester concentrations of pregnancy associated plasma protein A and placental protein 14 in Down's syndrome. *Br. Med. J.*, **305**, 28.

22

First trimester fetal nuchal translucency

M.L. BRIZOT, P. THEODOROPOULOS,
R.J.M. SNIJDERS AND K.H. NICOLAIDES

This chapter proposes screening for fetal trisomies based on the combination of fetal nuchal translucency (NT) thickness at 10–13 weeks of gestation and maternal age. In trying to introduce this new method of screening, it is essential to establish the prevalence of trisomies and the prevalence of increased NT thickness in chromosomally normal and trisomic fetuses at 10–13 weeks of gestation. Furthermore, an appropriate method of diagnosis should be available for the high-risk groups.

Prevalence of fetal trisomies at 10–13 weeks

Since the incidence of chromosomal abnormalities increases with maternal age, to calculate the prevalence of trisomies at 10–13 weeks of gestation it is necessary (i) to know the maternal age distribution of the population under investigation and (ii) to derive maternal age-specific risks for trisomies in the first trimester.

Maternal age distribution

The maternal age distribution of deliveries in England and Wales in 1991 is shown in Table 22.1 (Office of Population Census and Statistics). From this distribution it is possible to predict the relative contribution of trisomic fetuses by each maternal age group (Table 22.1). Approximately 1% of pregnant women are aged ≥ 40 years and this group contributues 12% of trisomic fetuses.

Since the early 1980s, the relative frequency of pregnancies in women $\geq$ 35 years increased from 5.1% in 1981 to 7.5% in 1991 (Fig. 22.1). Therefore a policy of offering invasive testing to women $\geq$ 35 years would have required a 50% expansion in the necessary facilities.

Table 22.1. *Maternal-age distribution of deliveries and distribution of Down's syndrome fetuses in England and Wales in* 1991

Maternal age (years)	All deliveries (%)	Down's syndrome fetuses (%)
< 24	36.3	19.4
25–29	35.4	23.2
30–34	20.9	24.2
35–39	6.4	21.0
≥ 40	1.0	12.1
Total	100.0	100.0

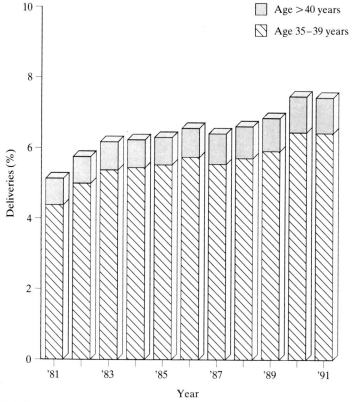

Fig. 22.1. Percentage of total deliveries to women aged 35–39 and ≥ 40 years (OPCS).

Maternal age-specific risks for trisomies in the first trimester

Snijders *et al.* (1994) established estimates of maternal age-related risks for fetal trisomies at 9–14 weeks of gestation. Analyses were confined to trisomies 21, 18 and 13, since they account for 67% of all chromosomal abnormalities; on the basis of currently available data they are the only ones for which estimates can be calculated. They calculated the incidence of trisomies 21, 18 and 13 in 15 793 women aged 35–45 years who underwent first-trimester karyotyping for the sole indication of maternal age ≥ 35 years. The values were compared to the incidence of trisomy 21 in livebirths which were calculated by Cuckle *et al.* (1987) on a total of 3 289 114 pregnancies published in eight large surveys.

The incidence of trisomy 21 at 10–14 weeks of gestation was 2.2 times as high as in livebirths. Since the ratio for the incidence of trisomy 21 at 9–14 weeks to that in livebirths was not significantly associated with maternal age, estimates for women below 35 years of age were derived by multiplying the livebirth incidence by 2.2. At 9–14 weeks, the relative frequency of trisomies 18 and 13, compared to that of trisomy 21, was found to be 41%. Therefore, the incidence for these trisomies was derived by multiplying estimates for trisomy 21 by 0.41.

Traditionally, counselling parents as to the risk of fetal chromosomal abnormalities has depended on the provision of the livebirth incidence of trisomy 21. The findings of Snijders *et al.* (1994) make it possible to give estimates for the three most common trisomies at 9–14 weeks of gestation, when screening and invasive testing for chromosomal abnormalities are performed. Furthermore, the data can be used to calculate the expected incidence of the three trisomies in any study group when new ultrasonographic or biochemical methods of first-trimester screening are being evaluated.

Nuchal fluid and chromosomal defects

Cystic hygromata, nuchal oedema and nuchal translucency

During the second and third trimesters of pregnancy, abnormal accumulation of fluid behind the fetal neck can be classified as nuchal cystic hygromata and nuchal oedema.

Cystic hygromata are bilateral, septated cystic structures, which are strongly associated with Turner syndrome (Table 22.2). They are thought to represent over-distension of jugular lymphatic sacs as a consequence of failure of communication with the internal jugular vein.

Table 22.2. *Summary of reported series on antenatally diagnosed cystic hygromata providing data on the presence of associated chromosomal defects*

Author	Gestational age (weeks)	n	Total		Turner's		Abnormal karyotype				
							Trisomy 21		Trisomy 18		Other
			No.	%	No.	%	No.	%	No.	%	
Chervenak et al., 1983	18–29	15	11	73	11	100	—	—	—	—	—
Newman and Cooperberg, 1984	16–26	3	2	67	1	50	1	50	—	—	—
Redford et al., 1984	17–26	5	4	80	2	50	1	25	1	25	—
Marchese et al., 1985	16–20	6	5	83	4	80	—	—	1	20	—
Nicolaides et al., 1985	16–22	8	6	75	5	83	—	—	1	17	—
Pearce et al., 1985	16–26	22	17	77	14	82	2	12	1	6	—
Carr et al., 1986	17–28	5	3	60	2	67	1	33	—	—	—
Garden et al., 1986	14–26	16	13	81	11	85	—	—	1	8	47XXY
Palmer et al., 1987	16–26	8	6	63	4	67	1	17	—	—	46 + 5p
Gembruch et al., 1988	13–26	29	17	48	10	59	6	35	1	6	—
Hegge et al., 1988	15–17	4	3	75	2	50	1	25	—	—	—
Pijpers et al., 1988	12–25	15	9	60	8	89	—	—	1	11	—
Abramowicz et al., 1989	12–31	17	10	59	6	60	3	30	1	10	—
Cohen et al., 1989	10–30	15	10	67	5	50	4	40	1	10	—
Edyoux et al., 1989	12–32	41	19	46	14	74	4	21	1	5	—
Miyabara et al., 1989	12–23	10	9	90	4	44	1	11	3	33	47 + 13, del 4p
Holzgreve et al., 1990	—	15	10	67	7	70	2	20	1	10	—
Langer et al., 1990	12–29	17	8	47	7	88	1	12	—	—	—
Rizzo et al., 1990	15–27	13	10	77	8	80	1	10	1	10	—
Tannirandorn et al., 1990	16–23	11	7	64	5	71	—	—	1	14	47 + 13
Azar et al., 1991	16–26	44	33	75	31	94	1	3	—	—	—
Bernstein et al., 1991	12–39	45	29	64	20	69	3	10	3	10	47 + 13, del Y, 46 + 15q
Droste et al., 1991	12–27	23	18	78	10	50	4	22	1	6	47 + 13, del 4p, del 13q
MacLeod and McHugo, 1991	16–21	15	10	67	3	30	3	30	2	20	47 + 13, 46 + 5q
Santolaya et al., 1992	13–40	15	10	66	7	70	3	30	—	—	—
Ville et al., 1992a	16–26	6	4	66	3	75	—	—	1	25	—
Bronshtein et al., 1993	13–17	25	18	72	?	?	?	?	?	?	—
Total	12–39	448	301	67	204	72	43	15	23	8	13 (5%)

Nuchal oedema is the result of subcutaneous accumulation of fluid that produces a characteristic tremor on ballotment of the fetal head. It may be considered as an early sign of hydrops fetalis, which has a diverse aetiology including trisomies, cardiovascular and pulmonary defects, skeletal dysplasias, congenital infection and metabolic and haematological disorders. In a series of 145 fetuses with nuchal oedema, 53 (37%) had chromosomal abnormalities, mainly trisomy 21, but also other trisomies, deletions or translocations, triploidy and Turner's syndrome (Nicolaides *et al.*, 1992a). Furthermore, the chromosomally normal fetuses had a very poor prognosis because in many cases there was an underlying skeletal dysplasia, genetic syndrome or cardiac defect; in 79 (87%) of the 91 cases there were additional defects.

Recent publications have suggested the possible association between abnormal nuchal fluid and chromosomal abnormalities in the first trimester of pregnancy. Although in some studies the condition was defined as a multiseptated, thin walled cystic mass similar to that seen in the second trimester, in others the term was used loosely to include nuchal thickening or oedema. We prefer the use of the term translucency because this is the ultrasonographic feature that is observed (Fig. 22.2).

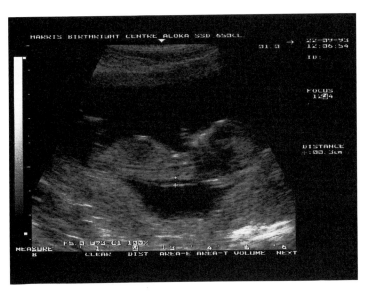

Fig. 22.2. Ultrasound picture of fetal nuchal translucency thickness of 3 mm at 11 weeks of gestation.

Table 22.3. Summary of reported series on first-trimester fetal nuchal translucency providing data on the presence of associated chromosomal defects

Author	Gestational age (weeks)	Nuchel translucency thickness (mm)	Total cases	Abnormal karyotype						
				Total	No. (%)	Turner	Trisomy 13	Trisomy 18	Trisomy 21	Other
Johnson et al., 1993	10–14	≥2.0	68	41	(60)	9	2	9	16	5[a]
Shulman et al., 1992	10–13	≥2.5	32	15	(47)	4	3	4	4	–
Nicolaides et al., 1992b	10–13	≥3.0	51	18	(35)	–	2	4	10	2[b]
Szabo and Gellen, 1990	11–12	≥3.0	8	7	(88)	–	–	–	7	–
Wilson et al., 1992	8–11	≥3.0	14	3	(21)	1	–	–	–	2[c]
Ville et al., 1992b	9–14	≥3.0	29	8	(28)	–	1	3	4	–
Nadel et al., 1993	10–15	≥4.0	63	43	(68)	10	1	15	15	2[d]
Savoldelli et al., 1993	9–12	≥4.0	24	19	(79)	1	1	2	15	–
Shulte-Valentin and Schindler, 1992	10–14	≥4.0	8	7	(88)	–	–	–	7	–
van Zalen-Sprock et al., 1992	10–14	≥4.0	18	5	(28)	1	–	1	3	1[e]
Cullen et al., 1990	11–13	≥6.0	29	15	(52)	4	–	2	6	3[f]
Suchet et al., 1992	8–14	≥10.0	13	8	(62)	7	–	–	–	1[g]
Total	8–15		357	189	53	37	10	40	87	16

[a] Unbalanced translocation 10[4; 10]; balanced translocation [1; 18]; 45,X/46,XY; 47,XXX/46,XX; unbalanced translocation 18[7; 18].
[b] 47,XY + fragment; trisomy 22.
[c] Two cases of triploidy.
[d] 45,X-15 + der(15) + t(Y; 15).
[e] 47,XY + 15/46,XX; 49,XXXXY; 47,XX-21 + der(21)t(q18;p21).
[f] 47,XXY.

Measurement and reproducibility of fetal NT thickness

Transabdominal ultrasound examination is performed to obtain a sagittal section of the fetus for measurement of fetal crown–rump length. The maximum thickness of the subcutaneous translucency between the skin and the soft tissue overlying the cervical spine is measured. Care is taken to distinguish between fetal skin and amnion because at this gestation both structures appear as thin membranes. This is achieved by waiting for spontaneous fetal movement away from the amniotic membrane; alternatively the fetus is bounced off the amnion by asking the mother to cough and/or by tapping the maternal abdomen.

In a study of 200 women we established that the intra- and inter-observer variabilities in measurement of NT thickness are 3% and 5%, respectively. In all cases with different measurements the difference was 1 mm.

Increased NT thickness and chromosomal abnormalities

Several prenatal ultrasonographic studies have documented a strong association between increased NT thickness and chromosomal abnormalities in the first trimester of pregnancy (Table 22.3). From the combined data of 12 series, 189 of 357 fetuses (53%) were chromosomally abnormal.

Prevalence of increased NT thickness at 10–13 weeks

The prevalence of increased NT thickness (≥ 3 mm) at 10–13 weeks was examined in a prospective study of 827 women with singleton pregnancies undergoing first-trimester fetal karyotyping because of advanced maternal age, parental anxiety or a family history of a chromosomal abnormality in the absence of balanced parental translocation (Nicolaides *et al.*, 1992b). The overall incidence of chromosomal defects was 3.4% (Table 22.4), and of trisomies 21, 18 or 13 was 2.4% ($n = 20$). NT ≥ 3 mm was found in 80% of fetuses with trisomies 21, 18 and 13 and in 4.1% of chromosomally normal fetuses.

In an expanded series of 1273 women having first-trimester fetal karyotyping, trisomies 21, 18 or 13 were found in 36 (2.8%) of the cases (Nicolaides *et al.*, 1994a). The NT thickness was ≥ 3 mm in 86.1% of the trisomic and in 4.5% of the chromosomally normal fetuses (Table 22.5). In the group with normal fetal karyotype, the incidence of NT ≥ 3 mm was independent of maternal age and it was therefore possible to derive

Table 22.4. *Incidence of fetal nuchal translucency >3 mm in 827 low-risk pregnancies at 10–13 weeks of gestation*

Karyotype	*n*	NT ≥ 3 mm
Normal	799	33
Abnormal	28	18
Trisomy 21	13	10
Trisomy 18	5	4
Trisomy 13	2	2
Trisomy 22	1	1
Trisomy fragment	1	1
Mosaic trisomy 21 or 8	2	0
47,XXX or 47,XXY	4	0
Total	827	51

NT, nuchal translucency.

Table 22.5. *Nuchal translucency thickness and fetal karyotype*

Nuchal translucency thickness (mm)	Total cases	Normal karotype	Abnormal karyotype			
			Trisomy 21	Trisomy 18	Trisomy 13	Other
<3	1185	1172	4	1	–	8[a]
≥3	88	55	21	8	2	2[b]
Total	1273	1227	25	9	2	10

[a] 46,XX,18p; 47,XXX (*n* = 2); 47XXY (*n* = 2); 47,XXX/46,XX; 47,XX + 21/46,XX; 47,XX + 8/16,XX.
[b] 47,XX + 22; 47,XY + fragment.

estimates of risks for fetal trisomies on the basis of maternal age and fetal NT thickness; NT < 3 mm was associated with a 4.5-fold reduction, whereas NT ≥ 3 mm was associated with 12-fold increase in maternal age-related risk.

In a series of 560 fetuses with NT ≥ 3 mm, which included cases that were identified from our prospective screening study and patients referred to our centre for karyotyping because of increased NT thickness, it was possible to derive risks for trisomies with increasing translucency thickness (Pandya *et al.*, 1994). Thus, translucencies of 3 mm, 4 mm, 5 mm and

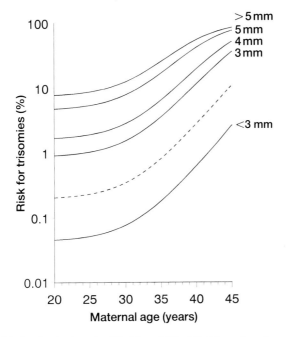

Fig. 22.3. Risk for fetal trisomies 21, 18 and 13 at 9–14 weeks of gestation based on maternal age alone (- - -) and with fetal nuchal translucency thickness (NT) of <3 mm, 3 mm, 4 mm, 5 mm and >5 mm, respectively.

≥6 mm were associated with 4-fold, 21-fold, 26-fold and 41-fold increase in maternal age-related risks, respectively (Fig. 22.3).

Advantages of screening by NT thickness

Presently available data suggest that 84% of trisomy 21 fetuses (or 86% of trisomy 21 or 18 or 13 fetuses) and 4.5% of chromosomally normal fetuses have NT thickness of ≥3 mm. In England and Wales, approximately 1% of deliveries are in women ≥ 40 years of age and from estimates of maternal age-related risks this group contributes approximately 12% of trisomy 21 infants (Table 22.1). On the basis of these data it is predicted that a policy which offers fetal karyotyping to women aged < 40 years if the fetal NT thickness is ≥3 mm and to all women aged ≥40 years could potentially identify more than 85% of trisomy 21 fetuses with a false-positive rate of approximately 5% (Table 22.6).

For the same false-positive rate (approximately 5%), the sensitivity of the new method of screening compares favourably with the respective

Table 22.6. *Observed number of trisomies 21, 18 and 13 in relation to fetal nuchal translucency thickness and the expected number on the basis of maternal age*

Nuchal translucency thickness (mm)	n	Observed			Expected			Observed to expected ratio		
		21	18/13	21/18/13	21	18/13	21/18/13	21	18/13	21/18/13
3	383	16	7	23	4.20	1.81	6.01	3.8	3.9	3.8
4	67	16	5	21	0.71	0.31	1.02	22.5	16.0	20.6
5	41	13	7	20	0.53	0.23	0.76	24.5	30.0	26.3
≥6	69	16	22	38	0.65	0.28	0.93	24.6	78.6	40.9
Total	560	61	41	102	6.09	2.63	8.72	10.0	15.6	11.7

values of 20–30% and 50–60% for screening by maternal age alone or maternal age and serum biochemistry (Haddow *et al.*, 1992; Phillips *et al.*, 1992; Wald *et al.*, 1992). Furthermore, the uptake of invasive testing for fetal karyotyping following the identification of a visible marker in the fetus is likely to be higher than with risks derived from maternal factors.

A major criticism of screening by ultrasound, in contrast to biochemical testing, is that scanning requires highly skilled operators. This is certainly true for many of the subtle markers of chromosomal abnormalities detectable at 18–20 weeks of gestation. However, the skill necessary for measurement of NT at 10–13 weeks is no greater than that required to obtain a reliable measurement of the crown–rump length, which is essential for accurate dating of pregnancy and correct interpretation of serum biochemistry results.

The sensitivity and specificity of NT $\geq$ 3 mm as a marker of chromosomal defects in routine transabdominal ultrasonographic examination of the whole population remains to be determined. Furthermore, the cost of implementing a routine ultrasound scan at 10–13 weeks in addition to the fetal abnormality scan at 20 weeks needs to be considered. Nevertheless, maternal serum biochemistry screening is being introduced widely and as part of this screening it is recommended that a scan should be performed before biochemical testing (Wald *et al.*, 1992). The available data suggest that this scan should be undertaken at 10–13 weeks of gestation and the fetal nuchal region should be examined.

Methods of diagnosis

Amniocentesis for fetal karyotyping is traditionally performed at 16 weeks of gestation and the results are available at 18–20 weeks. A randomised study reported that this technique is associated with a 1% risk of spontaneous abortion (Tabor *et al.*, 1986). In the early 1980s, first-trimester diagnosis became possible with the introduction of chorion villus sampling (CVS). Three randomised trials comparing the safety of first-trimester CVS and second-trimester amniocentesis reported conflicting results; the chances of having a successful pregnancy outcome after first-trimester CVS was 4.6% lower (MRC Working Party, 1991), 0.6% lower (Canadian trial, 1989) or 0.1% higher (Smidt-Jehnsen *et al.*, 1992). In these studies the need for repeat testing after CVS, because of inadequate sample, mosaic result or culture failure, was 3–10%. In the late 1980s, early amniocentesis (EA) was introduced and four studies with complete pregnancy follow-up have reported that the procedure-related rate of fetal loss was 3.3–6.6% (Nevin *et al.*, 1990; Penso *et al.*, 1990; Stripparo *et al.*, 1990; Hanson *et al.*, 1992).

We have recently completed a prospective study comparing amniocentesis and CVS for fetal karyotyping in the first trimester of pregnancy, involving 1301 women (Nicolaides *et al.*, 1994b). In this study women were given the option to choose between the available methods of non-invasive screening and invasive testing, and, in the analysis of data, comparisons were made between both the total groups, including those that chose to have EA or CVS, and the subgroups that were randomised into one of these procedures. The groups did not differ significantly in the various factors that could influence pregnancy outcome, such as maternal age, previous obstetric history, maternal smoking, weight, threatened miscarriage, fetal crown–rump length or placental position.

EA was performed in 731 cases and CVS was performed in 570 cases. Both procedures were performed by transabdominal ultrasound-guided insertion of a needle (20 gauge) using a free-hand technique. Successful sampling resulting in a non-mosaic cytogenetic result was the same for both EA and CVS (97.5%). Spontaneous loss (intrauterine and neonatal death) after EA was significantly higher than after CVS (total group: mean = 2.3%, 95% CI: 1.2–3.9; randomised subgroup: mean = 1.2%, 95% CI: 0.3–3.5). The gestation at delivery and birth weight of the infants after EA and CVS were similar and the frequencies of preterm delivery or low birthweight were not higher than would be expected in a normal population. In the EA group the incidence of talipes equinovarus (1.6%) was higher than in the CVS group (0.6%), but this difference was not significant.

Conclusion

There is substantial evidence that effective screening and diagnosis of fetal trisomies can now be achieved in the first trimester of pregnancy. Assessment of risk can be based on ultrasound examination at 10–13 weeks for measurement of NT thickness combined with maternal age. Those patients at high risk who choose to have prenatal diagnosis can be offered CVS and direct cytogenetic analysis which will provide results within a few days of sampling.

References

Abramowicz, J.S., Warsof, S.L., Doyle, D.L., Smith, D. & Levy, D.L. (1989). Congenital cystic hygroma of the neck diagnosed prenatally: outcome with normal and abnormal karyotype. *Prenatal Diagn.*, **9**, 321–27.

Azar, G.B., Snijders, R.J.M., Gosden, C. & Nicolaides, K.H. (1991). Fetal nuchal cystic hygromata: associated malformations and chromosomal defects. *Fetal Diagn. Ther.*, **6**, 46–57.

Bernstein, H.S., Filly, R.A., Goldberg, J.D. & Golbus, M.S. (1991). Prognosis of fetuses with a cystic hygroma. *Prenatal Diagn.*, **11**, 349–55.

Bronshtein, M., Bar Hava, I., Blumenfeld, I., Bejar, J., Toder, V. & Blumenfeld, Z. (1993). The difference between septated and nonseptated nuchal cystic hygroma in the early second trimester. *Obstet. Gynecol.*, **81**, 683–7.

Canadian Collaborative CVS-amniocentesis Clinical Trial Group (1989). Multicentre randomised clinical trial of chorion villus sampling and amniocentesis. *Lancet*, **i**, 1–6.

Carr, R.F., Ochs, R.H., Kenny, J.D., Fridey, J.L. & Ming, P.L. (1986). Fetal cystic hygroma and Turner's syndrome. *Am. J. Dis. Child.*, **140**, 580–3.

Chervenak, F.A., Isaacson, G., Blakemore, K.J. *et al.* (1983). Fetal cystic hygroma: cause and natural history. *N. Engl. J. Med.*, **309**, 822–5.

Cohen, M.M., Schwartz, S., Schwartz, M.F. *et al.* (1989). Antenatal detection of cystic hygroma. *Obstet. Gynecol. Surv.*, **44**, 481–90.

Cuckle, H.S., Wald, N.J. & Thompson, S.G. (1987). Estimating a woman's risk of having a pregnancy associated with Down's syndrome using her age and serum alpha-fetoprotein level. *Br. J. Obstet. Gynaecol.*, **94**, 387–402.

Cullen, M.T., Gabrielli, S., Green, J.J. *et al.* (1990). Diagnosis and significance of cystic hygroma in the first trimester. *Prenatal Diagn.*, **10**, 643–51.

Droste, S., Hendricks, S.K., von Alfrey, H. & Mack, L.A. (1991). Cystic hygroma colli: perinatal outcome after prenatal diagnosis. *J. Perinat. Med.*, **19**, 449–54.

Eydoux, P., Choiset, A., Le Porrier, N. *et al.* (1989). Chromosomal prenatal diagnosis: study of 936 cases of intrauterine abnormalities after ultrasound assessment. *Prenatal Diagn.*, **9**, 255–68.

Garden, A.S., Benzie, R.J., Miskin, M. & Gardner, H.A. (1986). Fetal cystic hygroma colli: antenatal diagnosis, significance, and management. *Am. J. Obstet. Gynecol.*, **154**, 221–5.

Gembruch, U., Hansmann, M., Bald, R., Zerres, K., Schwanitz, G. & Fodisch, H.J. (1988). Prenatal diagnosis and management in fetuses with cystic hygromata colli. *Eur. J. Obstet. Gynecol. Reprod. Biol.*, **29**, 241–55.

Haddow, J.E., Palomaki, G.E., Knight, G.J. *et al.* (1992). Prenatal screening for Down's syndrome with use of maternal serum markers. *N. Engl. J. Med.*, **327**, 588–93.

Hanson, F.W., Tennant, F., Hune, S. & Brookhyser, K. (1992). Early amniocentesis: outcome, risks, and technical problems at ≤12.8 weeks. *Am. J. Obstet. Gynecol.*, **166**, 1707–11.

Hegge, F.N., Prescott, G.H. & Watson, P.T. (1988). Sonography at the time of genetic amniocentesis to screen for fetal malformations. *Obstet. Gynecol.*, **71**, 522–5.

Holzgreve, W., Miny, P., Gerlach, B., Westerndrop, A., Ahlert, D. & Horst, J. (1990). Benefits of placental biopsies for rapid karyotyping in the second and third trimesters (late chorionic villus sampling) in high-risk pregnancies. *Am. J. Obstet. Gynecol.*, **162**, 1188–92.

Johnson, M.P., Johnson, A., Holzgreve, W. *et al.* (1993). First-trimester simple hygroma: cause and outcome. *Am. J. Obstet. Gynecol.*, **168**, 156–61.

Langer, J.C., Fitzgerald, P.G., Desa, D. *et al.* (1990). Cervical cystic hygroma in the fetus: clinical spectrum and outcome. *J. Pediatr. Surg.*, **25**, 58–61.

MacLeod, A.M. & McHugo, J.M. (1991). Prenatal diagnosis of nuchal cystic hygroma. *Br. J. Radiol.*, **64**, 802–7.

Marchese, C., Savin, E., Dragone, E. *et al.* (1985). Cystic hygroma: prenatal diagnosis and genetic counselling. *Prenatal Diagn.*, **5**, 221–7.

Miyabara, S., Sugihara, H., Maehara, N. *et al.* (1989). Significance of cardiovascular malformations in cystic hygroma: a new interpretation of the pathogenesis. *Am. J. Med. Genet.*, **34**, 489–501.

MRC Working Party on the Evaluation of Chorion Villus Sampling (1991). Medical Research Council European trial of chorion villus sampling. *Lancet*, **337**, 1491–9.

Nadel, A., Bromley, B. & Benacerraf, B.R. (1993). Nuchal thickening or cystic hygromas in first- and early second-trimester fetuses: prognosis and outcome. *Obstet. Gynecol.*, **82**, 43–8.

Nevin, J., Nevin, N.C., Dornan, J.C., Sim, D. & Armstrong, M.J. (1990). Early amniocentesis: experience of 222 consecutive patients, 1987–1988. *Prenatal Diagn.*, **10**, 79–83.

Newman, D.E. & Cooperberg, P.L. (1984). Genetics of sonographically detected intrauterine fetal cystic hygromas. *J. Can. Assoc. Radiol.*, **35**, 77–9.

Nicolaides, K.H., Rodeck, C.H., Lange, I. *et al.* (1985). Fetoscopy in the assessment of unexplained fetal hydrops. *Br. J. Obstet. Gynaecol.*, **92**, 671–9.

Nicolaides, K.H., Azar, G., Snijders, R.J.M. & Gosden, C.M. (1992a). Fetal nuchal oedema: associated malformations and chromosomal defects. *Fetal. Diagn. Ther.*, **7**, 123–31.

Nicolaides, K.H., Azar, G., Byrne, D., Mansur, C. & Marks, K. (1992b). Fetal nuchal translucency: ultrasound screening for chromosomal defects in first trimester of pregnancy. *Br. Med. J.*, **304**, 867–9.

Nicolaides, K.H., Brizot, M.L. & Snijders, R.J.M. (1994a). Fetal nuchal translucency: ultrasound screening for fetal trisomy in the first trimester of pregnancy. *Br. J. Obstet. Gynaecol.*, in press.

Nicolaides, K.H., Brizot, M.L., Patel, F. & Snijders, R.J.M. (1994b). Comparative study of chorion villus sampling and amniocentesis for fetal karyotyping at 10–13 weeks gestation. *Lancet*, in press.

Palmer, C.G., Miles, J.H., Howard-Peebles, P.N., Magenis, R.E., Patil, S. & Friedman, J.M. (1987). Fetal karyotype following ascertainment of fetal anomalies by ultrasound. *Prenatal Diagn.*, **7**, 551–5.

Pandya, P.P., Brizot, M.L., Kuhn, P., Snijders, R.J.M. & Nicolaides, K.H. (1994). First trimester fetal nuchal translucency thickness and risk for trisomies. *Obstet. Gynecol.*, in press.

Pearce, J.M., Griffin, D. & Campbell, S. (1985). The differential prenatal diagnosis of cystic hygromata and encephalocele by ultrasound examination. *J. Clin. Ultrasound*, **13**, 317–20.

Penso, C.A., Snadstrom, M.M., Garber, M.F., Ladoulis, M., Stryker, J.M. & Benacerraf, B.B. (1990). Early amniocentesis: report of 407 cases with neonatal follow-up. *Obstet. Gynecol.*, **76**, 1032–6.

Pijpers, L., Reuss, A., Stewart, P.A., Wladimiroff, J.W. & Sachs, E.S. (1988). Fetal cystic hygroma: prenatal diagnosis and management. *Obstet. Gynecol.*, **72**, 223–4.

Phillips, O.P., Elias, S., Shulman, L.P., Andersen, R.N., Morgan, C.D. & Simpson, J.L. (1992). Maternal serum screening for fetal Down syndrome in women less than 35 years of age using α-fetoprotein, hCG and unconjugated estriol: a prospective 2-year study. *Obstet. Gynecol.*, **80**, 353–8.

Redford, D.H., McNay, M.B., Ferguson-Smith, M.E. & Jamieson, M.E. (1984). Aneuploidy and cystic hygroma detectable by ultrasound. *Prenatal Diagn.*, **4**, 377–82.

Rizzo, N., Pittalis, M.C., Pilu, G., Orsini, L.F., Perolo, A. & Bovicelli, L. (1990). Prenatal karyotyping in malformed fetuses. *Prenatal Diagn.*, **10**, 17–23.

Savoldelli, G., Binkert, F., Achermann, J. & Schmid, W. (1993). Ultrasound screening for chromosomal anomalies in the first trimester of pregnancy. *Prenatal Diagn.*, **13**, 513–18.

Santolaya, J., Alley, D., Jaffe, R. & Warsof, S.L. (1992). Antenatal classification of hydrops fetalis. *Obstet. Gynecol.*, **79**, 256–9.

Schulte-Vallentin, M. & Schindler, H. (1992). Non-echogenic nuchal oedema as a marker in trisomy 21 screening. *Lancet*, **339**, 1053.

Shulman, L.P., Emerson, D., Felker, R., Phillips, O., Simpson, J. & Elias, S. (1992). High frequency of cytogenetic abnormalities with cystic hygroma diagnosed in the first trimester. *Obstet. Gynecol.*, **80**, 80–2.

Smidt-Jehnsen, S., Permin, M., Philip, J. *et al.* (1992). Randomised comparison of amniocentesis and transabdominal and transcervical chorion villus sampling. *Lancet*, **340**, 1237–44.

Snijders, R.J.M., Holzgreve, W., Cuckle, H. & Nicolaides, K.H. (1994). Maternal age-specific risk for trisomies at 9–14 weeks gestation. *Prenatal Diagn.*, in press.

Stripparo, L., Buscaglia, M., Longatti, L. *et al.* (1990). Genetic amniocentesis: 505 cases performed before the sixteenth week of gestation. *Prenatal Diagn.*, **10**, 3359–64.

Suchet, I.B., van der Westhuizen, N.G. & Labatte, M.F. (1992). Fetal cystic hygromas: further insights into their natural history. *Can. Assoc. Radiol. J.*, **6**, 420–4.

Szabo, J. & Gellen, J. (1990). Nuchal fluid accumulation in trisomy-21 detected by vaginal sonography in first trimester. *Lancet*, **336**, 1133.

Tabor, A., Philip, J., Madsen, M., Bang, J., Obel, E.B. & Nørgaard-Pedersen, B. (1986). Randomised controlled trial of genetic amniocentesis in 4606 low-risk women. *Lancet*, **i**, 1287–93.

Tannirandorn, Y., Nicolini, U., Nicolaidis, P.C., Fisk, N.M., Arulkumaran, S. & Rodeck, C.H. (1990). Fetal cystic hygromata: insights gained from fetal blood sampling. *Prenatal Diagn.*, **10**, 189–93.

van Zalen-Sprock, M.M., van Vugt, J.M.G. & van Geijn, H.P. (1992). First-trimester diagnosis of cystic hygroma – course and outcome. *Am. J. Obstet. Gynecol.*, **167**, 94–8.

Ville, Y., Borghi, E., Pons, J.C. & Lelorc'h, M. (1992a). Fetal karyotype from cystic hygroma fluid. *Prenatal Diagn.*, **12**, 139–43.

Ville, Y., Lalondrelle, C., Doumerc, S. *et al.* (1992b). First-trimester diagnosis of nuchal anomalies: significance and fetal outcome. *Ultrasound Obstet. Gynecol.*, **2**, 314–16.

Wald, N.J., Kennard, A., Densem, J.W., Cuckle, H.S., Chard, T. & Butler, L. (1992). Antenatal maternal serum screening for Down's syndrome: results of a demonstration project. *Br. Med. J.*, **305**, 391–4.

Wilson, R.D., Venir, N. & Farquharson, D.F. (1992). Fetal nuchal fluid – physiological or pathological? – in pregnancies less than 17 menstrual weeks. *Prenatal Diagn.*, **12**, 755–63.

23

Screening at 11–14 weeks of gestation: the role of established markers and PAPP-A

H. CUCKLE

In most centres, maternal serum screening for Down's syndrome is currently offered from 15 weeks of gestation, but evidence is accumulating to support a change in practice to earlier testing. For some markers the extent of elevation or reduction in affected pregnancies when expressed in multiples of the normal gestation specific median (MoMs) is largely independent of gestational age. Also there are new markers such as pregnancy-associated placental protein A (PAPP-A) that, although of no apparent value after 15 weeks of gestation, may be useful when measured earlier in pregnancy.

A change in policy whereby Down's syndrome screening is offered in the early weeks of pregnancy would be beneficial to women with affected pregnancies. Any consequent abortion would be less traumatic for the patient and the medical staff involved than current practice when terminations are carried out after 17 weeks. Whilst recognising this to be desirable, not all would consider a radical policy change such as screening at 6–10 weeks. An alternative approach that might be more acceptable is to gradually reduce the lower gestational limit at which a test is interpreted.

This has been tried in Leeds. As a first step, the gestational limit has been reduced to 13 weeks. Among the 4139 women tested since the change in policy, 878 (21%) were tested at 13–14 weeks and the modal gestational age for testing has been reduced from 16 to 15 weeks. As experience with screening at this gestational period increases, it is anticipated that the limit will be reduced again to 11 weeks.

In a retrospective analysis of stored maternal serum samples taken at 11–14 weeks of gestation, Crandall et al. (1993) measured α-fetoprotein (AFP), unconjugated oestriol (uE$_3$) and human chorionic gonadotrophin (hCG) levels. The screening detection and false-positive rates were comparable with those achieved with the same markers at later gestational ages. In this chapter, the feasibility of screening for Down's syndrome at this gestational period is discussed in relation to these and newer markers, particularly PAPP-A.

Current practice

Several factors contribute to the present policy of not offering the screening test before 15 weeks of gestation. These relate to AFP being a marker of neural tube defects (NTD), to the gestational ages when women usually present for testing and to early fetal loss in Down's syndrome. None of them represent an overwhelming reason for not screening at 11–14 weeks of gestation.

AFP and neural tube defects

It would not be possible to use a single blood sample for NTD as well as Down's syndrome screening if the test were done before 15 weeks. That is because maternal serum AFP (MSAFP) levels are not raised in the presence of open neural lesions before this time in pregnancy. However, the availability of routine high resolution, detailed ultrasound at 18–20 weeks of gestation has reduced the need for AFP testing to detect NTD and some centres only continue to measure AFP because of Down's syndrome screening. Moreover, the incidence of NTD is declining and will fall further once primary prevention programmes to increase folate intake are implemented.

Gestation at presentation

An early testing policy relies on women presenting for the test at a suitable gestation time. In the UK, many women do not attend their first antenatal clinic until 15 weeks or later. However, the timing of antenatal visits is determined by general practitioner referral patterns that can be changed. An appointment is requested by the general practitioner at a gestation which reflects the expectations of hospital staff. A change could be made provided there was a clear benefit to the patient, such as the ability to make an earlier diagnosis of Down's syndrome.

Early fetal loss in Down's syndrome

A third concern relates to the possibility that affected pregnancies with abnormal marker levels may include a disproportionate number that will miscarry. The rate of fetal loss is high in Down's syndrome and, if there is selective detection of non-viable cases, the screening results could be strongly biased. Whilst this applies to tests done after 15 weeks as well as earlier tests, the magnitude of any bias would be greater before 15 weeks since the rate of fetal loss is considerably higher. This is a strong reason for not immediately changing to screening at 6–10 weeks. Instead, by gradually reducing the lower gestation limit to between 11 and 14 weeks, the presence of any bias should become apparent.

Established markers

AFP, uE₃, hCG and free β-hCG

Centres planning to carry out prospective screening at 11–14 weeks gestation may need to modify the regression equations for the normal medians used to calculate MoMs and the parameters used to calculate an individual woman's risk of Down's syndrome.

Normal medians

There is evidence that the relationship found after 15 weeks of gestation between the normal median levels of AFP and uE_3 and the gestational age does not apply earlier in pregnancy. This can be seen from the retrospective study of Crandall *et al.* (1993) and from prospective experience in Leeds. Table 23.1 shows that the average weekly increase in AFP and uE_3 levels is much greater prior to 15 weeks than later. This

Table 23.1. *Weekly percentage increase in AFP and uE₃ median levels*

Gestation (weeks)	AFP (% increase)		uE₃ (% increase)	
	Los Angeles	Leeds	Los Angeles	Leeds
11	15	–	56	–
12	31	–	60	–
13	29	40	64	58
14	–	19	–	43
15	–	20	–	33
16	–	10	–	26
17	–	18	–	22

The Los Angeles study (Crandall *et al.*, 1993) included 92, 194, 350 and 200 women at 11–14 weeks, respectively; in Leeds (Cuckle *et al.*, 1994) the numbers were 210, 383, 1929, 1615, 529 and 199 at 13–18 weeks, respectively.

means that the widely used log-linear regression of level on gestation will not be the best fit over a wider gestational range and quadratic or higher-order regression may be more appropriate. Neither intact/total hCG nor free β-hCG present this kind of problem. The additive exponential curve is designed to fit the rapid fall-off in levels in early pregnancy to a plateau in mid-trimester.

Down's syndrome medians

There is not sufficient published data to compare the median level, in MoMs, among Down's syndrome pregnancies tested before 15 weeks of gestation and those tested later. The median levels for the two periods based on meta-analysis of published studies are shown in Table 23.2.

Table 23.2. *Established markers: median level according to gestational age*

Marker	Gestation (weeks)	No. of Down's syndrome	Median (MoM)
AFP	<15	114	0.73
	≥15	823	0.74
uE$_3$	<15	75	0.58
	≥15	363	0.73
hCG	<15	127	1.19
	≥15	530	2.04
Free β-hCG	<15	63	2.04
	≥15	477	2.30
Free α-hCG	<15	26	0.92
	≥15	126	1.40
SP1	<15	35	0.60
	≥15	261	1.46

Based on a meta-analysis of published studies. The median is the geometric mean of the individual median values either reported or obtained from a figure or table in the publication, weighted for the number of Down's in each study.

The <15-week results were derived from the 13 studies cited in Macintosh and Chard (1992) together with Bogart *et al.* (1989), Johnson *et al.* (1991), Kratzer *et al.* (1991), Aitken *et al.* (1993), Crandall *et al.* (1993), Macintosh *et al.* (1993) and Macri *et al.* (1993), after discounting cases included in more than one study.

The ≥15-week results were derived from the 38 studies cited in Wald and Cuckle (1992), together with Spencer (1991), Crossley *et al.* (1991), Ryall *et al.* (1992), Spencer and Macri (1992), Graham *et al.* (1992), Spencer *et al.* (1992), Spencer (1993), Stone *et al.* (1993), Wald *et al.* (1993) and Nørgaard-Pedersen *et al.* (1994).

If the low level of MSAFP found in Down's syndrome is a result of reduced fetal production, the levels before 15 weeks will not be as low as later in pregnancy. This is because the yolk sac is an important contributor to maternal AFP in early pregnancy. However there is a remarkable similarity in the median AFP level in the two gestational periods.

Before 15 weeks of gestation, the median uE_3 level in Down's syndrome is lower than later in pregnancy. This value is largely attributable to a single pre-15-week study with a median of 0.35 MoM (Cuckle *et al.*, 1988). Maternal serum samples in this study were tested after modifying the second-trimester Amerlex kit and that could have made it non-specific for uE_3. If so, the results would differ from those obtained using other assay techniques. Excluding this study, the median level prior to 15 weeks is 0.68, a figure that is not significantly lower statistically than the 0.73 found later in pregnancy. More data will be needed before it can be certain that the median uE_3 level is not lower at 11–14 weeks of gestation, but, meanwhile, it is reasonable to use the post-15-week value in risk calculation.

There is a clear effect of gestational age on the median level of hCG in Down's syndrome whereas this is not the case for free β-hCG. The median hCG level prior to 15 weeks is so close to the normal median as to preclude its use as a marker. Whilst hCG is likely to be of more value at 11–14 weeks than in very early pregnancy, laboratories planning to lower the gestational limit for accepting tests should use free β-hCG. There is already a detection advantage after 15 weeks of gestation for assays that measure the free β-subunit of hCG over those measuring either the intact molecule or total hCG. The small difference in median free β-hCG levels before and after 15 weeks is probably a chance effect and, as with uE_3, those screening at 11–14 weeks could use the post-15-week median.

Other parameters

Table 23.3 shows the standard deviations and correlation coefficients found for AFP, uE_3 and free β-hCG among unaffected pregnancies tested in Leeds at 13–14 weeks of gestation compared with 15–18 weeks. There are no material differences between these sets of parameters except for uE_3, which had a greater standard deviation in the earlier period than later (0.164 and 0.142, respectively: 0.007 difference in variance). Crandall *et al.* (1993) also found a wide spread of uE_3 values at 11–14 weeks. On the basis of the reported inter-quartile ranges, the standard deviation was 0.189. The slope of the regression equation relating $\log_{10}$ MoM to maternal weight is similar in the two gestational periods (see Table 22.3).

Table 23.3. *AFP, uE$_3$ and free β-hCG: standard deviation, correlation coefficient and slope of maternal weight regression according to gestational age*

		Gestation (weeks)	
Parameter[a]	Marker[b]	13–15	16–18
Standard deviation	AFP	0.170	0.142
	uE$_3$	0.164	0.141
	Free β-hCG	0.254	0.248
Correlation coefficient	AFP–uE$_3$	0.231	0.280
	AFP–free β-hCG	0.054	0.099
	uE$_3$–free β-hCG	−0.145	−0.099
Slope (/10 kg)	AFP	−0.030	−0.043
	uE$_3$	−0.014	−0.013
	Free β-hCG	−0.038	−0.039

[a] Based on 6030 women tested in Leeds (878 at 13–14 weeks and 5125 at 16–18 weeks of gestation). The standard deviations were calculated from the 10th–90th percentile range divided by 2.563; the correlation coefficients and slopes were calculated after excluding marker values exceeding 3 standard deviations from the mean. The median maternal weight at 13–15 weeks was 63.5 kg and at 16–18 weeks it was 63.2 kg.
[b] Log$_{10}$ values.

Therefore standard deviations and correlation coefficients which have been adjusted to take account of routine maternal weight correction can be expected to apply at all gestations.

In view of the similarity before and after 15 weeks of gestation in the average level in Down's syndrome pregnancies, it is reasonable to use published parameters designed for later in pregnancy. The only modification would be to increase the standard deviation for uE$_3$ by adding 0.007 to the published variance.

Other established markers

Of the four markers discussed so far, AFP has the lowest screening efficiency. Since AFP is of no value in NTD screening prior to 15 weeks, some centres would want to consider substituting a better marker when screening for Down's syndrome at 11–14 weeks. Others may want to retain AFP but add a fourth marker.

Table 23.2 shows the median level of free α-hCG and pregnancy specific β_1-glycoprotein (Schwangerschafts protein, SP1) levels in Down's syndrome according to gestation. The well-established elevation in levels of both markers after 15 weeks is not seen at earlier gestations. Although there are relatively few results prior to 15 weeks, they are not encouraging. The suggestion that the average SP1 level in affected pregnancies is low at some time prior to 15 weeks and high later in pregnancy is intriguing but it is not known at what gestation the change occurs. Therefore, neither marker can be considered for screening at 11–14 weeks.

PAPP-A

Brambati and colleagues (1991) were the first to show that the maternal serum level of PAPP-A was reduced on average in pregnancies with Down's syndrome. In 13 cases tested at 6–9 weeks of gestation, the median level was less than 0.4 MoM. The observation has now been confirmed in several studies based largely on blood samples taken before 15 weeks of gestation, whilst those investigating the marker later in pregnancy have failed to find a material reduction in levels. The results of all eight published studies are summarised in Table 23.4.

The potential of PAPP-A measurements at 11–14 weeks of gestation can be investigated using data from five studies in which the marker was measured at the Royal London Hospital. The assay method was described in detail elsewhere (Sinosich *et al.*, 1982). The studies included a total of 94 Down's syndrome and 1074 unaffected pregnancies ranging from 5 to 20 weeks of gestation (Cuckle *et al.*, 1992; Wald *et al.*, 1992b; Brambati *et al.*, 1993; Muller *et al.*, 1993; van Lith *et al.*, 1994).

Table 23.4. *PAPP-A: median level in Down's syndrome pregnancies from eight studies*

Study	No. of Down's cases	Gestational range (weeks)	Median (MoM)
Wald *et al.*, 1992a	19	9–12	0.23
Brambati *et al.*, 1993	14	6–11	0.30
Hurley *et al.*, 1993	7	9–12	0.33
Brambati *et al.*, 1991	13	6–9	<0.40
Muller *et al.*, 1993	17	9–14	0.43
Cuckle *et al.*, 1992	18	14–19	0.87
Knight *et al.*, 1993	30	15–19	1.01
Wald and Voller, 1993	16	15–19	1.02

Table 23.5. *PAPP-A: median level in unaffected pregnancies according to gestational age*

Gestation (weeks)	No. of women	Median PAPP-A (IU/l)	
		Observed	Regressed[a]
5	5	47	46
6	28	102	98
7	102	180	197
8	156	372	376
9	268	779	677
10	164	1000	1200
11	88	1780	1850
12	27	1830	2800
13	18	3620	4010
14	44	7080	5430
15	40	6820	6930
16	23	9090	8360
17	8	10 800	9520
18	0	–	10 240
19	6	9470	10 400
20	5	7680	9980

[a] Log_{10} PAPP-A $= -0.3607 + 0.4664x - 0.01242x^2$, where x is gestation in completed weeks.

The normal median level at each completed week of gestation is shown in Table 23.5. As others have found (Westergaard *et al.*, 1983; Ruge *et al.*, 1990), the increase in maternal serum PAPP-A levels, which is steep even on a logarithmic scale, gradually reduces to a plateau by about 20 weeks. Quadratic regression of median $\log_{10}$ PAPP-A on gestation, weighted for the number tested at each week, fitted the data well. The extent of fit can be seen in Table 23.5 which compares the observed and fitted levels.

The regression equation was used to calculate the MoM value for each Down's syndrome and unaffected pregnancy. Table 23.6 shows the median PAPP-A level, in MoMs, according to gestation. As expected, the lowest level in affected pregnancies was before 11 weeks and the highest after 15 weeks. Nonetheless, at 11–14 weeks there was a statistically significant reduction in the distribution of levels in the 28 Down's syndrome pregnancies compared with the 177 unaffected pregnancies ($p < 0.0001$; Wilcoxon Rank Sum Test). The frequency distribution of $\log_{10}$ PAPP-A at 11–14 weeks of gestation in both affected and unaffected pregnancies

Table 23.6. *PAPP-A: median and quartile levels in Down's syndrome and unaffected pregnancies according to gestational age*

Gestation (weeks)	Pregnancy	No. of women	PAPP-A (MoM) Median	PAPP-A (MoM) Inter-quartile range
5–10	Down's	49	0.29	0.22–0.62
	Unaffected	721	1.00	0.62–1.52
11–14	Down's	28	0.42	0.17–0.66
	Unaffected	177	0.93	0.59–1.37
15–20	Down's	17	0.76	0.54–1.30
	Unaffected	82	1.08	0.71–1.42

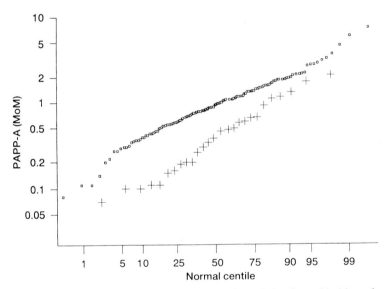

Fig. 23.1. Probability plot of maternal serum PAPP-A levels at 11–14 weeks of gestation in 28 Down's syndrome (+) and 177 unaffected pregnancies (□).

approximated well to a Gaussian fit over the 0.2–2.0 MoM range. This can be observed by examining the probability plot of the MoMs (Fig. 23.1); a straight line shows that the fit is good. The spread of values was wider in the Down's syndrome pregnancies as indicated by the steeper slope of the line. On the basis of the inter-quartile ranges, the standard deviations of $\log_{10}$ PAPP-A are 0.436 and 0.271 in affected and unaffected pregnancies, respectively.

Table 23.7. *AFP, uE$_3$, free β-hCG and PAPP-A at 11–14 weeks of gestation: estimated detection rate given a fixed false-positive rate[a]*

False-positive rate (%)	Detection rate (%)			
	AFP	uE$_3$	Free β-hCG	PAPP-A
3	26	28	49	43
4	30	32	53	47
5	32	36	57	50
6	35	38	59	52
7	37	41	62	54

[a] Using the single marker level and maternal age to calibrate risk; the rates are based on the age discrimination of 1989–90 maternities in England and Wales (OPCS, 1991 and 1992).

There are no published data to compare directly the screening efficiency of PAPP-A at 11–14 weeks with each of AFP, uE$_3$ and free β-hCG. However, an indirect comparison can be made using statistical models to estimate the detection rate for a fixed false-positive rate. This is done in Table 23.7 using the parameters of PAPP-A derived above together with the post-15-week medians for the other markers in Table 23.2 and published parameters (Wald *et al.*, 1992b, 1993; Wald and Densem, 1994) modified for uE$_3$. This analysis shows that, as a single marker, PAPP-A has greater screening efficiency than either AFP or uE$_3$ and is almost as efficient as free β-hCG.

In practice, the decision to replace AFP by PAPP-A when screening at 11–14 weeks or to use it as an additional marker to AFP and free β-hCG with or without uE$_3$ will be dependent on the correlations between the markers. This information is still lacking, but the results so far are encouraging.

Conclusion

Provided that detailed ultrasound is available to detect NTD there is no practical reason to limit Down's syndrome screening to women presenting after 15 weeks of gestation. A gradual change in policy to include tests at 11–14 weeks is feasible. The markers of choice at this time in pregnancy are AFP, uE$_3$ and free β-hCG. There may be a need to modify the equations used in calculating MoMs for AFP and uE$_3$ but the only parameter used in risk estimation that requires changing is the standard deviation of uE_3. There are grounds to believe that PAPP-A may also be a useful marker at 11–14 weeks. It could be used instead of AFP or as a fourth marker, but more information will be needed on the correlation with the established markers. Screening for Down's syndrome earlier in pregnancy than hitherto would be beneficial, particularly for those women who consequently have a therapeutic abortion.

References

Aitken, D.A., McCaw, G., Crossley, J.A. *et al.* (1993). First-trimester biochemical screening for fetal chromosome abnormalities and neural tube defects. *Prenatal Diagn.*, **13**, 681–89.

Bogart, M.H., Golbus, M.S., Sorg, N.D. & Jones, O.W. (1989). Human chorionic gonadotropin level in pregnancies with aneuploid fetuses. *Prenatal Diagn.*, **9**, 379–84.

Brambati, B., Lanzani, A. & Tului, L. (1991). Ultrasound and biochemical assessment of the first-trimester pregnancy. In *The Embryo: Normal and Abnormal Development and Growth*, ed. M. Chapman, J.G. Grudzinskas & T. Chard, pp. 181–94. Berlin: Springer-Verlag.

Brambati, B., Macintosh, M.C.M., Teisner, B. *et al.* (1993). Low maternal serum levels of pregnancy associated plasma protein A (PAPP-A) in the first trimester in association with abnormal fetal karyotype. *Br. J. Obstet. Gynaecol.*, **100**, 324–6.

Crandall, B.F., Hanson, F.W., Keener, S., Matsumoto, M. & Miller, W. (1993). Maternal serum screening for α-fetoprotein, unconjugated oestriol and human chorionic gonadotropin between 11 and 15 weeks of pregnancy to detect fetal chromosome abnormalities. *Am. J. Obstet. Gynecol.*, **168**, 1864–9.

Crossley, J.A., Aitken, D.A. & Connor, J.M. (1991). Free β-hCG and prenatal screening for chromosome abnormalities. *J. Med. Genet.*, **28**, 570.

Cuckle, H.S., Wald, N.J., Barkai, G. *et al.* (1988). First trimester biochemical screening for Down's syndrome. *Lancet*, **ii**, 851–2.

Cuckle, H., Lilford, R.J., Teisner, B., Holding, S., Chard, T. & Grudzinskas, J.G. (1992). Pregnancy associated plasma protein A in Down's syndrome. *Br. Med. J.*, **305**, 425.

Cuckle, H., Lilford, R. & Jones, R. (1994). Maternal serum screening for Down's syndrome before 15 weeks. *Am. J. Obstet. Gynecol.*, in press.

Graham, G.W., Crossley, J.A., Aitken, D.A. & Connor, J.M. (1992). Variation in the levels of pregnancy-specific β-1-glycoprotein in maternal serum from chromosomally abnormal pregnancies. *Prenatal Diagn.*, **12**, 505–12.

Hurley, P.A., Ward, R.H.T., Teisner, B., Iles, R.K., Lucas, M. & Grudzinskas, J.G. (1993). Serum PAPP-A measurements in first-trimester screening for Down's syndrome. *Prenatal Diagn.*, **13**, 903–8.

Johnson, A., Cowchock, F.S., Darby, M., Wapner, R. & Jackson L.G. (1991). First trimester maternal serum alpha-fetoprotein and chorionic gonadotropin in aneuploid pregnancies. *Prenatal Diagn.*, **11**, 443–50.

Knight, G.J., Palomaki, G.E., Haddow, J.E., Miller, W., Bersinger, N.A. &

Schneider, H. (1993). Pregnancy associated plasma protein A as a marker for Down syndrome in the second trimester of pregnancy. *Prenatal Diagn.*, **13**, 222–3.

Kratzer, P.G., Golbus, M.S., Monroe, S.E., Finkelstein, D.E. & Taylor, R.N. (1991). First-trimester aneuploidy screening using serum human chorionic gonadotropin (hCG), free α-hCG and progesterone. *Prenatal Diagn.*, **11**, 751–65.

Macintosh, M.C.M. & Chard, T. (1992). First trimester biochemical screening for Down's syndrome. *Contemp. Rev. Obstet. Gynaecol.*, **4**, 185–90.

Macintosh, M.C.M., Brambati, B., Chard, T. & Grudzinskas, J.G. (1993). First-trimester maternal serum Schwangerschafts protein 1 (SP1) in pregnancies associated with chromosomal anomalies. *Prenatal Diagn.*, **13**, 563–8.

Macri, J.N., Spencer, K., Aitken, D. *et al.* (1993). First-trimester free beta (hCG) screening for Down's syndrome. *Prenatal Diagn.*, **13**, 557–62.

Muller, F., Cuckle, H., Teisner, B. & Grudzinskas, J.G. (1993). Serum PAPP-A levels are depressed in women with fetal Down syndrome in early pregnancy. *Prenatal Diagn.*, **13**, 633–6.

Nørgaard-Pedersen, B., Alfthan, H., Arends, J. *et al.* (1994). A new simple and rapid dual assay for AFP and free β-hCG in screening for Down's syndrome. *Clin. Genet.*, in press.

OPCS (Office of Population Censuses and Surveys) (1991 & 1992). *Birth Statistics Series FM*1, Nos. 18 & 19. London: Her Majesty's Stationery Office.

Ruge, S., Pedersen, J.F., Sorensen, S. & Lange, A.P. (1990). Can pregnancy-associated plasma protein A (PAPP-A) predict the outcome of pregnancy in women with threatened abortion and confirmed fetal viability? *Acta Obstet. Scand.*, **69**, 589–95.

Ryall, R.G., Staples, A.J., Robertson, E.F. & Pollard, A.C. (1992). Improved performance in a prenatal screening programme for Down's syndrome incorporating serum-free hCG subunit analyses. *Prenatal Diagn.*, **12**, 251–61.

Sinosich, M.J., Teisner, B., Folkersen, J., Saunders, D.M. & Grudzinskas, J.G. (1982). Radioimmunoassay for pregnancy-associated plasma protein A. *Clin. Chem.*, **28**, 50–3.

Spencer, K. (1991). Evaluation of an assay of the free β-subunit of choriogonadotropin and its potential value in screening for Down's syndrome. *Clin. Chem.*, **37**, 809–14.

Spencer, K. (1993). Free α-subunit of human chorionic gonadotropin in Down syndrome. *Am. J. Obstet. Gynecol.*, **168**, 132–5.

Spencer, K. & Macri, J.N. (1992). Early detection of Down's syndrome using free beta human choriogonadotropin. *Ann. Clin. Biochem.*, **29**, 349–50.

Spencer, K., Coombes, E.J., Mallard, A.S. & Milford-Ward, A. (1992). Free beta human choriogonadotropin in Down's syndrome screening: a multicentre study of its role compared with other biochemical markers. *Ann. Clin. Biochem.*, **29**, 506–18.

Stone, S., Henley, R., Reynolds, T. & John, R. (1993). A comparison of total and free β-hCG assays in Down syndrome screening. *Prenatal Diagn.*, **13**, 535–7.

van Lith, J., Grudzinskas, J.G., Mantingh, A. *et al.* (1994). Maternal serum PAPP-A levels in pregnancies with chromosomally normal and abnormal fetuses. *Br. J. Obstet. Gynaecol.*, in press.

Wald, N. & Cuckle, H. (1992). Biochemical screening. In *Prenatal Diagnosis and*

Screening, ed. D.J.H. Brock & C. Rodeck, pp. 563–77. Edinburgh: Churchill Livingstone.

Wald, N.J. & Densem, J.W. (1994). Use of unconjugated oestriol in screening for Down's syndrome. *Prenatal Diagn.,* in press.

Wald, N.J. & Voller, A. (1993). Pregnancy associated plasma protein A in Down's syndrome. *Br. Med. J.,* **305**, 425.

Wald, N.J., Cuckle, H.S., Densem, J.W., Kennard, A. & Smith, D. (1992a). Maternal serum screening for Down's syndrome: the effect of routine ultrasound scan determination of gestational age and adjustment for maternal weight. *Br. J. Obstet. Gynaecol.,* **99**, 144–9.

Wald, N., Cuckle, H.S., Grudzinskas, J.G. *et al.* (1992b). First trimester concentrations of pregnancy associated plasma protein A and placental protein 14 in Down's syndrome. *Br. Med. J.,* **305**, 28.

Wald, N., Densem, J., Stone, R. & Cheng, R. (1993). The use of free β-hCG in antenatal screening for Down's syndrome. *Br. J. Obstet. Gynaecol.,* **100**, 550–7.

Westergaard, J.G., Sinosich, M.J., Bugge, M., Madsen, L.T., Teisner, B. & Grudzinskas, J.G. (1983). Pregnancy-associated plasma protein A in the prediction of early pregnancy failure. *Am. J. Obstet. Gynecol.,* **145**, 67–9.

24

Mid-trimester biochemistry in prediction of third trimester complications

J.L. SIMPSON, L. SHULMAN, J. DUNGAN, O. PHILLIPS AND S. ELIAS

Introduction

Maternal serum screening is employed to identify pregnancies at risk for fetal abnormalities, namely neural tube defects (NTD) and autosomal trisomy. However, relatively few women with abnormal serum values actually have an affected fetus. Are outcomes of women with abnormal serum values but without identifiable fetal anomalies at amniocentesis different from outcomes in the general obstetric population? Increasingly, we are learning that unexplained serum abnormalities are associated with increased likelihood of fetal loss and other pregnancy complications.

In this chapter we shall review data associating perinatal outcome with maternal serum human chorionic gonadotropin (hCG) or unconjugated estriol (uE$_3$) values, or combinations thereof. In addition, preliminary information concerning third-trimester screening is presented.

Elevated α-fetoprotein (AFP)

Maternal serum α-fetoprotein screening (MSAFP) during the second trimester has long since become an integral part of obstetrical care. By definition approximately 3–4% of all MSAFP assays are defined as having elevated MSAFP. Pursuing women with these elevated values will detect 80–85% of all NTD cases. However, most women with unexplained values do not have NTD: specifically only about 1 per 15 women undergoing amniocentesis for 'unexplained' MSAFP elevations. Unexplained mid-trimester MSAFP elevations have proved to be associated with pregnancy loss and other adverse perinatal outcomes. Unexplained MSAFP elevations have been associated with increased risk for low birth weight (LBW), intrauterine growth retardation (IUGR), preterm delivery, placental

325

abruption, preeclampsia and congenital anomalies other than open NTDs and anterior abdominal wall defects. In addition, unexplained MSAFP elevations have been associated with placental abnormalities that are evident on ultrasound and at delivery.

Low birth weight

The initial studies demonstrating an association between LBW and unexplained elevated MSAFP were by Brock and colleagues (1979). Among women who had unexplained elevated MSAFP values of 2.3 MoM or greater, 10.7% were delivered of infants weighing less than 2500 g, compared with 4.2% of the general population, i.e. with normal MSAFP values. Wald *et al.* (1977) showed that mean birth weight of infants born to women with unexplained MSAFP elevations (≥ 3.0 MoM) was 334 g less than the birth weight of infants born to women with MSAFP values between 0.75 and 1.49 MoM. Among women who had elevated MSAFP values ≥ 2.5 MoM, Burton (1988) found that 15% were delivered of LBW infants compared to only 7.2% among women with normal MSAFP values. Neither of these three studies could differentiate between preterm deliveries resulting in LBW infants and full-term deliveries with IUGR. Crandall *et al.* (1991) reported that 11% of continuing pregnancies with unexplained MSAFP elevations showed IUGR, and Davis *et al.* (1991) reported that elevated MSAFP was associated with preterm delivery but not with growth retardation. Overall, unexplained elevations of MSAFP seem to be associated with an increased risk for LBW infants. Yet, Ghosh *et al.* (1986) demonstrated that elevated MSAFP values would identify only 7% of LBW infants. Accordingly, MSAFP is not a sensitive screening tool for detecting women at increased risk for delivering LBW infants.

Fetal demise

An association also exists between elevated MSAFP and fetal demise. For example, Nelson *et al.* (1987) reported that among women with elevated MSAFP values 3–5% were found to be carrying a non-viable fetus; in the group of women with MSAFP values ≥ 5.0 MoM, 20% of women will experience fetal demise. When Robinson and co-workers (1989) also stratified their study group by MSAFP MoM values, risks of fetal deaths were 6% for women with MSAFP values 2.5–2.9 MoM, 9% for values 3.0–3.9 MoM and 24% for values > 4.0 MoM. This study also helped

Table 24.1. *Fetal deaths with*
mid-trimester MSAFP greater than
2.0 MoM

Gestation (weeks)	Fetal deaths	
	No.	%
20–23	17/139	12.2
24–27	16/102	15.7
28–31	15/83	18.1
32–37	24/166	14.5
>37	6/122	4.9

Percentage of fetal demises at various stages
of gestation having mid-trimester
MSAFP > 2.0 MoM.
Data of Waller *et al.*, 1991.

verify that unexplained elevations of MSAFP increased the risk of fetal demise in pregnancies in which a fetus was known to be viable at the time of initial evaluation. That is, the association cannot be explained simply by selection bias in which inadvertent samples occurred in women already having experienced a demise (missed abortion). Burton (1988) reported a 4% loss rate after 20 weeks of gestation among women with unexplained elevated MSAFP values, again with fetal viability confirmed at the time of ultrasound elevation following the abnormal maternal serum screening result. Overall, probably the most thorough study is that of Waller *et al.* (1991). This group conducted a case control study based on data in the California MSAFP screening program. After excluding multiple gestations and birth defects, mid-trimester MSAFP levels were compared between 612 pregnancies ending in fetal demise (at least 3 weeks after screening) and 2501 pregnancies ending in livebirths. For MSAFP levels > 3.0 MoM the odds ratio for fetal death was 11:1 (95% CI: 4.7–26.1). Table 24.1 shows loss rates, stratified by the time in gestation when the loss occurred.

Given the above, it is not surprising that unexplained elevations in MSAFP also appear to be associated with an increased risk for stillbirths and neonatal deaths. Burton (1988) reported a neonatal death rate of 2.1% in women with unexplained MSAFP elevations compared with 0.5% in controls. Robinson *et al.* (1989) reported a relative risk of 4.7 for neonatal death in cases of unexplained, elevated MSAFP. The risk seems to increase as MoM increases.

If obstetric complications are identified at the time of serum screening, the risk of fetal loss associated with unexplained elevated MSAFP is further increased. Haddow *et al.* (1986) reported the relative risk of fetal loss in women with unexplained elevated MSAFP values (≥ 2.0 MoM) to be 5.8, but an additional history of vaginal bleeding increased this risk to 12.6. Oligohydramnios also may worsen prognosis in cases of otherwise unexplained, elevated MSAFP (Dyer *et al.*, 1987; Richards *et al.*, 1988). Los and colleagues (1992) proposed that elevated MSAFP levels in oligohydramnios was the result of damage to the fetal membranes with subsequent leakage of amniotic fluid into decidual tissue and, hence, eventual resorption in the maternal circulation.

As with LBW, the overall predictive value of elevated MSAFP for fetal demise or neonatal death is low. Even defining the 'normal' cut-off value as 1.8 MoM, Schnittge and Kjessler (1984) were able to identify only 30% of cases of fetal demise or neonatal death. Burton (1988) reported that only 8% of fetal/neonatal losses could be predicted on the basis of elevated MSAFP values. Although unexplained, elevated MSAFP is associated with increased risk for fetal/neonatal loss, it follows that most losses occur among women with normal or low MSAFP values.

Other pregnancy complications

Associations between elevated MSAFP and other obstetric complications have also been reported. Walters *et al.* (1985) found that 13% of women with elevated MSAFP developed preeclampsia, compared to only 1% in controls (i.e. with normal MSAFP). A significant increase in pregnancy-induced hypertension among women with elevated MSAFP compared to women with normal MSAFP values (28% versus 16%) has been reported (Hamilton *et al.*, 1985; Milunsky *et al.*, 1989). Clayton-Hopkins *et al.* (1982) found that women with chronic hypertension had higher MSAFP levels than normotensive women, suggesting that vascular pathology associated with hypertensive states may be responsible for elevated maternal serum AFP. Several studies have demonstrated increased placental abruption among women with elevated MSAFP (Persson *et al.*, 1983; Purdie *et al.*, 1983; Milunsky *et al.*, 1989). Other more descriptive studies also hint at such a relationship (Zelopo *et al.*, 1992).

When the outcomes of 201 women with unexplained, elevated MSAFP (≥ 2.0 MoM) were compared with 211 women with normal MSAFP, an association was obtained between unexplained, elevated MSAFP and LBW (adjusted risk ratio (ARR) 3.7), preterm delivery (ARR 3.6),

IUGR (ARR 4.0), preeclampsia (ARR 3.8) and placental abruption (ARR 4.8) (Williams *et al.*, 1992). For LBW, preterm delivery and IUGR, the adjusted risk ratios were even higher when both unexplained, elevated MSAFP and ultrasound-detected placental abnormalities co-existed. Among 44 pregnancies characterized by MSAFP values of 8.0 MoM or greater, the elevation in 8 cases was associated with one of the above obstetrical complications or a placental abnormality (Killam *et al.*, 1991).

Anomalies other than neural tube defects

Women with unexplained elevated MSAFP values may also be at increased risk for congenital abnormalities other than NTD. Milunsky *et al.* (1989) observed a 2.5% frequency of major non-NTD malformations among offspring of women with elevated MSAFP; none of the defects was chromosomal. Crandall and colleagues (1983) reported that 21% of the abnormalities detected by elevated MSAFP were a result of chromosome abnormalities. Burton (1988) found that 6.2% of women having elevated MSAFP but normal amniotic fluid α-fetoprotein (AFAFP) were carrying a fetus with at least one major malformation, compared to 1.4% for women having both normal MSAFP and normal AFAFP. From the same group, Warner and colleagues (1990) later reported that the frequency of chromosome abnormalities associated with unexplained elevated MSAFP was almost 1%, a frequency comparable to that in 36-year-old women. This information is relevant to decisions whether amniocentesis should be offered to women with unexplained elevated MSAFP values.

In conclusion, it is apparent from the various studies that elevated MSAFP – explained or unexplained – is associated with a spectrum of adverse perinatal outcomes. Whether the associations hold true in all populations still remains unclear. Our observation in a high-risk population (inner city clinic) failed to show further risk for elevated MSAFP compared to that found in our general clinic population, which was already at increased risk (Phillips *et al.*, 1992).

Low α-fetoprotein

Shortly after Merkatz and colleagues (1984) reported that low MSAFP was associated with an increased incidence of Down's syndrome, our group and others began to investigate whether unexplained low levels of MSAFP were associated with adverse perinatal outcome. Several groups had reported very high frequencies (over 40%) of perinatal loss among women with low MSAFP (Stein *et al.*, 1981; Davenport and Macri, 1983). However, these reports failed to remove from the cohort either pregnancies affected by chromosome abnormalities or pregnancies in which fetal demise had occurred before sampling. Our group did both and found that the risk of fetal loss and other perinatal abnormalities among women with unexplained (i.e. normal fetal ultrasound and karyotypic evaluation) low MSAFP differed little from the general population (Simpson *et al.*, 1986). Burton (1988) also reported only a slight increased risk of fetal loss compared with these early studies (Stein *et al.*, 1981; Davenport and Macri, 1983), as did Milunsky and colleagues (1986) (relative risk 3.3 for fetal demise). In our study and the last two, fetal demise at the time of sampling was excluded. Therefore, some increased fetal loss rate may be associated with low MSAFP, but not nearly as high as initially proposed.

Less information is available concerning pregnancy complications in women having low MSAFP, but at present there is little evidence that low MSAFP presages such complications (Milunsky, 1986; Simpson *et al.*, 1986; Burton, 1988).

Elevated human chorionic gonadotropin

Elevated maternal serum hCG levels were first reported to be associated with fetal aneuploidy by Bogart *et al.*, (1987). Others later confirmed the usefulness of this analyte in detecting fetal aneuploidy (Wald *et al.*, 1988; White *et al.*, 1989; Heyl *et al.*, 1990), and hCG is now routinely incorporated in many fetal Down's syndrome screening programs.

Elevated levels of hCG (>5.0 MoM) were found to be associated with pregnancy complications (Gravett *et al.*, 1992): among 3000 consecutive pregnancies, seven showed unexplained elevated hCG levels (>5.0 MoM). Four of the seven (57%) delivered prematurely; two of these four had preeclampsia and HELLP syndrome (hemolysis, elevated liver enzymes, low platelets), one had abruptio placenta, and one had preterm labor. The remaining three pregnancies had normal outcomes. One of the four pregnancies with adverse outcome also had an unexplained elevated MSAFP (>2.5 MoM); however, no other risk factors co-existed in these women.

Moderately elevated hCG (>2.5 MoM) has been found associated with adverse pregnancy outcome (Gonen *et al.*, 1992). Of 6011 pregnancies,

417 (6.9%) had elevated serum hCG levels (≥ 2.9 MoM). An explanation for the elevations was found in 133 (2.2%), either over-estimation of gestational age, multiple pregnancies or fetal karyotypic abnormalities. In the remaining 284 (4.7%) with unexplained, elevated hCG, pregnancy outcome was compared to a randomly selected control group (hCG levels 0.2–2.5 MoM). An increased risk for 'hypertensive pregnancy disorders' was observed: 33 cases (12.2%) versus 7 controls (3.2%) for an odds ratio of 4.4 ($p < 0.001$). For those with hCG > 4.0 MoM, the odds ratio was 6.8. IUGR was also associated with elevated hCG: 28 cases (10.3%) versus 11 controls (5%) (odds ratio 2.5; $p < 0.05$); however, growth retardation was dependent on the presence of hypertension. No association was found for diabetes mellitus, abruptio placentae, premature rupture of membranes (PROM), fetal distress, preterm delivery, fetal loss, neonatal death or low Apgar scores.

Tanaka *et al.* (1993) also found an association between unexplained hCG elevation (≥ 2.0 MoM) and fetal growth retardation. Small-for-gestational age infants were detected in 8 of 42 (19%) women with elevated hCG, compared to 23 of 596 (3.9%) controls ($p < 0.001$). A significantly higher risk was also found for fetal death, PROM and abruptio placenta ($p < 0.05$); however, there were only 2 cases in each category. No association between 'pregnancy-induced hypertension' and elevated hCG levels was observed, but again numbers were very small. In addition, many cases had more than a single adverse outcome, but data were not partitioned to assess this effect.

In contrast to the above studies, no association between unexplained elevated hCG levels (≥ 2.5 MoM) and adverse pregnancy outcome was found by Santolaya *et al.* (1992). Of 3116 patients, 134 had hCG levels ≥ 2.5 MoM. Using a matched control design, no association was found with any of 41 pregnancy complications and outcome variables, including fetal loss, premature delivery and LBW.

In summary, most, but not all, studies have found some association between adverse outcome and unexplained elevated hCG. Unfortunately, available studies have many potential pitfalls, including inadequate sample size, failure to take into account potential confounding variables and failure to use proper controls. Although it has been proposed that placental hCG may directly reflect placental function and that abnormal hCG levels, therefore, might presage such pregnancy complications as abruptio placenta and preeclampsia (Gravett *et al.*, 1992), further studies are clearly necessary before concluding that elevated hCG is a predictor of adverse perinatal outcome.

Low human chorionic gonadotropin

Patients with low hCG levels (≤ 0.4 MoM, $n = 246$) showed no association with any of 41 adverse pregnancy outcomes (Santolaya *et al.*, 1992). By contrast, Mason *et al.* (1993) found an increased risk of fetal loss (blighted ovum, missed abortion and miscarriage) in women with low levels of hCG (< 0.4 MoM, $n = 6$). That the low levels of serum hCG merely reflected a pregnancy demise already present when the blood sample was drawn was not excluded.

Low unconjugated estriol (uE_3)

Prior to availability of electronic fetal monitoring, obstetricians frequently assessed fetal well-being by serial urinary estriol (E_3) excretion. Persistently low values or a precipitous drop in urinary E_3 were considered ominous. Thus, an association between low *serum* uE_3 and adverse pregnancy outcome would not be too surprising. Indeed, Mason *et al.* (1993) found that the combination of low uE_3 (< 0.4 MoM) and low hCG was associated with fetal loss. Among 207 pregnancies with low uE_3 (≤ 0.4 MoM) alone, Santolaya *et al.* (1992) found an association between fetal loss and low birth weight, compared with matched controls. In the same study, no relationship was found between *elevated* uE_3 (> 1.6 MoM) and any of 41 pregnancy complications studied.

Overall, an association may exist between low uE_3 and fetal death; an association with other adverse prenatal outcomes remains unproven. Larger studies are necessary before definitive conclusions can be made.

Positive serum screening for Down's syndrome (triple analyte screening)

Maternal serum screening for fetal Down's syndrome involves using AFP, uE_3, hCG and maternal age to calculate an adjusted risk for having an affected fetus (Cuckle and Wald, 1990, 1993). This approach is accepted as producing approximately 60% sensitivity in detection of fetal Down's syndrome. The false-positive (amniocentesis) rate for triple analyte screening is 3–5%. The question arises whether 'false-positive' triple analyte screening is also associated with adverse perinatal outcome.

Predicting whether an association exists is not simple because the mechanism underlying the abnormal concentrations of serum analytes in aneuploid pregnancies is unknown. Altered maternal serum levels presumably reflect fetal production because pathologic changes in placentae of trisomic fetuses have not been demonstrated universally. The prevailing hypothesis is that the fetoplacental unit is less 'mature' developmentally in fetuses with Down's syndrome, so that these particular analytes are produced at rates appropriate for normal fetuses of earlier gestational age.

Our group analyzed the pregnancy outcomes of 99 women having positive maternal serum screening for fetal Down's syndrome but carrying chromosomally normal fetuses. (Dungan *et al.*, 1994). The control group (negative triple analyte serum screening) was matched for age, race, parity and presence or absence of vaginal bleeding. We observed no significant differences in the frequency of fetal death, IUGR, preeclampsia, or fetal anomalies (Dungan *et al.*, 1994). By contrast, a smaller series showed a 3-fold *increase* in adverse perinatal outcome in 59 women having positive triple analyte screening: 34% showed abnormalities that included fetal wastage, preterm delivery, preterm labor, premature rupture of membranes (PROM) and preeclampsia (Rissman *et al.*, 1992).

Large prospective studies examining the association between pregnancy complications and positive Down's syndrome screening are needed. Until these are completed, increased obstetric surveillance does not seem necessary for pregnancies showing abnormal triple analyte screening but not having Down's syndrome.

Positive Down's syndrome serum screening and elevated MSAFP

Beekhuis *et al.* (1992) examined pregnancy outcomes in women having both positive serum screening for Down's syndrome *and* elevated MSAFP. The sample consisted of women with both serum AFP $\geq$ 2.0 MoM and serum hCG $\geq$ 2.0 MoM. Eleven women fulfilled both criteria, although size of the original patient base was not given. There were four fetal deaths (20, 21, 22, and 26 weeks). Three other women had fetuses with severe congenital abnormalities necessitating pregnancy terminations. Of the remaining four pregnancies, three showed normal liveborn children, albeit one delivered prematurely. The fourth pregnancy ended in premature labor with delivery of a 26-week fetus, which subsequently died. Overall, only two of the 11 pregnancies were normal. All fetal karyotypes were normal.

University of Tennessee experience: cohort studies assessing abnormal second-trimester MSAFP and evaluating role of third-trimester MSAFP

Although women with unexplained, elevated MSAFP in the second trimester clearly seem to have an increased risk of subsequent fetal loss and certain other pregnancy complications, limitations exist in the current data. Few studies are cohort in nature and no intervention trials have been reported. Therefore, there is no consensus in the obstetric community concerning the form the widely recommended 'increased obstetric surveillance' should take (Elias *et al.*, 1990).

One difficulty is that not only is increased obstetric surveillance potentially expensive and of uncertain value, but a relatively low positive predictive value exists between unexplained MSAFP elevation and pregnancy complications. To define detection rates for second trimester MSAFP, we and colleagues at the Foundation for Blood Research (Scarborough, ME) are conducting cohort studies. In these studies we seek to assess the potential use of serial second and third trimester MSAFP. After first gathering normative MSAFP data in the late second and third trimesters (Simpson *et al.*, 1991, 1992, unpublished data), we obtained MSAFP in both second and third trimesters and then correlated results with respect to presence or absence of various adverse perinatal outcomes and pregnancy complications.

The MSAFP variance at a given week of gestation is indeed higher at 24–36 weeks of gestation than at 15–20 weeks (Simpson *et al.*, 1991). However, for screening purposes the principal concern is with variance around the median. Prior to weight adjustments, $\log_{10}$ S.D. is 0.1955; after weight adjustment $\log_{10}$ S.D. is 0.187, a value not dissimilar to that in the second trimester (0.185) (Simpson *et al.*, 1992). Therefore, MSAFP population distributions around the median are similar in the second and third trimester.

In our cohort, the outcome most strongly associated with elevated second trimester MSAFP was PROM (Simpson *et al.*, unpublished data). Forty percent of all PROM cases occurred among the 6% of subjects having elevated (≥ 2.0 MoM) second trimester MSAFP. Women with elevated MSAFP showed an odds ratio of near 10 for PROM. Preterm birth, IUGR and LBW all show similar associations with second trimester MSAFP elevations, albeit to a lesser extent. However, for all outcomes, the association decreased to non-significance in the third trimester. Elevated MSAFP in both second and third trimester was relatively specific for LBW (4 of 11 cases), but quite insensitive (4 of 68). In contrast to observations cited by others, preeclampsia, oligohydramnios, and polyhydramnios were not associated with second trimester MSAFP elevations in our cohort.

Therefore, neither MSAFP values later in gestation (24–36 weeks) nor serial MSAFP values added predictive value over that derived on the basis of a single second-trimester (15–20 weeks) MSAFP. These data are consistent with those of Wenstrom *et al.* (1992), who reported that the *initial* second trimester MSAFP value was more highly correlated with pregnancy outcome than was a second or third MSAFP sample assayed later in the same trimester. Our findings do not necessarily mean that third trimester MSAFP is without value in all circumstances, but it is clear that little additional information is gained by studying 24–36 week MSAFP.

It is not clear why the 15–20 week MSAFP value correlates less well with adverse pregnancy outcomes than does the second trimester MSAFP. We had predicted that if abnormal placentation or disruption of the amniotic cavity/decidual interface leads to elevated MSAFP in the second trimester, such processes would continue into the third trimester.

Recommended clinical management (1993)

After detecting an abnormal maternal serum analyte value in the second trimester, prudence probably dictates serial assessment of fetal growth and assessment for the risk factors predicting preterm birth. The patient should be counseled on the potential for adverse pregnancy outcome, if for no other reason than to increase both patient and physician awareness of factors dictating early intervention. Women with elevated second trimester MSAFP should specifically be followed for evidence of IUGR, evaluated for risk factors indicative of preterm birth and counseled concerning symptoms and signs that may precede this complication. However, no specific clinical protocol can be recommended.

References

Beekhuis, J.R., van Lith, J.M.M., DeWolf, B.T.H.M. *et al.* (1992). Increased maternal serum alpha-fetoprotein and human chorionic gonadotropin in compromised pregnancies other than for neural tube defects or Down syndrome. *Prenatal Diagn.*, **12**, 643–7.

Bogart, H.M., Pandian, M.R. & Jones, O.W. (1987). Abnormal maternal serum chorionic gonadotropin levels in pregnancies with fetal chromosome abnormalities. *Prenatal Diagn.*, **7**, 623–30.

Brock, D.J., Barron, L. & Duncan, P. (1979). Significance of elevated mid-trimester maternal plasma alpha-fetoprotein values. *Lancet*, **1**, 1281–2.

Burton, B.K. (1988). Outcome of pregnancy in patients with unexplained elevated or low levels of maternal serum alpha-fetoprotein. *Obstet. Gynecol.*, **72**, 709–13.

Clayton-Hopkins, J.A., Olen, P.N. & Blake, A.P. (1982). Maternal serum alpha-fetoprotein levels in pregnancy complicated by hypertension. *Prenatal Diagn.*, **2**, 47–54.

Crandall, B.F., Robinson, R.D., Lebherz, T.B. *et al.* (1983). Maternal serum alpha-fetoprotein screening for the detection of neural tube defects. *West J. Med.*, **138**, 524.

Crandall, B.F., Robinson, L. & Grau, P. (1991). Risks associated with an elevated maternal serum alpha-fetoprotein level. *Am. J. Obstet. Gynecol.*, **165**, 581.

Cuckle, H.S. & Wald, N.J. (1990). Screening for Down syndrome. In *Prenatal Diagnosis and Prognosis*, ed. R.J. Lilford, p. 67–92. London: Butterworth.

Cuckle, H.S. & Wald, N.J. (1993). hCG, estriol, and other maternal blood markers of fetal aneuploidy. In *Maternal Serum Screening for Fetal Genetic Disorders.* ed. S. Elias & S. Simpson, p. 87–107. New York: Churchill Livingstone.

Davenport, D.M. & Macri, J.N. (1983). The clinical significance of low maternal serum α-fetoprotein. *Am. J. Obstet. Gynecol.*, **146**, 657–61.

Davis, R.O., Goldenberg, R.L., Boots, L. *et al.* (1992). Elevated levels of midtrimester maternal serum alpha fetoprotein are associated with preterm delivery but not with fetal growth retardation. *Am. J. Obstet. Gynecol.*, **167**, 596–601.

Dungan, J.S., Shulman, L.P., Phillips, O.P. *et al.* (1994). Positive serum screening for fetal Down syndrome does not predict adverse pregnancy outcome in absence of fetal aneuploidy. *J. Soc. Gynecol. Investig.*, **1**, 55–8.

Dyer, S.N., Burton, B.K. & Nelson, L.H. (1987). Elevated maternal serum alpha-fetoprotein levels and olgiohydramnios: poor prognosis for pregnancy levels. *Am. J. Obstet. Gynecol.*, **157**, 336–9.

Elias, S., Simpson, J.L. & Golbus, M.S. (1990). Update on MSAFP statement. (Letter). *Am. J. Hum. Genet.*, **48**, 847.

Ghosh, A., Tang, M.H.Y., Tai, D. *et al.* (1986). Justification of maternal serum alpha-fetoprotein screening in a population with low incidence of neural tube defects. *Prenatal Diagn.*, **6**, 83–7.

Gonen, R., Perez, R., David, M. *et al.* (1992). The association between unexplained second-trimester serum hCG elevation and pregnancy complications. *Obstet. Gynecol.*, **80**, 83–5.

Gravett, C.P., Buckmaster, J.G., Watson, P.T. *et al.* (1992). Elevated second trimester maternal serum β-hCG concentrations and subsequent adverse pregnancy outcome. *Am. J. Med. Genet.*, **44**, 485–6.

Haddow, J.E., Knight, G.J., Kloza, E.M. & Palomaki, G.E. (1986). Alpha-fetoprotein, vaginal bleeding and pregnancy risk. *Br. J. Obstet. Gynecol.*, **93**, 589–93.

Hamilton, M.P.R., Abdalla, H.I. & Whitfield, C.R. (1985). Significance of raised maternal serum alpha-fetoprotein in singleton pregnancies with normally formed fetuses. *Obstet. Gynecol.*, **65**, 465–70.

Heyl, P.S., Miller, W. & Canick, J.A. (1990). Maternal serum screening for aneuploid pregnancy by alpha-fetoprotein, hCG, and unconjugated estriol. *Obstet. Gynecol.*, **76**, 1025–31.

Killam, W.P., Miller, R.C. & Seeds, J.W. (1991). Extremely high maternal serum alpha-fetoprotein levels at second trimester screening. *Obstet. Gynecol.*, **78**, 257–61.

Los, F.J., Beekhuis, J.R., Marrink, J. *et al.* (1992). Origin of raised maternal serum alpha-fetoprotein levels in second-trimester oligohydramnios. *Prenatal Diagn.*, **12**, 39–45.

Mason, G., Lindow, S., Ramsden, C. *et al.* (1993). Low maternal serum oestriol and chorionic gonadotropin in the prediction of adverse pregnancy outcome. *Prenatal Diagn.*, **20**, 223–5.

Merkatz, I.R., Nitowsky, H.M., Macri, N. *et al.* (1984). An association between low maternal serum alpha-fetoprotein and fetal chromosomal abnormalities. *Am. J. Obstet. Gynecol.*, **148**, 886–94.

Milunsky, A. (1986). The prenatal diagnosis of neural tube and other congenital defects. In *Genetic Disorders and the Fetus: Diagnosis, Prevention and Treatment*, 2nd edn, ed. A. Milunsky, p. 453–519. New York: Plenum Press.

Milunsky, A. Jick, S.S., Bruell, C.L. *et al.* (1989). Predictive values, relative risks, and overall benefits of high and low maternal serum alpha-fetoprotein screening in singleton pregnancies: new epidemiologic data. *Am. J. Obstet. Gynecol.*, **161**, 291–7.

Nelson, L.M., Benson, J. & Burton, B.K. (1987). Outcomes in patients with unusually high maternal serum alpha-fetoprotein levels. *Obstet. Gynecol.*, **157**, 572–6.

Persson, P.H., Kullander, S., Gennser, G. *et al.* (1983). Screening for fetal malformations using ultrasound and measurements of alpha-fetoprotein in maternal serum. *Br. Med. J.*, **286**, 747.

Phillips, O.P., Simpson, J.L., Morgan, C.D. *et al.* (1992). Unexplained elevated maternal serum alpha fetoprotein (MSAFP) is not necessarily predictive of adverse perinatal outcome in an indigent urban population. *Am. J. Obstet. Gynecol.*, **166**, 978–82.

Purdie, P.W., Young, J.L., Guthrie, K.A. & Picton, C.E. (1983). Fetal growth achievement and elevated maternal serum alpha-fetoprotein. *Br. J. Obstet. Gynecol.*, **90**, 433–6.

Richards, D.S., Seeds, J.W., Katz, V.L. *et al.* (1988). Elevated maternal serum alpha-fetoprotein with oligohydramnios: ultrasound evaluation and outcome. *Obstet. Gynecol.*, **72**, 337–41.

Rissman, A., Fine, B. & Pergament, E. (1992). Triple screening and adverse outcome; a new dimension in prenatal diagnosis. *Am. J. Hum. Genet.*, **51**, A263.

Robinson, L., Grau, P. & Crandall, B.F. (1989). Pregnancy outcomes after increasing maternal serum alpha fetoprotein levels. *Obstet. Gynecol.*, **74**, 17–19.

Santolaya, J. Jessup, J. Nieb, B. *et al.* (1992). The significance of elevated and low levels of maternal serum alpha fetoprotein, human chorionic gonadotropin and unconjugated estriol in the midtrimester of pregnancy. *Am. J. Hum. Genet.*, **51**, A1039.

Schnittge, A. & Kjessler, B. (1984). Alpha-fetoprotein screening in obstetric practice and the use of differential action limits. *Acta Obstet. Gynecol. Scand.*, **119**(Suppl.), 33–41.

Simpson, J.L., Baum, L.D., Depp, R. *et al.* (1986). Maternal serum alpha-fetoprotein (MSAFP) screening: low and high values for detection of genetic abnormalities. *Am. J. Obstet. Gynecol.*, **156**, 593–7.

Simpson, J.L., Elias, S., Morgan, C.D. *et al.* (1991). Does unexplained second trimester (15–20 weeks' gestation) maternal serum α-fetoprotein elevation presage adverse perinatal outcome? *Am. J. Obstet. Gynecol.*, **164**, 829–36.

Simpson, J.L., Palomaki, G.E., Elias, S. *et al.* (1992). Elevated second trimester maternal serum alpha fetoprotein (MSAFP) is more predictive of certain pregnancy complications than elevated third trimester MSAFP. American Society of Human Genetics, 42nd Annual Meeting, San Francisco, C.A. *Am. J. Hum. Genet.*, **51**(S), 65.

Simpson, J.L., Palomaki, G., Elias, S. *et al.* (1994). Third trimester maternal serum alpha fetoprotein (MSAFP): correlation between values in second trimester (15–20 weeks) and later in gestation (24–36 weeks) value. in press.

Stein, S.M., Watt, M.S. & Scrimgeour, J.B. (1981). Very low maternal plasma alpha-fetoprotein concentration: an indication for follow-up. *Br. J. Obstet. Gynaecol.*, **88**, 635–9.

Tanaka, M., Natori, M., Kohn, H. *et al.* (1993). Fetal growth in patients with elevated maternal serum hCG levels. *Obstet. Gynecol.*, **81**, 341–3.

Wald, N., Cuckle, H., Stirrat, C.M. *et al.* (1977). Maternal serum alpha fetoprotein and low birth weight. *Lancet*, **2**, 268–70.

Wald, N.J., Cuckle, H.S., Densem, J.W. *et al.* (1988). Maternal serum screening for Down syndrome in early pregnancy. *Br. Med. J.*, **297**, 883–7.

Waller, D.K., Lustig, L.S., Cunningham, G.C. *et al.* (1991). Second trimester maternal serum alpha-fetoprotein levels and the risk of subsequent fetal death. *N. Engl. J. Med.*, **325**, 6–10.

Walters, B.N.J., Lao, T., Smith, V., DeSwiet, M. (1985). Alpha-fetoprotein elevation and proteinuric pre-eclampsia. *Br. J. Obstet. Gynecol.*, **92**, 341–4.

Warner, A.A., Pettenati, M. & Burton, B.K. (1990). Risk of fetal chromosome anomalies in patients with elevated maternal serum alpha-fetoprotein. *Obstet. Gynecol.*, **75**, 64–6.

Wenstrom, K.D., Sipes, S.L., Williamson, R.A. *et al.* (1992). Prediction of pregnancy outcome with single versus serial maternal serum α-fetoprotein tests. *Am. J. Obstet. Gynecol.*, **167**, 1529–33.

White, I., Papiha, S.S. & Magnay, D. (1989). Improving methods of screening for Down's syndrome. *N. Engl. J. Med.*, **320**, 401–2.

Williams, M.A., Hickok, D.E., Zingheim, R.W. *et al.* (1992). Elevated maternal serum alpha-fetoprotein levels and midtrimester placental abnormalities in relation to subsequent adverse pregnancy outcomes. *Am. J. Obstet. Gynecol.*, **167**, 1032–7.

Zelopo, C., Nadel, A., Friogoletto, F.D. *et al.* (1992). Placental accreta/percreta/increta: a cause of elevated maternal serum alpha-fetoprotein. *Obstet. Gynecol.*, **80**, 693–4.

Index

339